Palliative Care and Ethics

Palliative Care and Ethics

Edited by Timothy E. Quill
and
Franklin G. Miller

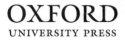

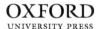

OXFORD
UNIVERSITY PRESS

Oxford University Press is a department of the University of Oxford.
It furthers the University's objective of excellence in research, scholarship,
and education by publishing worldwide.

Oxford   New York
Auckland   Cape Town   Dar es Salaam   Hong Kong   Karachi
Kuala Lumpur   Madrid   Melbourne   Mexico City   Nairobi
New Delhi   Shanghai   Taipei   Toronto

With offices in
Argentina   Austria   Brazil   Chile   Czech Republic   France   Greece
Guatemala   Hungary   Italy   Japan   Poland   Portugal   Singapore
South Korea   Switzerland   Thailand   Turkey   Ukraine   Vietnam

Oxford is a registered trademark of Oxford University Press
in the UK and certain other countries.

Published in the United States of America by
Oxford University Press
198 Madison Avenue, New York, NY 10016

Library of Congress Cataloging-in-Publication Data
Palliative care and ethics: edited by
Timothy E. Quill and Franklin G. Miller.
   p. ; cm.
Includes bibliographical references.
ISBN 978–0–19–931667–0
I.   Quill, Timothy E., editor of compilation.   II. Miller, Franklin G., editor
of compilation.
[DNLM: 1. Palliative Care—ethics—Europe.   2. Palliative Care—ethics—United
States.   3. Terminal Care—ethics—Europe.   4. Terminal Care—ethics—United States.
WB 310]
R726'179.7—dc23   2013035545

9 8 7 6 5 4 3 2 1
Printed in the United States of America
on acid-free paper

CONTENTS

SECTION IV: Difficult Decisions Near the Very End of Life

CONTRIBUTORS

Amy P. Abernethy, M.D., Ph.D. is Associate Professor of Medicine in the Division of Medical Oncology at Duke University School of Medicine where she co-directs both the Duke Center for Learning Health Care and the Duke Cancer Care Research Program. She is current president of the American Academy of Hospice and Palliative Medicine.

Yesne Alici, M.D. is Assistant Attending Psychiatrist, Psychiatry Service, Department of Psychiatry and Behavioral Sciences, Memorial Sloan-Kettering Cancer Center and Assistant Professor of Psychiatry, Weill Cornell Medical College.

James L. Bernat, M.D. is the Louis and Ruth Frank Professor of Neuroscience and Professor of Medicine and Neurology at the Geisel School of Medicine at Dartmouth.

J. Andrew Billings, M.D. is the founder and former Director of the Massachusetts General Hospital Palliative Care Service and is Co-Director of the Harvard Medical School Center for Palliative Care and physician at the Cambridge Health Alliance. He was a founding member and former President of the American Academy of Hospice and Palliative Medicine.

Susan D. Block, M.D. is Chair of the Department of Psychosocial Oncology and Palliative Care at Dana-Farber Cancer Institute and Brigham and Women's Hospital, Co-Director of the Harvard Medical School Center for Palliative Care, and Professor of Psychiatry and Medicine at Harvard Medical School.

Renee D. Boss, M.D. is an Assistant Professor of Neonatal-Perinatal Medicine and Palliative Care at Johns Hopkins University School of Medicine, and Associate Faculty at the Johns Hopkins Berman Bioethics Institute.

William S. Breitbart, M.D. is Interim Chairman, Chief, Psychiatry Service, Department of Psychiatry and Behavioral Sciences, and Attending Psychiatrist, Pain and Palliative Care Service, Department of Medicine, Memorial Sloan-Kettering Cancer Center and Professor of Psychiatry, Weill Cornell Medical College. He is a former President of the International Psycho-oncology Society, and the Academy of Psychosomatic Medicine.

Howard Brody, M.D., Ph.D. is the Director of the Institute for the Medical Humanities and John P. McGovern Centennial Chair in Family Medicine, University of Texas Medical Branch at Galveston who was given the Lifetime Achievement Award of the American Society for Bioethics and Humanities in 2009.

Eduardo Bruera, M.D. is the Chair of the Department of Palliative Care and Rehabilitation Medicine at the University of Texas MD Anderson Cancer Center where he currently holds the F. T. McGraw Chair in the Treatment of Cancer.

Nathan Cherny, M.D. is a Professor of Medicine at Shaare Zedek Medical Center in Jerusalem, Israel where he is also the Norman Levan Chair of Humanistic Medicine and Director of the Cancer Pain and Palliative Medicine Service.

David C. Currow, B.Med., M.P.H. is a Professor of Palliative and Supportive Services, Flinders University, Adelaide, Australia, where he is also the Chief Cancer Officer and the Chief Executive Officer of the Cancer Institute, New South Wales, Australia.

Maxine de la Cruz, M.D. is an Assistant Professor in the Department of Palliative Care and Rehabilitative Medicine at the University of Texas MD Anderson Cancer Center.

Peggy L. Determeyer, M.B.A., M.Div. is a Staff Chaplain at Memorial Hermann Medical Center in Houston, Texas where she also serves on the hospital bioethics committee and is involved in ethics consultation and education.

Vikki A. Entwistle, M.A., Ph.D. is a Professor of Health Services Research and Ethics at the University of Aberdeen, Scotland, UK.

Ronald M. Epstein, M.D. is a Professor of Family Medicine, Psychiatry, Oncology, and Nursing at the University of Rochester Medical Center where he also serves as Director of the Center for Communication and Disparities Research.

Linda Ganzini, M.D., M.P.H. is a Professor of Psychiatry and Medicine at Oregon Health & Science University and Director of the Interprofessional Fellowship in Palliative Care at the Portland Veterans Affairs Medical Center where she also serves as a consult-liaison psychiatrist.

Robert Gramling, M.D., D.Sc. is an Associate Professor of Family Medicine, Public Health Sciences and Nursing at the University of Rochester Medical Center, and Co-Director of Research in the Division of Palliative Care.

Nancy Hutton, M.D. is a Professor of Pediatrics at the Johns Hopkins University School of Medicine, Medical Director of Harriet Lane Compassionate Care, the pediatric palliative care program of the Johns Hopkins Children's Center, and also the director of an interdisciplinary, comprehensive program for children with HIV and AIDS.

Thomas W. LeBlanc, M.D., M.A. is an Assistant Professor of Medicine in the Division of Hematologic Malignancies and Cellular Therapy at the Duke University School of Medicine, and a Faculty Associate in the Trent Center for Bioethics, Humanities and History of Medicine.

Diane E. Meier, M.D. is the Director of the Center to Advance Palliative Care, and the Vice Chair for Public Policy at the Department of Geriatrics and Palliative Medicine of the Icahn School of Medicine at Mount Sinai.

Franklin G. Miller, Ph.D. is a senior faculty member of the Department of Bioethics at the National Institute of Health, a fellow of the Hastings Center, and a faculty affiliate at the Kennedy Institute of Ethics.

Kanan Modhwadia, M.D. is a Clinical Fellow, Psychiatry Service, Department of Psychiatry and Behavioral Sciences, Memorial Sloan-Kettering Cancer Center.

Sally A. Norton, Ph.D., R.N. is an Associate Professor of Nursing, Medical Humanities and Family Medicine at the University of Rochester Medical Center, and Director for Research for its Palliative Care Program.

Jane L. Phillips, R.N., Ph.D. is a Professor of Palliative Nursing at the University of Notre Dame, Australia and the Co-Director of The Cunningham Centre for Palliative Care based at Sacred Heart Hospice in Sydney, Australia.

Timothy E. Quill, M.D. is a Professor of Medicine, Psychiatry and Medical Humanities at the University of Rochester Medical Center where he also directs its Palliative Care Program. He is the immediate Past-President of American Academy of Hospice and Palliative Medicine.

Emily B. Rubin, J.D., M.D. holds a law degree from the University of Virginia and is currently a first year fellow in pulmonary and critical care medicine at the University of Pennsylvania.

Robert D. Truog, M.D. is a Professor of Medical Ethics, Anaesthesiology & Pediatrics at Harvard Medical School, a Senior Associate in Critical Care Medicine at Boston Children's Hospital, Director of Clinical Ethics at Harvard

Medical School, and Executive Director of the Institute for Professionalism and Ethical Practice.

Charles F. von Gunten, M.D. is the Vice President of Medical Affairs of Hospice and Palliative Care for the OhioHealth System based in Columbus, Ohio, and the Editor-in-Chief of the *Journal of Palliative Medicine*.

Deborah Waldrop, Ph.D. is a Professor of Social Work at the University at Buffalo where she is also Associate Dean for Faculty Development.

Emily G. Warner, J.D. is Senior Policy Analyst at the Center to Advance Palliative Care at the Icahn School of Medicine at Mount Sinai.

Heleen Weyers, Ph.D. is an Associate Professor of Sociology of Law in the Department of Legal Theory at the University of Groningen (the Netherlands).

SECTION I

Introduction and Overview

1

Introduction

Timothy E. Quill and Franklin G. Miller

Improvements in public health and new successes in medical treatment for potentially fatal diseases have led to significant increases in life expectancy over the past few decades. The unstated hope in these successes is that people will live longer, healthier lives, and then have relatively short periods of sickness after which they will die peacefully and comfortably. The theory is called the "compression of morbidity,"[1] and it theoretically makes sense and seems desirable. Unfortunately, the reality faced by most patients in the developed world can be significantly different. Patients are indeed on average living healthy a little bit longer, but (for better or worse, and sometimes both) many of these same patients are subsequently living lives dominated by varying degrees of sickness, suffering, and disability for substantially longer periods of time.[2, 3] And at the end of what can be a sustained period of serious morbidity, patients (if they are still cognitively able to participate) and their families are asked to face daunting decisions about using medical technology to try to extend life a little longer, or allowing patients to die without such interventions.

The fields of palliative care and hospice have emerged out of this background. Hospice had its beginning in England in the 1960s, and became established in the United States in the early 1980s.[4] Hospice encouraged the development of programs that would systematically attend to relieving pain and other symptoms for dying patients, and simultaneously help them and their families prepare for a meaningful death. The U.S. Medicare hospice medical benefit would pay for symptom-relieving medications for terminally ill patients aged 65 years, and provide added medical care and support to enhance quality of life, if possible in the patient's own home, for the rest of his or her life. Hospices were paid a fixed amount each day to provide all of this care (medications, hospital beds, durable goods, as well as nursing and home health aide support) so that aggregate costs could be controlled and better allocated.[5] Private insurers subsequently supported very similar programs for younger terminally ill patients.

However, to be admitted to hospice, patients and their families had to accept some hard realities: (a) the patient was deemed by a physician to be more likely than not to die in the next 6 months (in reality, half of hospice patients now die within less than 3 weeks of being admitted, and many live only a few hours or days), and (b) the patient's medical treatment would be limited to "comfort measures only," and he or she had to "give up" on medical treatments directed toward controlling or curing the underlying disease. (Of course, many treatments achieve both goals simultaneously, such as the basic treatments for congestive heart failure, so sometimes the sharp distinction between these types of treatments is hard to find in the real world of clinical medicine.) All treatment would be directed toward relieving symptoms and providing support, with the goal of helping enrolled patients "live as well as they can for as long as they can" for the time that remains. In our death-denying society, heavily oriented toward aggressive disease-fighting treatment, both of these stipulations are very difficult for many physicians, patients, and families to accept.[6] This probably accounts for the fact that about 60% of potentially eligible patients who eventually die are never admitted to hospice, and many of the approximately 40% who are referred are on the brink of death before being enrolled.

Against this background, palliative care formally emerged as a field of medicine in the early 1990s.[7] Like hospice, palliative care focused on careful attention to pain and symptom management and added family support; however, unlike hospice, palliative care allowed for patients to simultaneously receive any and all possibly effective medical treatments directed toward their underlying disease(s). Also unlike hospice, palliative care was not set up as an independent health care benefit, but rather as a limited consultative supplement to usual medical and surgical treatments. On the plus side, palliative care did not require that patients "give up" on disease-directed medical treatments to receive symptom-oriented treatments and added support (which clearly makes sense). But on the negative side, palliative care could be viewed as just another specialty lining up to maximally treat (and financially charge for) their piece of the care for seriously ill patients. Palliative care initially started as a hospital-based consult service, but more and more programs are developing outpatient and home-based practices to provide outpatient consultation and longitudinal follow-up.

Implementation of the overlapping fields of palliative care and hospice by medical systems raise a host of complex and sometimes troubling ethical issues. These ethical challenges and opportunities will be the focus of this book. By way of introduction, we will present a longitudinal case of a patient who was very ill with advanced congestive heart failure for several years before he ultimately died. Throughout the description of his clinical course, we will pose some of the related ethical questions that will be addressed in depth in subsequent chapters of this book by some of the most well-known and experienced palliative care/hospice and bioethics experts in North America and Western Europe. This initial case is intended to whet the reader's appetite, and to give an overarching sense of what we are planning to accomplish in the book.

The subsequent chapters will be divided into four broad categories: (a) overview of hospice and palliative care; (b) challenges within current systems of care; (c) addressing dimensions of suffering; and (d) difficult decisions near the end of life. Most chapters use clinical cases to illustrate salient ethical and policy challenges, indicating where there is consensus and common ground, as well as areas where controversy and differences of opinion exist. We have given chapter authors relatively free reign in their selection of cases and subtopics, so there is a wide range of clinical dilemmas and ethical positions illustrated without adherence to a strict formula or ethical stance. A brief overview of topics to be addressed within each chapter is presented toward the end of this introductory chapter.

Although the treatment and care of cancer patients has loomed large in the history of hospice and palliative care, these services are increasingly being provided to a much wider range of patients with all kinds of serious acute and chronic illnesses. We have selected a patient with advanced congestive heart failure for our introductory case presentation in part to illustrate this broader applicability.

Case Presentation

Albert Jones is a 68-year-old African-American man with advanced congestive heart failure. His left ventricular ejection fraction is less than 20%, and he has been recently hospitalized for the second time in the last 6 months. He has adult–onset diabetes mellitus, hypertension, hypercholesterolemia, obesity, and drinks two beers per day. He quit smoking 2 years ago when he first developed congestive heart failure. Mr. Jones has always wanted "everything" done medically, and has not done any advance care planning. He has been evaluated and was declined for heart transplantation unless he is able to lose 100 pounds (he weighs 350 pounds plus whatever excess fluid he has accumulated at any given time). His cardiologist participates in a large left ventricular assist device (LVAD) program, and Mr. Jones was told he might be a candidate for a "destination" LVAD (an external mechanical pump connected to his heart put in to prolong his life and improve his cardiac function without the prospect of transitioning to cardiac transplant). His cardiologist felt that his prognosis was poor without the LVAD—most likely 6 to 12 months, but it could be longer if he were able lose weight and adhere to his medications and diet; however, he could also die tomorrow if he had a severe arrhythmia or a major new ischemic event. With the LVAD, if he survived the initial implantation process without major complication, these odds could be significantly improved.

Some Clinical Questions with Ethical Implications

The first section of this book includes an Introduction and Overview of hospice and palliative care. Some clinical questions with ethical implications relative to the care of Mr. Jones addressed in this section include: (a) When would be the best time to involve either palliative care or hospice in his care, and how is it paid for? (b) If the palliative care team is involved, how should they interface with his heart failure treatment team in making major decisions about his medical treatments and options? (c) If Mr. Jones were referred to hospice, can all of his heart failure medications (even the expensive intravenous ones) be continued as part of the symptomatic treatment of his heart failure? (d) What are the financial incentives for referring such patients to hospice versus continuing in the traditional medical payment system?

The second section looks at Challenges within Current Systems of Care. Additional questions raised that are potentially relevant to Mr. Jones' care include: (a) Should all heart failure clinicians learn how to do basic palliative care as part of their overall skills, reserving specialty level palliative care for the most challenging cases, or should all seriously ill patients have access to specialty palliative care? (b) What is the appropriate public policy for allocating and paying for very expensive treatments that have a small but significant potential to improve survival and quality of life for a small number of patients?[8] (c) Who among the many teams of healthcare providers involved in Mr. Jones' care is (or should be) responsible for making major medical decisions and ensuring informed decision making? (d) If there is a difference of opinion among the professional care providers about how best to proceed with Mr. Jones' treatment, how should these differences be sorted out and resolved?

Return to the Case Presentation

Mr. Jones has experienced increasing difficulty walking, gets easily fatigued, and feels short of breath most of the time, rating his baseline dyspnea (shortness of breath) at 7 on a 10-point scale (anchored by 0 = none and 10 = extremely severe). When previously hospitalized for congestive heart failure exacerbations, he became at times mentally confused, so his clinicians were reluctant to use opioids for symptomatic dyspnea treatment. They also discovered that he had a history of cocaine abuse in his past, although he had not "used" for many years. His cardiologist commented that if he was "dying of cancer that would be another story, but he may live for many years with this condition, and I am afraid we might do more harm than good (prescribing opioids)." When asked about depression, Mr. Jones snapped back, "Wouldn't you be in my shoes?" and then with prompting rated his depression as 6/10 on the same scale. He had been living alone for the past 30 years since a divorce, and he and his family were beginning to wonder if this was still feasible given his declining functional status and intermittent confusion. On the other hand, he had always said he would "rather be dead than to live in a nursing home."

ADDITIONAL QUESTIONS

The third section of this book considers Clinical Questions with Ethical Implications related to how clinicians should address the many relevant dimensions of patient suffering. Some of the questions raised in this case include: (a) How aggressive should clinicians be in managing pain (and dyspnea) with opioids when patients may well live many years? (b) How large is the risk of respiratory depression when using opioids to treat dyspnea for patients like Mr. Jones, and how would a clinician decide if that risk was worth taking? (c) If Mr. Jones developed an agitated delirium at this point in his illness, how should his clinicians ethically decide about whether to treat it symptomatically versus aggressively searching for a potentially correctable underlying cause? (d) Isn't it normal for Mr. Jones to experience some depression and/or anxiety in this setting and, if so, how should clinicians decide whether antidepressant medications and/or psychotherapy should be recommended?

Return to the Case

Mr. Jones was discharged home on intravenous milrinone (an expensive medication that can symptomatically help congestive heart failure but does not prolong life). He was hesitant to set any limits on his treatment, including requesting cardiopulmonary resuscitation (CPR) in the event of cardiac arrest. His doctors were fearful of giving him opioids to lessen his shortness of breath because his respiratory status seemed too fragile, so he was relatively uncomfortable and anxious much of the time. He did not qualify for hospice care at home because of the expense of the milrinone (despite the fact it is a palliative medication that improves quality of life without extending it) and because of his desire to potentially return to the acute hospital and to receive further aggressive therapy if and when he got sicker in the future. Traditional home care services did not have any way to supplement his care at home beyond what was needed to deliver and monitor his milrinone. Because he was still receiving disease-directed treatments, no systematic effort was made to help him prepare for the possibility that death could come sooner rather than later. He felt very anxious about being home alone (as was the medical team), so one of his daughters took a temporary leave of absence from work to help take care of him. Neither he nor his daughter talked about their hopes and fears, and both were overwhelmed with the day-to-day logistics of his treatment.

About 3 weeks after discharge, Mr. Jones became acutely short of breath, and his daughter called 911. He was intubated (a breathing tube was put down his throat to allow for mechanical assistance with breathing) by the ambulance crew, who found him to be unresponsive, severely hypoxic, and hypotensive. He was admitted to the cardiac intensive care unit where he gradually improved over the next 3 days. He was weaned off the ventilator, but needed high-flow oxygen and medications to raise his blood pressure to maintain adequate oxygenation and perfusion of his organs. His kidney function deteriorated substantially. He was alert, but the medical team was uncertain how much he could participate in complex "life-and-death" decision making. His daughter and several other family members were invited to a family meeting to discuss options for how to proceed. The medical team felt his prognosis was very poor. They believed he might be able to be stabilized for a short period of time with intensive medical support, but the prospect for his being able to be discharged home was extremely unlikely. The odds of him being stabilized enough to go to a skilled nursing facility were also low, but that was more in the realm of possibility if he were to continue to respond to treatment.

More Questions

As Mr. Jones becomes more ill and appears to be nearing the end of his life, additional questions arise that are considered in the third and fourth sections of the book. Questions include: (a) How much should Mr. Jones himself be directly involved in medical decision making at this point given his current very limited capacity to fully understand his complex circumstances and options? (b) If he is not involved, how does "substituted judgment" work when patients have given potentially incompatible directives in the past (wanting "everything" but never wanting to go to a nursing home)? (c) If a decision were made to withdraw treatment, should Mr. Jones be heavily sedated upfront for treatment withdrawal, or should clinicians wait for symptoms to develop and then give the least amount of medications that can control symptoms? (d) If Mr. Jones and/ or his family still wanted "everything" done in this circumstance,[9] would some or all further life-sustaining treatments be "futile" and therefore not required to be offered?

Final Challenges of the Case

At the beginning of the family meeting, the clinical teams (palliative care and pulmonary/critical care) reviewed Mr. Jones' clinical situation with his family. They communicated that his heart failure had progressed, his blood pressure was very low, he was unable to breathe adequately without mechanical ventilation, and his kidneys were also "failing." They could potentially prolong his life a little bit with very aggressive medical intervention in the intensive care unit, but he was likely dying no matter what they did in terms of medical interventions. His family appeared to understand his dire medical condition, but reiterated that Mr. Jones had always wanted "everything" to be done to help him live longer. The medical team acknowledged that this was indeed consistent with his expressed prior preferences, but also gently suggested that he had also hated being in the hospital and had hoped to die at home. Mr. Jones himself was mildly sedated to tolerate the ventilator. He appeared relatively comfortable, but was completely unable to participate in decision making.

In searching for a way forward, the family was not at all comfortable with the prospect of withdrawing treatment. They suggested that "he would never want that" and "we could not live with such a decision." The team then recommended that they continue to do "everything that might help him" (current supports be continued for now including mechanical ventilation, pressors, diuretics, and blood work), but that "no new invasive treatments be added that would only hurt him" (dialysis would not be feasible because of his low blood pressure, and cardiopulmonary resuscitation would not be recommended at the very end because of its invasiveness and the high likelihood it would be unsuccessful). The team also said they would do their best to keep him as comfortable as possible no matter what decision was made about aggressive medical treatment, and suggested that the family should visit him as often as they could because his time alive was likely quite limited. The family was hesitant to make a do-not-resuscitate decision, but agreed to "think it over." They did agree with the plan to continue current life supports and to simultaneously try to keep him comfortable.

The intensive care unit team was unhappy with the outcome of the meeting because they felt that further invasive treatment was "futile" and should not be offered. The prospect of having to do cardiopulmonary resuscitation on this man when it was so unlikely to be successful from the beginning seemed abusive both to the patient and to the staff in their eyes. There was some frustration with the palliative care team for not "getting the DNR" in this circumstance in which it seemed clearly indicated. There was also some exploration about how long the "code" would have to be, and the palliative care team suggested that if he had not responded within one cycle of genuine cardiopulmonary resuscitation then it could be stopped based on medical futility. The teams agreed to continue discussions with the family about setting limits on his resuscitation status.

The palliative care team continued to meet several times per day with the family who understood and accepted that Mr. Jones was likely dying. His family spent most of the day at his bedside, and appreciated both the efforts to prolong his life as well as the efforts to keep him comfortable. When the subject of resuscitation came up, they reiterated their view that he would want "everything" tried to keep him alive, and that they would be haunted if they set this limit against his wishes. The palliative care team wrote a clear note in the medical record documenting these discussions, but also recommending that cardiopulmonary resuscitation be stopped after one cycle based on medical futility if the patient was not responding. They also recommended that the family stop being asked about their resuscitation preferences unless they brought it up because they had made their preferences clear.

Forty-eight hours later, Mr. Jones experienced a cardiopulmonary arrest. A brief attempt at cardiopulmonary resuscitation was stopped after one cycle, and the patient was pronounced dead. The family felt very satisfied with the care, and felt Mr. Jones' wishes had been honored every step of the way. The medical team remained uneasy and uncertain about having unilaterally limited their resuscitation effort, but generally felt they had made the best out of a very difficult situation.

Additional Issues and Questions

Additional ethical issues raised in the final phase of this case include the following: (a) Are there circumstances in which it is ethically permissible to unilaterally set limits on treatment when patients and families request that "everything" be done?[9] (b) Are clinicians obligated to talk with patients and families about all possible treatments, including those that are near futile, or is it proper to exercise some clinical judgment about which treatments to discuss? (c) What are the criteria for stopping cardiopulmonary resuscitation, and how much should patients and families be involved in the details of this decision? And (d) Can medical futility be defined, and can "near futile" treatments be unilaterally be withheld as a matter of policy?

Because patients like Mr. Jones are commonly seen in every medical center in the country, clinicians who care for seriously ill patients regularly confront these and other palliative care questions with significant ethical overtones. The sorts of questions posed so far in this case are the tip of the iceberg in terms of what kinds of ethical dilemmas lie just beneath the surface of day-to-day medical and palliative care practice. Mr. Jones and his family wanted his life to be extended for as long as possible even if it required that he experience added suffering. Other patients with different values and priorities may make completely opposite tradeoffs. For them, minimizing suffering might be given the highest priority, especially if recovery is not in the realm of possibility. Such patients may want to explore some or all of the "last resort" options described in chapters 14 to 17, including palliative sedation, voluntarily stopping eating and drinking, and physician-assisted death. Many legal and ethical questions surrounding these practices are explored these later chapters.

Most major academic medical centers now have trained palliative care consultants to help other clinicians and caregivers address the many dilemmas faced by patients like Mr. Jones. Unfortunately, palliative care involvement would still be the exception rather than the rule given the relatively small number of trained clinicians and the large number of severely ill patients facing these challenges in very diverse clinical settings.[7] Similarly, the availability of trained ethics consultants is even more limited and uneven, and there are no national consensus criteria for professional qualifications and training. Even with palliative care and ethics training, there are no easy solutions or widely agreed upon approaches to many of the ethical issues patients with advanced serious illness, their families, and their clinicians are facing on a regular basis.[10] Our plan is for this book to articulate and explore many of these ethical and policy issues to inform and guide clinicians who care for seriously ill patients and their families.

Overview of Subsequent Chapters

We are fortunate to have some of the best known palliative care clinician scholars and bioethicists in the North America and Western Europe to help us probe these questions. Chapter authors were given considerable latitude in choosing specific questions and in undertaking ethical and policy analyses within the palliative care domain they have chosen to explore. Although our chapter authors have published extensively in the domain they are covering, each chapter is an original work that reflects the current state of the art and science of the interface between palliative care and ethics in their area. We have challenged our authors to search for depth of ethical thought and reasoning within their domain rather than pursuing a single, common approach to all chapters. The aim is to generate new ideas and promote careful analysis using a variety of potential strategies, leading to debate and disagreement in some cases, and challenging established ways of thinking in others.

In this section we briefly identify the chapter authors, and provide a glimpse of the subtopics covered in their section.

- **Chapter 2: Hospice. Charles F. von Gunten** reviews the history and structure of the Medicare Hospice Benefit in the United States, the implications of organizing hospices as "for profit" and "not for profit," and the influence that tracking of hospital mortality statistics has had on in-hospital hospice referral. He closes the chapter by presenting some paradigmatic ethical challenges posed by several individual hospice cases he and his team have encountered.

- **Chapter 3: Palliative Care. Susan D. Block** reviews the key ethical dimensions that relate to the concepts of palliative care access, value, and care. The current status of palliative care access and barriers to enhanced availability are reviewed. Quality and cost, two central elements of value, are key dimensions of palliative care. The importance of a humanistic caring relationship between clinician and patient is described as a core element of ethical practice within palliative care.

Section II. Ethical Challenges within Current Systems of Care

- **Chapter 4: Emerging Complexities in Pediatric Palliative Care. Renee D. Boss** and **Nancy Hutton** illustrate how the standard bioethical principles of autonomy, justice, beneficence, and nonmaleficence often fall short in giving useful guidance to pediatric palliative care, leaving families, clinicians, and ethics consultants struggling to determine what is in the "best interests" of the young child. Building on four cases, this chapter highlights several unique ethical complexities in pediatric palliative care across life stages (perinatal period, infancy, childhood, and adolescence) and different medical diagnoses (congenital anomalies, extreme prematurity, intentional trauma, HIV/AIDS). Parental decision making, adolescent autonomy, and the use of emerging technologies are discussed.

¤ **Chapter 5: Patient-Centered Ethos in an Era of Cost Control: Palliative Care and Healthcare Reform. Diane E. Meier** and **Emily Warner** review how many of the reforms in the U.S. Patient Protection and Affordable Care Act aim to reduce costs while improving quality. However, efforts to reduce costs can cause consumer concerns about rationing and a loss of patient autonomy, despite government attempts to define, measure, and incentivize high-quality care. The success of palliative care elucidates how cost reduction can exist alongside patient autonomy by providing the highest-value care possible for the patient. By engaging patients in the definition of quality, and minimizing the noneconomic costs of care to the patient, treatment plans can be matched to patient goals, increasing efficiency and, ultimately, reducing costs.

¤ **Chapter 6: Palliative Care, Ethics, and Interprofessional Teams. Sally A. Norton, Deborah Waldrop**, and **Robert Gramling** examine ethical challenges faced by interprofessional palliative care teams, and how such challenges are viewed differently through varying disciplinary lenses. The ethical principles that guide the central roles of social workers, nurses, and physicians in palliative care programs are compared. The importance and intrinsic nature of team culture is described. Four clinical cases are presented to highlight areas of conflict and resolution within palliative care teams. The chapter ends with description of the important elements of high-quality teamwork and strategies for resolving conflicts.

Section III. Addressing Dimensions of Suffering

¤ **Chapter 7: Pain Relief and Palliative Care. Nathan Cherny** explores these ethical issues using a case-based approach, and addresses individual and public health duties and responsibilities that derive from the right of palliative care patients to adequate relief of pain. Finding a balance between access to adequate pain relief and preventing addiction and diversion is addressed. The rule of double effect is examined, as is the use of sedation at the end of life in the context of intractable pain.

¤ **Chapter 8: Management of Dyspnea. Thomas W. LeBlanc, David C. Currow, Jane L. Phillips**, and **Amy P. Abernethy** discuss dyspnea, which is one of the most prevalent, variable, and difficult to manage symptoms arising in hospice/palliative care clinical practice; its complexity introduces a host of ethical issues. Despite its prevalence, dyspnea remains under-recognized and under-treated, and its impact on patients and caregivers is far-reaching. This chapter briefly reviews the physiology of dyspnea and highlights various complexities of dyspnea management using several case studies to demonstrate and explore common ethical difficulties in this clinical setting.

◻ **Chapter 9: Diagnosis and Treatment of Delirium. Maxine de la Cruz** and **Eduardo Bruera** examine clinical and ethical issues relating to delirium, a neuropsychiatric condition characterized by reduced level of consciousness and cognition and psychomotor disturbance. Altered mentation can result in overexpression of symptoms by the patient, misinterpretation of symptoms by the family and medical providers, and questions about patient participation in decision making. Diagnosis and treatment of delirium are critical to the delivery of optimal care for patients. There are a series of potential ethical challenges regularly faced as patients become dehydrated and confused toward the end of life, calling for decisions to be made about evaluation/treatment versus pure palliation.

◻ **Chapter 10: Psychosocial and Psychiatric Suffering. Yesne Alici, Kanan Modhwadia,** and **William S. Breitbart** assert that suffering is a complex part of human existence inevitably encountered in palliative care settings. "Despair," a "loss of essence of what makes one human," may be a more informative description than "suffering" for the goals of psychiatric, psychosocial, and existential palliative care. Assessment and management of psychiatric disorders such as depression, anxiety, and delirium are integral to good palliative care. Hopelessness, loss of meaning, loss of dignity, demoralization, loss of spiritual well-being, desire for hastened death, and suicidal ideation are unrecognized, but common sources of suffering and despair. An overview of the main sources of psychiatric and psychosocial suffering encountered in palliative care settings including assessment and management recommendations is provided.

◻ **Chapter 11: Capacity and Shared Decision Making in Serious Illness.** Decisions in the context of serious and life-limiting illness involve preferences and values of patients with varying levels of capacity to participate in care. Clinical decisions are often influenced by family members and clinicians with varying degrees of familiarity with the patient and his or her values. This chapter by **Ronald M. Epstein** and **Vikki Entwistle** explores how clinicians can appropriately promote shared decision making in these settings. The authors propose ways in which effective communication can help address ethical problems in serious and life-limiting illness, and offer several recommendations for clinical practice in palliative care and other settings.

Section IV. Difficult Decisions Near the Very End of Life

◻ **Chapter 12: Withholding and Withdrawing Life-Sustaining Treatments.** Many of the most difficult and challenging aspects of palliative care revolve around decisions to withhold or withdraw life-sustaining treatments. **Robert D. Truog** begins this chapter with a general examination of whether there are ethical, psychological, or practical differences between decisions to withhold or withdraw a treatment. Relevant distinctions between different types of therapies that may be withheld or withdrawn are reviewed, focusing especially upon cardiac pacemakers and artificial nutrition and hydration. Finally, the chapter explores several key principles for symptom management in end-of-life care, with particular attention to strategies for withdrawal of mechanical ventilation, and some pearls and pitfalls associated with the use of sedatives and analgesics at the end of life.

¤ **Chapter 13: Medical Futility: Content in the Context of Care. Peggy L. Determeyer** and **Howard Brody** discuss the overarching concept of medical futility. Although the precise definition of "medical futility" has generated much debate, the basic idea is simple—interventions that predictably will not work to achieve the agreed-upon goals. Ultimately, they contend, it is not possible to eliminate the concept of medical futility. Three core ethical values are relevant to futility determinations—patient autonomy, professional integrity, and respectful treatment of patients and families. The best way to balance the three core values is through protocols and procedures in healthcare institutions that maximize opportunities for respectful, effective communication while recognizing the ultimate prerogative of clinicians not to provide interventions that violate their integrity.

¤ **Chapter 14: Palliative Sedation.** Palliative sedation is a recent concept in clinical medicine with multiple meanings, each with different ethical implications. **J. Andrew Billings** parses the various definitions of this "treatment of last resort," focusing on the use of sedation to obliterate consciousness of physical and psychosocial suffering in the imminently dying patient. Normative ethics of palliative sedation to unconsciousness are outlined with particular attention to justifiable killing, the rule of double effect, and rights-based arguments. Finally, clinical skills necessary for evaluating candidates for palliative sedation are presented with suggestions for safeguards against misuse.

¤ **Chapter 15: Voluntarily Stopping Eating and Drinking. Emily B. Rubin** and **James L. Bernat** address the option of voluntarily stopping eating and drinking (VSED) as a palliative option of last resort for patients with terminal or complex chronic illness. The chapter discusses the arguments in support of VSED as a legal and ethical way to hasten death when a patient with advanced illness is ready to die, the ethical distinctions between VSED and physician-assisted death, some of the benefits and disadvantages of VSED as a means of hastening death, safeguards that clinicians should seek to enforce when patients consider VSED, and some of the practical challenges and potential limitations of the practice.

¤ **Chapter 16: Physician-Assisted Death. Timothy E. Quill** and **Franklin G. Miller** use a case-based approach to address seven questions regarding physician-assisted death: (a) What language best describes the practice? (b) How much and what kind of suffering should be required? (c) Is there a moral bright line between withdrawing life supports and physician-assisted suicide (PAS) or voluntary active euthanasia (VAE)? (d) Are the differences between PAS and VAE important? (e) Are the differences between palliative sedation to unconsciousness and PAS/VAE important? (f) Are other legally available last resort options enough? (g) Is self-administration a guarantee of voluntariness?

¤ **Chapter 17A: Lessons from Legalized Physician-Assisted Death in Oregon and Washington. Linda Ganzini** describes the situation in four states, Oregon, Washington, Montana, and Vermont, that have defined a legal pathway for their citizens to choose physician-assisted death (PAD). Substantial data from Oregon available since 1997 demonstrate that two in 1,000 deaths are from PAD, and that those choosing it are more highly educated and more likely to suffer from cancer, human immunodeficiency virus, or amyotrophic lateral sclerosis compared with other Oregon deaths. Ninety percent of Oregonians who die by lethal prescription are enrolled in hospice. Hospices have varied in their accommodation to PAD, although none would discharge a patient who made this choice.

¤ **Chapter 17B: Physician-Assisted Death in Western Europe: The Legal and Empirical Situation. Heleen Weyers** provides an overview of the legal and empirical situation of physician-assisted death and other end-of-life practices in Western Europe. Special attention is paid to the system of control with respect to euthanasia in the Netherlands and Belgium. The argument is made that although this system is not perfect, it provides much more control and transparency than other systems do.

References

1. Fries, J.F., *Aging, natural death, and the compression of morbidity.* N Engl J Med, 1980. **303**(3): p. 130–5.

2. Lynn, J., et al., *Prognoses of seriously ill hospitalized patients on the days before death: implications for patient care and public policy.* New Horiz, 1997. **5**(1): p. 56–61.

3. *A controlled trial to improve care for seriously ill hospitalized patients. The study to understand prognoses and preferences for outcomes and risks of treatments (SUPPORT). The SUPPORT Principal Investigators.* JAMA, 1995. **274**(20): p. 1591–8.

4. Stoddard, S., *Hospice in the United States: an overview.* J Palliat Care, 1989. **5**(3): p. 10–9.

5. Fowler, N.M. and J. Lynn, *Potential medicare reimbursements for services to patients with chronic fatal illnesses.* J Palliat Med, 2000. **3**(2): p. 165–80.

6. Casarett, D.J. and T.E. Quill, *"I'm not ready for hospice": strategies for timely and effective hospice discussions.* Ann Intern Med, 2007. **146**(6): p. 443–9.

7. Morrison, R.S. and D.E. Meier, *Clinical practice. Palliative care.* N Engl J Med, 2004. **350**(25): p. 2582–90.

8. Rogers, J.G., Bostic, R.R., Tong, K.B., Adamson, R., Russo, M., Slaughter, M.S., *Cost-Effective Analysis of Continuous Flow Left Ventricular Assist Devices as Destination Therapy.* Circulation: Heart Failure, 2011.

9. Quill, T.E., R. Arnold, and A.L. Back, *Discussing treatment preferences with patients who want "everything."* Ann Intern Med, 2009. **151**(5): p. 345–9.

10. Demme, R.A., et al., *Ethical issues in palliative care.* Anesthesiol Clin, 2006. **24**(1): p. 129–44.

2

Hospice

Charles F. von Gunten

In the United States, a program of hospice care is the best-funded widely available approach to the care of terminally ill patients in the world. However, like all policy approaches to healthcare, it has its merits and unintended consequences. The purpose of this chapter is first to summarize the history and background of hospice care in the United States. This sets the stage for understanding its role in the continuum of healthcare in the United States. We will then describe who is well served, and who is less well served by hospice care as it is structured in the United States. That leads to a comparison of the "for-profit" and "not-for-profit" hospices, as well as a consideration of the "expanded access" approaches that some large hospices have taken to serve more patients as contrasted with that of small hospice programs. Then, we will review the policy implications of whether a hospital death with hospice care is, or should be, counted differently from a death in another part of the healthcare system as a measure of healthcare quality. Finally, some vignettes from hospice care are used to illustrate the ethical challenges to the relief of suffering that persist within hospice programs.

Brief History of Hospice and Hospice Care

In the United States, the word "hospice" has several meanings:

(1) A federal system of reimbursement for a distinct program of end-of-life care
(2) A place to go to die
(3) A home-based, team approach to caring for a dying person and his or her family
(4) A philosophy or approach to care of sick people

The word "hospice" shares the same Latin root as the words hospital and hospitality. From the beginning of the Dark Ages to the Enlightenment in Europe, primarily religious institutions staffed inpatient facilities where the sick could be treated until they recovered or died (1). By the 12th century, there were distinctions between hospitals, in which patients could potentially be cured, and hospices, in which the dying poor were sent. Such institutions disappeared after the Protestant Reformation. However, in the 19th century in France and England, the practice was revived in a few centers (2).

In the 1940s, Cicely Saunders, trained as a nurse then working as a social worker, observed poor care of the dying in hospitals in London. She trained as a physician in order to be more effective in advocating for better care of the dying in hospitals or existing hospices. She founded St. Christopher's Hospice in a southern suburb of London England in 1967 as the culmination of nearly 20 years of direct observation of the care of terminally ill people (2). The challenges for changing existing patterns of care were so great that she needed to found her own separate institution; she was unsuccessful in influencing change in existing hospitals or hospices.

The multiple meanings of the word "hospice" can be traced to her work. She founded a place using an established name "hospice," but articulated and demonstrated a new set of principles for care of patients dying primarily of cancer. It was also a site for training people to apply the principles in their own countries with different funding and service delivery models. She was quite clear that the approaches would be applied differently in different places. The principles she articulated and demonstrated have come to be known as "hospice care." In francophone cultures, where the term "hospice" is still used for residential facilities for care of the terminally ill, the term "palliative care" was coined to refer to the same approach as hospice care, but a changed label for the purpose of gaining acceptance in French-speaking Canada.

In the United States, the publication of *On Death and Dying* by Dr. Elisabeth Kübler-Ross in 1969 capped a decade of general discussion about poor end-of-life care in the United States (3). Dr. Kübler-Ross was an academic psychiatrist at the University of Chicago Medical School. The combination of intense public marketing and personal appearances throughout the nation with a message critical of standard medicine set an important tone. Cicely Saunders was also a charismatic speaker. Many people who heard her in the United States went to visit St. Christopher's, and then came back to the United States to try to implement what they had seen. Those inspired by their own experiences, and motivated by Drs. Kübler-Ross and Saunders, united behind a vision of care that was defined by being different from standard healthcare. The polemic used a characterization of "standard care" that dying patients could either be subjected to invasive, uncomfortable, impersonal, and useless medical care or they could be abandoned by that standard care. A different and separate approach was proposed as an alternative. These public advocates, notable for being driven primarily by nursing and lay volunteers, achieved two federal government initiatives.

THE NATIONAL HOSPICE STUDY

In 1979, The National Hospice Demonstration Project was initiated as a research study funded by the US federal government to study the phenomenon of hospice care in the United States (4). The study aimed to select hospices from each of three models that had emerged in the United States: (1) Hospital-based hospice programs. The majority only had a dedicated inpatient unit without a significant home care component. (2) Home health agency hospice programs without a dedicated hospice inpatient unit, and (3) Independent hospice programs exclusively serving terminally ill patients, with or without a special inpatient unit, staffed primarily by volunteers (professional and lay). The Healthcare Financing Administration chose 26 existing hospice programs as demonstration projects out of 233 applicants in late 1979 and provided them with funding for their work. The chosen hospice programs were located in 16 states. A comparison sample of 14 hospice programs were chosen from among the three types as controls who did not receive federal demonstration project funding. The chosen hospices were not randomly selected. During the course of the National Hospice Study, 13,374 patients were admitted to participating demonstration and nondemonstration hospice programs between 1980 and 1982. Broadly, the study showed that patients who chose hospice care did not suffer any deprivation of care, often (although not always) required a lower level of expenditure, and usually were able to spend more time at home.

THE MEDICARE HOSPICE BENEFIT

The US Congress enacted legislation in 1982 authorizing a hospice care benefit to all beneficiaries of the federal healthcare plan designed to cover the hospital needs of people over the age of 65 and those who are disabled. The benefits are summarized in Table 2.1. They did this while the National Hospice Study was still in progress. However, the results influenced the development of the regulations that implemented the congressional action.

The standards and criteria that had been developed by the National Hospice Organization received enough dissemination and favorable reaction in the US Congress that they became part of the Medicare Hospice Benefit (5). This broad benefit led to rapid growth of hospice care in the United States. This federal funding led to the establishment of a hospice industry in the United States. In 2010 there were 5,150 hospice organizations receiving $12 billion from the US government for the terminal care of about 1.58 million Americans (6). About 36% are nonprofit; 6% are government owned, and the remainder are for-profit. Eighty-five percent of all hospice care is paid for from this benefit. Its terms influence the other 15% of payers. Therefore, the Medicare Hospice Benefit is the driving force behind all US hospice care.

Briefly, for hospice care to be covered under the Medicare Hospice Benefit, two broad criteria must be met. First, the patient must have a prognosis of less than 6 months (later changed to less than 6 months if the disease follows its usual course) as determined by two physicians. Second, the treatment plan for the terminal illness needs to be palliative. Table 2.2 summarizes some prognostic criteria for cancer, which was the model illness for which hospice care was developed. Once a patient is eligible and elects hospice care, the hospice agency receives a fixed amount of

TABLE 2.1
Medicare Hospice Benefit

Covered Services (100%—No Co-pay)

- ¤ Nursing care: to provide intermittent (usually 1–3 times/week) assessment, support, skilled services, treatments, and case management services
- ¤ 24-hour availability for assessment and management of changes, crises, and other acute needs
- ¤ Social work: supportive counseling, practical aspects of care (other community services), and planning (healthcare surrogates, advance directives)
- ¤ Counseling services, including chaplaincy
- ¤ Home health aide and homemaker services
- ¤ Speech therapy, nutrition, physical therapy, and occupational therapy services
- ¤ Bereavement support to family after the death
- ¤ Medical oversight of the plan of care by the hospice medical director
- ¤ All medications and supplies for management and palliation of the advanced illness (hospices may collect a small co-pay for medications)
- ¤ Durable medical equipment (e.g., hospital bed, commode, wheelchair)
- ¤ Short-term general inpatient care for problems that cannot be managed at home, such as pain, dyspnea, delirium, acute needs requiring skilled care
- ¤ Short-term respite to permit family caregivers to take a break
- ¤ Continuous care at home for short episodes of acute need

Services Not Covered by the Medicare Hospice Benefit

- ¤ Continuous nursing or nurse aide care
- ¤ Medications unrelated to the advanced illness
- ¤ Doctor visits for direct medical care (billed to Medicare separately)
- ¤ Residential (nonacute) care in a facility

TABLE 2.2
Cancer: Prognostic Factors, Median Survival Assuming Maximal Medical Therapy

Factor		Median Survival
Karnofsky performance status	50–60	90 days
Karnofsky performance status	20–30	50 days
Karnofsky performance status	10–20	17 days
ECOG/Zubrod/WHO Score	3	3 months
ECOG/Zubrod/WHO Score	4	1 month
Hypercalcemia		1 month
Brain mets (multiple)	No Rx	1 month
Brain mets (multiple)	Corticosteroids	3 months
Brain mets (multiple)	Radiation therapy	6 months
Malignant pleural effusion		4 months
Serum albumin	<2.5 mg/dl	<6 months
Unintentional weight loss	10%	<6 months
Dyspnea		<6 months
Anorexia		<6 months
Delirium		6 weeks

ECOG, Eastern Cooperative Oncology Group; WHO, World Health Organization.

money per patient per day for care. In the United States, this was the first federal example of a managed care plan in which the hospice agency carried the "risk" for caring for the population of patients rather than being reimbursed on a cost basis, as was the standard for Medicare coverage.

Once the patient enrolls in a hospice care, the patient and his or her family are assigned to a team that, at a minimum, must be comprised of a nurse, counselor (usually social worker), chaplain, and nurse's aide. Other services can be provided depending on the plan of care for the particular patient and family. The team meets at least every other week to discuss the care of the patient and his or her family. The frequency and duration of the visits to the patient and family are determined by the team and the circumstances in a written plan of care.

Distinctive Contributions of Hospice to Continuum of Care for Dying Patients

The most important contribution that hospice care has made to the continuum of care for dying patients in the United States is to provide a uniform package of services designed to provide care to the patient and family as a unit in the general categories of physical care (including sympton control), psychological care (emotional support), social care (including family systems and practical aspects of living at home), and spiritual care provided under a single regulatory structure in the setting in which they live. In contrast with standard Medicare funding that requires a 20% contribution from the patient and only focuses on the patient's medical care, federal funding of hospice care with no copayment means that hospice care is now available in all inhabited areas of the country, rural and urban. In addition, the data is quite clear that hospice care provides better quality of care than standard care for dying patients from the perspective of their surviving families (7).

The most important unintended consequence of the model for paying for hospice care in the United States is the requirement that a patient choose hospice care and explicitly opt out of standard care of the terminal illness. A patient must enroll in hospice care and explicitly disenroll from care of the terminal illness by standard care paid for by standard Medicare and provided by standard doctors, hospitals, and outpatient environments. A patient must join what is essentially a different healthcare system when hospice care begins.

Who Gets Referred to Hospice before Death and Who Does Not?

The single most important feature of hospice care in the United States is that a patient must be labeled as terminally ill in a formal way by two physicians, and acknowledged by the patient insofar as the patient and family must sign up for a different approach to care. The patient then is cared for by a hospice program that only provides palliative care with the expectation that the patient will soon die. This feature has three implications for who is referred (and accepts referral) for hospice care. First, the patient must have an identifiable illness for which a physician can say there is a prognosis of less than 6 months if the disease follows its normal course. The model disease is solid tumor cancer. As a general model, a patient is treated with surgery, chemotherapy, and radiation for a disease like lung cancer or colon cancer until there is a point when such efforts are futile. At that point in time, a decision can be made to stop standard care and begin hospice care.

Second, two physicians must establish a prognosis that is less than 6 months if the disease follows its normal course. For a variety of reasons, the subject of prognostication has not been a major focus of medical care for more than 100 years. Whereas there was a time when the physician could, at best, answer the patient's questions of "What is wrong with me?" (diagnosis) and "What will happen to me?" (prognosis), the last 100 years have been preferentially focused on the question of "What can you do for me?" (treatment) (8).

In addition, there is a broad concern that the physician should not tell the patient the true prognosis out of a perceived duty to sustain hope for recovery. Further, there is a frequent belief among physicians that if they tell a patient about a poor prognosis, there will be a self-fulfilling prophecy and the patient will die sooner because the patient has given up hope. Coupled with poor science about prognostication, and little dissemination of the small amount of data that suggest that patients do not die from the news, it is not surprising that referral for hospice care comes late, if at all, in the course of illness.

In the example of cancer, an enormous industry for cancer treatment has arisen in the United States. Coupled with the business ethics of offering services that patients can choose analogous to shopping for a commodity in the local department store, the determination of "treatable" is no longer just a medical professional decision. Oncologists commonly describe the situation of having no treatments that will be effective for a patient, but administering further chemotherapy because the patient and family want it or they don't want to give up.

For cancer, the core data behind prognosis have been unchanging over the last 40 years (9). The ability to maintain usual patterns to perform the usual activities of daily living is closely related to prognosis. When a patient must spend more than 50% of waking hours in bed, the patient has 1 to 3 months left to live. For a patient who is bed bound because of cancer, the prognosis is about 1 month. As a generalization, there is a "tipping point" when the plateau of usual health and stamina changes and the downhill course is 4 to 6 weeks in duration. For the patient with cancer who "tips," it takes some weeks for that to register with the managing physicians, the recommendation for hospice care to be made and accepted, and the arrangements for hospice care to begin.

Even for cancer care, physicians are routinely and systematically more optimistic in their prognostication as compared with actual survival. Because patient care in the United States is generally divided up between specialists, there is also confusion as to who decides or is responsible for determining and communicating the prognosis. In addition, the patient and family need to accept the prognosis. It shouldn't be surprising that the average length of time spent in hospice care is measured in days to weeks, and 20% to 50% of eligible patients with cancer are never referred for hospice care (6).

For diseases other than cancer, the situation becomes more complicated. In contrast with cancer, there is no distinction between "curative" and "palliative" measures for patients with advanced heart failure, emphysema, motoneuron diseases, and dementia. In addition and in contrast to the course of cancer, there is a less predictable course over years of exacerbations and remediations of acute events; in one of which the patient dies (10).

Third, the patient and family must accept the prognosis. American culture is known for its consumer-oriented, individualistic features. There is a broad belief that what a patient believes will influence his or her outcomes irrespective of medical facts. Simultaneously, there has been an erosion of the professional ethic that mandates that the physician only provide care which the physician believes will help to a business ethic of "give the lady what she wants."

As a consequence of these three features, only about 40% of all Americans who die are referred for hospice care, with a range of time in hospice care measured from hours to months. About one-third of all patients referred for hospice care die within 7 days of admission. About 50% die within 14 days. There is a trend toward shorter lengths of stay looking at data year to year (6).

Incentives with For-Profit Hospices and Not-For-Profit Hospices

A feature of healthcare in the United States that distinguishes it from nearly all other countries is its use of a healthcare market instead of a healthcare system to meet the healthcare needs of its population. Healthcare organizations can be either for-profit or not-for-profit. Payers can make no distinction between the tax status of the healthcare providers. The success of for-profit hospice programs, like other for-profit businesses, is the return of a profit margin after all business expenses and income taxes are paid. In the United States, the profit margin for hospice programs has been on the order of 5% to 18% of gross income (11).

In contrast, not-for-profit hospice programs, like other not-for-profit organizations, have a preferential status in which they are not required to pay any income taxes. This is granted to organizations that are assumed to be providing a public good that would otherwise be provided by government at higher cost and lower efficiency, or wouldn't be provided at all. Not-for-profit hospices generally have a profit after expenses of –10% to 5%.

In other words, the difference between the two tax statuses of hospice programs is stark. Efforts to understand how two different corporate tax statuses can have two different financial outcomes while working under the same set of regulations for a single payer, and getting the same amount of money for each day of care from the United States federal government has yielded the following conclusions. There is no evidence that the quality of care between the two is different (12). However, for-profit hospice programs hire less skilled staff with higher caseloads per staff member (13). They also enroll patients with diseases that have longer life expectancy, notably patients with dementia living in residential care facilities. Such individuals frequently don't have family and therefore require fewer of the interventions of the hospice team. In other words, their care is less expensive.

The most recent development in for-profit hospice programs is for a long-term care company to also establish its own hospice program. Consequently, patients living in the company's facilities are covered both by Medicaid, the program that pays for two-thirds of the nation's costs of the elderly in nursing homes, and Medicare Hospice Benefit. It is an ongoing area of investigation to determine if there is a measure of double-dipping in such arrangements in which the federal government is paying twice for care that should be covered in only one of the payment mechanisms.

The data aside, it should be clear from the underlying principles that it is in the interest of for-profit hospice programs to care for patients with fewer needs and longer lengths of stay. Although the same principles presumably apply to a non-profit hospice, there is less of a reward for doing so. Contributing to this conflict of interest is the principle of choice. In contrast with Emergency Medical Treatment and Active Labor Act (EMTALA) laws that require hospitals to provide care for any patient who appears in their emergency rooms, there is no such requirement for hospice programs. They are free to accept or reject taking patients just as patients are free to reject the recommendation to seek hospice care as an alternative to standard care.

From an ethical and legal point of view, a for-profit business must return a profit to its owners as its primary goal. To do less is reasonable grounds to fire the employees. Service provision is secondary—it is done only insofar as it leads to the primary goal. In contrast, from an ethical and legal perspective, a community-owned not-for-profit must return value to its community at a total than is more than the government could have purchased using tax revenue. Consequently, it is difficult to defend the current situation where for-profit hospice companies comprise more than half of all hospice programs in the United States. Such a situation is unthinkable in the rest of the countries of the world.

Ethical Challenges and Opportunities of Expanded Access Models to Hospice

The federal guidelines governing hospice care require the hospice to pay for all costs of care related to the terminal illness. A barrier both to referral, and to the acceptance of the recommendation to enroll in hospice care, is the issue of giving up standard approaches to care and accepting only palliative care for the disease state. Because there is no regulatory barrier, some hospice programs have taken an expanded view of what constitutes palliative care of an illness. For example, all chemotherapy and radiotherapy for advanced cancer can be palliative if it actually works to shrink the cancer—if the cancer is better, the patient feels better. Because the hospice pays for expenses out of a pool of money from all patients enrolled, larger hospices have more money from which to spend on treatments like radiotherapy, chemotherapy, transfusions, medical devices, and the like. This in turn leads to lower barriers to enrollment. Consequently open access programs aim for longer lengths of stay and larger enrollments of patients.

Small hospices with restrictive admission policies are financially prohibited from such approaches. One patient with one expensive treatment would financially sink the average 60-person census hospice program. For the hospice program with 2,000 patients enrolled, it represents budget dust.

Critics of open access argue that such policies obscure the differences between hospice care and standard care. For patients who are nearing the end of life, continuing anti-disease therapies requires a more skilled nursing workforce, and a workforce that can tolerate caring for patients who may have more ambiguous or downright unrealistic goals despite the medical intent of the therapies. Advocates suggest that the interdisciplinary hospice team is well poised to manage the evolving goals of care of patients and their families while they are enrolled, rather than waiting for them to make firm choices before enrollment in an environment that doesn't provide such rich support.

Implications and Incentives of Hospice Deaths Not Counting in Hospital Mortality Measures

As the agenda to improve quality in American healthcare has taken hold, one of the measures of a hospital's quality is the number of deaths that occur in that hospital. Death in this model is presumed to be a medical failure and an error. Even adjusted for severity of illness, it is publicly reported that hospitals with lower mortality are better than those with higher mortality.

A patient can be enrolled in hospice care even when he or she is occupying a hospital bed. But, because that represents a discharge from the hospital and an admission to the hospice, that transaction is recorded. In some measures of hospital mortality, those deaths while enrolled in the hospice program don't count toward the hospital's quality measure. Similarly, a patient who is nearing death in the hospital can also be moved to a hospice unit, or to home, or to a nursing home under hospice care for the last hours to days and improve a hospital's mortality statistics (14).

It should be obvious that two hospitals that pursue the same overall approaches to care might have very different mortality statistics based on the availability and willingness of hospice programs to formally admit these short stay patients. Overall, hospice programs lose money on any patients who are enrolled less than 10 days. On the hospice side, the goal in taking short stay patients is to cultivate positive relationships with the hospital to hope to have more patients who will stay longer in the future. In fact, in the competition for relationships with a hospital, there is little to stop a hospice from giving favorable treatment to the discharge planners that make those choices—lunches, treats, and so on—in other words, the same behaviors that pharmaceutical companies have manifested with physicians for whom they wish to influence prescribing behaviors.

The purpose of reporting death rates is to improve overall quality of care. It does seem that counting the deaths that would have naturally occurred because of the underlying disease does not fit the goal of trying to prevent avoidable deaths. Therefore, it would make sense that deaths of patients enrolled in hospice care (and administratively discharged to hospice care from the hospital), or who come to the hospital to die, should not count against a hospital's scorecard. On the other hand, one could imagine "gaming" the system in which a patient who should have recovered, who is now dying and referred for hospice care, would hide a preventable death. Interestingly, those who rate hospitals are now moving toward a calculation of mortality index that relies more on conditions present at admission as a way to avoid this conundrum.

Hospice Approaches to Cases of Severe Suffering Despite Good Care

The overriding goal of care in the hospice setting is to relieve suffering in any of the four dimensions of physical (including symptoms), psychological (emotional distress such as anxiety), social (the consequences of disadvantaged living situations and distressed family relationships), and spiritual (existential distress).

There are a variety of situations in which suffering persists despite best application of a team-based approach. The following are a series of cases in which an ethics consultation had been requested. They are chosen because there aren't easy solutions to them—they represent challenges that persist despite being in a purposely designed system for the relief of the suffering of the dying and their families. They illustrate the range of ethical issues that arise in hospice care that are not within the sphere of policy, but rest squarely in the challenges of clinical medicine.

WHO DECIDES WHETHER THE PATIENT IS SUFFERING?

A 4-year-old child with cerebral palsy was admitted to an inpatient hospice unit for evaluation of pain. The patient has had a gastrostomy tube for feeding since birth. The child has had fevers to 105°F caused by aspiration pneumonia and possible body temperature dysregulation caused by the cerebral palsy. The patient has experienced recurrent episodes of pancreatitis because of an inoperable cyst in the bile duct and gastrostomy feeding. The child was observed to bang her head against objects, spin in bed, squirm, grunt, and scream. The hospice team thinks the child is in pain and requires pain medication. The pediatricians caring for the patient say this is all "normal" for many patients with severe cerebral palsy and they interpret the behaviors as self-stimulating or self-soothing. The patient has a history significant for a ventriculoperitoneal shunt for congenital hydrocephalus. The child has a developmental age of about 4 months. The child's foster mother is a former neonatal intensive care unit (ICU) nurse who has experience with 10 foster children with severe developmental abnormalities. She does not know whether the child is in pain or not.

Ethical Issues:

- Who decides the patient is suffering when the patient cannot speak for himself or herself? Is it the primary doctors, the nurses, the foster mother, or the hospice team? In this case, if the hospice staff is prevented from doing what they think is right, can the child be discharged from hospice care back to "usual" care? The child is thought to have a life expectancy of less than 6 months if the disease runs its normal course, so she clearly qualifies for hospice; the child is likely to die relatively suddenly from either pneumonia or sepsis. In this case, there was never a complete resolution. However, the child remained in hospice care, and there was a commitment to continued conversation about perceptions on the part of all involved in providing the care.

- This case illustrates a number of issues for hospice programs as they are designed in the United States. First, hospice care is organized as a choice. Patients can disenroll from hospice care if they want. In contrast, patients cannot disenroll from standard care; if the patient presents for standard medical care, the care must be given. Yet, the data are clear that hospice care yields the best outcomes for patients and family who are dying. In other words, there are ethical challenges of the hospice program being separate from standard care. Another aspect of choice is the hospice can choose which patients to enroll; and can find that, by not pursuing the hospice's plan of care, the family is choosing to disenroll.

- There is moral distress for hospice staff if their convictions about "good care" conflict with those of other healthcare professionals—in this case, the pediatricians. One way to end the distress is to discharge the patient from hospice care back to standard care. However, as in this case, if the patient's overall needs are best met within a hospice program, then the distress of the hospice staff must be addressed in other ways. Group discussion of the effects of the family and pediatrician decisions can be helpful, as well as framing the risks of compromising principles while remaining enrolled in hospice care versus the risk of abandonment if the patient is disenrolled.

- We have no better medical measure of the presence of pain than what the patient reports. The medical literature is quite clear that family, nurses, and doctors do not accurately report pain. Yet, in this case, all we have is behavior that is interpreted in various ways by the different adult caregivers. This illustrates the challenge of assessing pain in any patient who is cognitively impaired, such as those with dementia.

¤ In general, those working in hospice care believe that, when in doubt, erring on the side of administering medications for pain and symptom control is preferable to the risk of not treating the symptoms. However, others don't have those same values; some believe that symptom control medications are best minimized or avoided entirely rather than to medicate unnecessarily.

Discussion

Although there was no simple resolution of this case, the decision was made to keep the child enrolled in hospice care because that seemed to best meet the needs of the child and her foster mother. There were frequent meetings to openly discuss the moral distress that the hospice nurses and staff experienced. The pediatricians attended some of those meetings; a spirit of open communication and an acknowledgment of the difficulty accurately assessing pain in this patient were established. Rather than dividing into two camps of "the patient is in pain; the patient is not in pain," an approach of time-limited trials of pain treatment approaches to see if behavior was affected, and agreeing that the comfort of all affected by the child was also important, mother as well as staff.

FAMILY WON'T PERMIT THE RELIEF OF SUFFERING

An 89-year-old woman with dementia, stage D congestive heart failure, and renal failure was transferred to the hospice inpatient unit from the hospital for treatment of delirium and pain. The patient had a previous episode of delirium precipitated by gabapentin for pain control that made her confused, and that resolved after the drug was withdrawn. The patient's daughter reports her mother said she "never wanted to be confused like that again." The daughter was refusing permission for any medications for management of pain and delirium. The hospice team was concerned the patient was suffering and the daughter was not permitting standard of care. The patient looked like she would live hours to days with poor oxygen saturation, agitated delirium, ashen color, and little urine output.

The daughter felt she owed her life to her mother because her mother advocated the daughter be one of the first pediatric open heart patients for atrial septal defect. The sons would not get involved because they wanted to maintain a good relationship with the sister.

Ethical Issues:

¤ There is general agreement that family members are usually the best able to provide substituted judgment for patients who lack decision-making capacity. But there is little guidance about which family members are best. In the absence of a document naming one decision maker, it leaves the assessment open to judgment. Generally, the family member who knows the patient best would be chosen, but in cases such as this there may be countertransference issues that get in the way of proper decision making. In this case, there was no doubt that the daughter loved the patient, and was trying to "do the right thing," but there was a clear difference of opinion as to what should be done.

¤ Commonly, when there are multiple family members, the main surrogate decision maker may not be representing the best interests of the patient. In such cases, it is important not to be drawn into a "win" or "lose" dyad, but to commit to continued discussion that focuses as much as possible about what the family believes the patient would have wanted (substituted judgment).

¤ The courts have repeatedly said they prefer medical decisions be made close to the bedside—that courts are the least well-suited to establishing what is right. For that reason, and others, our hospice has a formal ethics consult team that was requested by the hospice team. Such an approach is preferable to going to court by far.

Discussion

The daughter was clearly suffering. As in the first case, a way to move forward is to try to climb down from the polarity of the positions that "the patient is suffering and the daughter is a barrier" versus "the evil hospice staff just want to drug the patient without regard to the consequences to the patient." A climate of mutual respect and concern was established and a concerted effort to have the daughter feel like she had been heard. In addition, efforts at bereavement support for the daughter were initiated. As in so many cases, time is an ally. The skill of the hospice staff was not to try to resolve the issue, but work with the daughter. The hospice's ethics team was consulted and provided a third, neutral voice that helped facilitate the communication of the daughter with the hospice team.

WHAT IF RELIGIOUS BELIEF CONFLICTS WITH THE MEDICAL
RELIEF OF SUFFERING?

A 76-year-old Christian Scientist has metastatic breast cancer to leptomeninges, bone, skin, and liver. She has open painful chest wounds because of the cancer in the skin. Moving her extremities causes severe pain because of the bone metastases. She cries and moans, complaining of the pain. She has been treated with standard surgery, hormonal therapy, and chemotherapy. She is being treated with fentanyl patch 150 µg/h. However, she won't take breakthrough pain medications and won't let her baseline pain medication dose be increased. Her family says the patient has told them she does not want any pain medications under any circumstances. The hospice staff reports that she told the medical team differently. She is being seen by a Christian Science practitioner who tells her she shouldn't be taking any pain medications or she won't get into heaven because of her lack of faith. When the hospice team is present, the patient says she has pain and wants treatment. The son John, her decision maker, is conflicted, but leans toward the Christian Science recommendation. His wife, the daughter-in-law, agrees with the Christian Science practitioner. The hospice team feels the patient's comfort is not being honored because of the influence of family and Christian Science practitioners.

Ethical Issues:

◻ The Christian Science view of suffering is different from standard allopathic healthcare, and also sometimes clashes with the culture of hospice. Hospice generally has to accommodate in such circumstances because it is the patient's values that count most. Christian Science is a recognized form of healthcare paid for by the government under Medicare.

◻ In this particular case, the patient was giving mixed messages—one to the hospice staff when alone and a different one when the family is present (common scenario). It is routine for people to say one thing in some situations, and something different in other situations. Sometimes this reflects simple politeness, and other times it is a part of significant ambivalence, and still others it represents family conflict. Yet, who decides whose version of "standard healthcare" prevails when the patient herself vacillates? The hospice team needs to explore and try to understand the underlying dynamics, and ultimately try to keep the patient in the center of decision making.

◻ Are patients allowed to make "bad decisions" on hospice, such as refusing effective pain management? The answer must be yes. Yet, it is very challenging to team members, especially when patients seem to be influenced by others.

Discussion

In this case, the patient's request for breakthrough medications by directly requesting it from the nurse made it very visible to others. In an inpatient setting (in contrast to home) the patient must report pain and ask for breakthrough medications. A patient-controlled analgesia pump at the bedside where the patient could push a button for additional medication represented an alternate way for her to be more private about her choices. In addition, a concerted effort by chaplaincy to help her address her feelings about the role of religion in her life in a nonjudgmental manner was very helpful in this case.

CAN A PATIENT BE SEDATED TO UNCONSCIOUSNESS FOR EXISTENTIAL DISTRESS?

A 71-year-old former litigation attorney has esophageal cancer with bone metastases. He was admitted to hospice care complaining of severe neck pain and nausea.

Those physical symptoms are controlled. However, he must wear a cervical collar to sustain the pain relief and spends most of his day in bed. He still walks to the bathroom and showers sitting in a chair. He expresses severe frustration with his loss of function. He finds his current situation "intolerable." Although the physical pain and nausea are reasonably well-controlled, it is existential distress that "this is no life worth living" and he would "go to Oregon if I could" for assisted suicide that leads to a request for sedation. The hospice team wonders if his existential distress could be relieved by further work with chaplaincy, psychiatry, and counseling. They have seen it happen with other patients.

Ethical Issues:

◘ Can the rationale for sedation for physical symptoms be extended to suffering from existential distress? The usual rationale for sedation is that the suffering is refractory to standard treatment. Palliative sedation is most easily understood and accepted for the treatment of severe, refractory physical suffering, yet there is no standard treatment for existential distress, and there would be much less consensus about the permissibility of palliative sedation for pure existential distress (see chapter 15).

◘ It is nearly routine for patients to consider suicide and hastened death at some point in their illness experience. Most ultimately reject it, but a few pursue the possibility in earnest (see chapter 16). A much smaller number find their existential angst is relieved with time and attention—but how long is enough?

◘ Although some healthcare staff are concerned that sedation represents a form of hastened death, it is well established in ethical discourse and supported by Supreme Court decision that sedation may be used to relieve distress. For physical distress, such as pain or shortness of breath, there is uniformity of opinion and broad support for the practice of sedation. For existential distress, there is uniformity that hospice teams need to try to understand and address the underlying issues, and get help if it is beyond their expertise, but there is less uniformity resolving it with heavy sedation.

◘ Of course most suffering represents a mix of physical and existential, so the mere presence of existential aspects of a patient's suffering should not disqualify him or her from access to aggressive symptom control measures. But the more dominant the existential issues, the more there would be need for a multidisciplinary, multidimensional evaluation to ensure it is as fully understood and addressed as possible.

In this case, acknowledging the distress and permitting the patient some control over the use of benzodiazepines "just to sleep" helped diffuse the sense of stand-off. Instituting other modalities of treatment such as aromatherapy, guided imagery, and hypnosis were also helpful. After a full assessment, the medical staff affirmed that they could initiate sedation if the patient decided that further awareness was intolerable. Discussions with staff to discuss their feelings, and to air their distress in a nonjudgmental manner were also helpful. As his cancer progressed, and he spent more of his time in bed asleep, the issue became less acute. He eventually died relatively peacefully using standard palliative treatments.

FINAL THOUGHTS

Hospice care is an organized approach to the provision of palliative care near the end of life. Like most solutions, it solves some problems, but not all. Within the parameters of the federal legislation under which all Medicare-certified hospice programs operate, there is still considerable variability. Although it is a comfort to know that "open access" can be pursued under existing regulations, it means that some hospice programs will not or cannot do that. But, even with the best hospice care, there are ethical issues presented by challenging cases. These four cases illustrate a few, but by no means all, of these challenges. A theme underlying resolution is to retreat from an effort to determine what is right and what is wrong to one of thoughtful dialogue to better understand positions, interests, worries, and concerns of patients, their families, the medical team, and the hospice team. This pattern of diplomacy seems to make room for solutions that will work for the present time in the particular case. If common ground cannot be found, seeking involvement of the ethics committee can provide a way out for staff that felt morally distressed or backed into a corner. When there is a general acknowledgment that we are engaged in a process and an achievement of right or wrong is not possible, there is the ability to see how we might manage care, at least for today—leaving tomorrow for later. Further, it helps not to try to establish policy or precedent, but to try to do the right thing, all things considered, for this patient and family today.

Acknowledgment

Steven Oppenheim, MD, Chief Medical Director and Charles R. Lewis, MD, former Chair of the Ethics Committee at San Diego Hospice and the Institute for Palliative Medicine provided the cases for this chapter.

References

1. Aries P. Western attitudes toward death from the middle ages to the present. The Johns Hopkins University Press, Baltimore, 1974, p76.
2. Saunders C. History of hospice care. In: *Oxford Textbook of Palliative Medicine*, 2nd ed. Oxford University Press, New York, 1998.
3. Kübler-Ross E. *On death and dying: what the dying have to teach doctors, nurses, clergy and their own families.* Macmillan Publishing, Inc., New York, 1969.

4. Mor V, Greer DS, Kastenbaum R. The hospice experiment: an alternative in terminal care. In: The Hospice Experiment. Eds: V. Mor, D. Greer, R. Kastenbaum. Johns Hopkins University Press, Baltimore, 1988, p7.

5. Hospice Standards. National Hospice Organization, Arlington, Virginia, 1979.

6. National Hospice and Palliative Care Organization Facts & Figures. Released January 2012. http://www.nhpco.org/i4a/pages/index.cfm?pageid=5994 (accessed August 14, 2012).

7. Teno JM, Clarridge BR, Casey V, Welch LC, Wetle T, Shield R, Mor V. Family perspectives on end-of-life care at the last place of care. JAMA 2004;291:88–93.

8. Christakis NA. Death foretold: prophecy and prognosis in medical care. University of Chicago Press, Chicago, 1999.

9. Glare P. Prognostic factors in terminal cancer. In: Prognostic Factors in Cancer, 3rd ed. Eds: MK Gospodarowicz, B O'Sullivan, LH Sobin. Wiley-Liss, a John Wiley & Sons, Inc. Publication. Hoboken, New Jersey, 2006, p63.

10. Field MJ, Cassel CK, eds. Approaching death: improving care at the end of life. Institute of Medicine. National Academy Press, Washington, D.C., 1997.

11. Von Gunten CF. Profit or not-for-profit: who cares? J Palliat Med 2008;11:954.

12. Wachterman MW, Marcantonio ER, Davis RB, McCarthy EP. Association of hospice agency profit status with patient diagnosis, location of care and length of stay. JAMA 2011;205:472–9.

13. Cherlin EJ, Carlson MDA, Herrin J, Schulman-Green D, Barry CL, McCorkle R, Johnson-Hurzeler R, Bradley EH. Interdisciplinary staffing patterns: do for-profit and nonprofit hospices differ? J Palliat Med 2010;389–94.

14. Cassel JB, Jones AB, Meier DE, Smith TJ, Spragens LH, Weissman D. Hospital mortality rates: how is palliative care taken into account? J Pain Sympt Manage 2010;40:914–25.

3

Palliative Care

Susan D. Block

Palliative care is a subspecialty discipline within medicine, an emerging component of the healthcare system, and a practice of caring for patients and their families at a time of great vulnerability. Essential to providing excellent support for people in the last phases of life are specialized expertise, a system to support people living with serious illness and to provide for their care, and an appreciation of the moral dimensions of this care. In this chapter, I will explore the challenges facing the field of palliative care as we work to meet these goals.

The field of palliative medicine has evolved rapidly during the past 20 years, and in many ways was fueled by the ethical challenges that arose with increasing sophistication of technical medical care and the unintended side effects it produced. Patient concerns about unnecessary suffering and control over their treatment at the end of life, clinicians' conflicts over ethical dilemmas about the appropriate use of life-sustaining treatments, and payor initiatives to constrain healthcare costs have all contributed to the current intense focus, within many healthcare systems and organizations, on improving care for patients at the end of life.

Access to palliative care services, the elements of "high-value" care, and the meaning of "care" from both a clinical and social perspective are critical ethical considerations and will be the focus of this chapter. This chapter will focus on how these variables affect care in the United States.

Access

Equitable access to palliative care services, including hospice care, is a basic element of ethical practice, and is viewed as a core element of professionalism.[1] Optimally, access to care would occur in the context of strong and trusting relationships.[2]

ACCESS TO PALLIATIVE CARE SERVICES

Over the past 10 years, there has been dramatic growth in the availability of palliative care services in hospitals. In 2009, 63% of hospitals with at least 50 beds had a palliative care program.[3] An increasing number of palliative care programs are developing outpatient programs to broaden provision of palliative care beyond the hospital setting.

ACCESS TO HOSPICE SERVICES

Hospice programs provide care to approximately 44% of the 2.35 million people who died in the United States in 2011 from causes other than accidental death or suicide.[4] Geographic access to hospice has improved substantially, with 88% of the US population within 30 minutes by automobile and 98% within 60 minutes of a hospice provider.[5]

DISPARITIES IN ACCESS TO PALLIATIVE CARE

Ethnic and racial disparities are regularly seen in access to opioids, hospice care, and advance care planning. Age (very old or young), homelessness, lack of a spouse or other caregiver, poverty, mental illness, nursing home residence, and substance abuse are all found to be associated with less access to palliative care services. Additionally, patients without cancer diagnoses also experience reduced palliative care access.[6]

Patients living in the West and Midwest were more likely to have access to palliative care, whereas patients in the South had lower access. Those receiving care in for-profit systems had less access compared with services in private hospitals.

Limited data are available about the prevalence of palliative care programs in public hospitals. In 2008, only 54% of public hospitals and 40% of community hospitals that serve as the only providers of care for their communities (and where many of the 47 million uninsured patients go for care) offered palliative care services, demonstrating a marked deficit in access to these services for the underserved patients who tend to use these institutions for care.[7] In California, in 2008, only 20% of public hospitals provided palliative care services. There are many barriers to the appropriate provision of palliative care in the public hospital setting. The business model for palliative care, challenging as it is in private institutions, is even more so in public hospitals. The patient population is poor and underserved, has fewer resources, and relies more heavily on social and hospital services. Language, race, and ethnic diversity add to the challenges in assuring access to palliative care services.[8]

We are currently unable to generate accurate national data about the overall proportion of dying patients who receive palliative care services in hospitals, nursing homes, and home or institutional hospice. Even without these data, it is clear that patients who are hospitalized in small hospitals, and patients hospitalized in 37% of larger hospitals, as well as patients cared for in public hospitals, those cared for in many for-profit hospitals, although they may have access to hospice services, lack access to palliative care services in the hospital, where one-third of all deaths take place.[9]

PALLIATIVE CARE SPECIALIST WORKFORCE

Palliative care is provided both by hospice and palliative medicine specialists, and by nonpalliative care specialists, including primary care physicians, oncologists, intensivists, hospitalists, and other clinicians. The current US hospice and palliative care specialist physician need, based on recent calculations, is approximately 15,297 full-time equivalents (FTEs). Currently, in the United States, there are approximately 4,400 hospice and palliative medicine physicians, comprising 1,700 to 2,200 FTEs. Thus, we currently have only 11% to 15% of the hospice and palliative medicine physicians needed to provide full access to hospice and palliative medicine (HPM) services.[10] Additional data on palliative care access show that the ratio between oncologists and newly diagnosed cancer patients (1:141) and cardiologists and those with cardiac disease (1:71) are dramatically lower than ratios of palliative care physicians to patients with serious and life-threatening illness (1:1,200).[11] We do not know what would be an appropriate ratio of palliative care specialists to patients with serious illness. The ratio of palliative care specialists to patients is likely to worsen substantially with the aging of the population, and the closing, in 2012, of the "grandfathering" rule allowing non–fellowship-trained palliative care physicians to achieve certification. There are currently 85 accredited Hospice and Palliative Medicine graduate medical education programs, producing fewer than 180 fellowship-trained physicians a year. This level of production is below the replacement level for retiring physicians, meaning a net loss of palliative medicine specialists each year. This current workforce crisis, and its anticipated worsening, has worrisome implications for access to palliative care services. There is no national plan to increase access, train more physicians or other healthcare professionals, or require palliative care competencies of other physicians to fill these gaps. Indeed, other specialties (e.g., oncology) are planning on relying on palliative care physicians to meet their workforce gaps.[12]

A number of policy approaches have been suggested to address these issues, including directing Graduate Medical Education payments for Hospice and Palliative Medicine training (as was done for geriatrics), developing mid-career training programs in palliative care for practicing physicians that can lead to some form of certification, creating career development awards in palliative care, and creating centers of excellence in palliative care education with federal support.[10] There appears to have been minimal forward movement on these proposals, however. The lack of an effective national strategy, on the part of the professional organizations and the federal government, to address palliative care workforce shortages is a major barrier to access and quality of care, now and for the future.

Palliative care specialists, barring dramatic changes, will not be able to meet all the palliative care needs in this country. We need to develop a set of scalable initiatives that will disseminate palliative care structures, processes, competencies, and metrics broadly across the healthcare system.

GENERALIST PALLIATIVE CARE TRAINING

Improving medical education in palliative care at all levels, and across most specialties is a key step in expanding access. Although there has been some progress on this agenda, efforts and impact still fall far short of needs. A large national study of students, residents, and faculty, conducted in 1999–2000, showed many gaps (e.g., addressing patient fears, spirituality, cultural issues managing their own feelings about patient deaths, helping bereaved families) in students' and residents' preparation to care for patients at the end of life. More than 40% of residents felt unprepared to teach other learners (e.g., students) about end-of-life care. Direct clinical observation and feedback about difficult end-of-life discussions did not occur regularly.[13]

Within the past 10 years, the Liaison Committee on Medical Education has instituted a standard requiring teaching about end-of-life care for all medical students, although there is no specificity about what should be taught. The Accreditation Council for Graduate Medical Education has integrated requirements for teaching about palliative care issues in many residencies, and there is increasing specificity in these requirements. Between 1998 and 2006, more graduating students reported that teaching time about death and dying was adequate (71% vs. 80%, $p <. 001$), perceived adequacy of teaching time in pain management increased from 34% to 55% ($p <. 001$), and perceived quality of overall training in palliative care improved from 60% to 75% ($p <. 001$), suggesting modest improvements in training as well as demonstrating significant shortcomings in addressing basic topics.[14]

National palliative care competencies for graduating medical students and for residents completing internal medicine and family medicine residencies have been developed[15] and begin to translate vague standards into specific expectations. Palliative care competencies are not routinely assessed at the medical student or residency level (except for those enrolled in HPM fellowships). Although students and residents may complete training with better palliative care competencies than was the case in the past, physician practice patterns and competency levels are likely to be inadequate to address the access and quality issues for patients.

SYSTEMIC INTERVENTIONS TO IMPROVE QUALITY AND ACCESS

How do we better disseminate best practices in palliative care to nonpalliative care clinicians to enhance access and quality? Well-developed clinical care pathways and checklists that can be used by nonexperts to guide the care of patients with palliative care needs[16] have had significant international impact. Faculty development programs, such as the *Program in Palliative Care Education and Practice* at Harvard Medical School, designed to improve the teaching of palliative care in medical schools and residency programs to better meet growing demands for high-quality educational experiences, can help improve the capacity and competencies of the palliative care teaching workforce.[17,18] States are increasingly requiring physicians to participate in continuing medical education requirements focused around pain and palliative care; this strategy targets practicing physicians and may enhance practitioner competencies, thereby improving access. Hospital systems are exploring creative options to expand the palliative care competencies of their physicians, including providing "mini-sabbaticals" for clinicians to learn focused competencies in palliative care related to their disciplines.

System-wide interventions that can promote access include external standards that could be promulgated by organizations like The Joint Commission, or by hospital system leadership, requiring hospitals over a certain size to have a palliative care program. Metrics that evaluate the proportion of dying patients each year who are seen by palliative care or hospice in the last year of life can inform systems about how many patients are being served, and serve as an impetus for quality improvement.

Value

Access to healthcare for all persons requires processes to assure that healthcare resources are used appropriately, and a system-wide willingness to address cost containment. Care at the end of life is an arena in which there are many opportunities to improve value. Costs are high (25% of the Medicare budget is spent on the last year of life; 9% is spent on the last month of life) and cost is not associated with quality of end-of-life care[19] (Dartmouth Atlas). Patients receive nonbeneficial care, fail to receive care in the setting of their choice (usually the home), do not receive the care that they say they want, and experience unnecessary suffering. Their families, too, struggle with emotional and financial burdens of caretaking without adequate support.[20–29]

As our healthcare system moves from a fee-for-service model to accountable care, palliative care has the potential to contribute significantly to addressing these problems, thus both improving care and reducing costs.

The quality and costs of palliative care services are institutional or system responsibilities, not the sole province of palliative care clinical programs, as most end-of-life care continues to take place outside of palliative care clinical programs, even those that are highly developed and integrated. Palliative care programs alone will be unable to assure high-quality care for all patients within a healthcare organization. In addition to the need to offer high-quality inpatient and outpatient and community-based services, system-wide initiatives, to address issues such as advance care planning, manage transitions across settings, evaluations of the patient experience at the end of life across all services, clinician education, bereavement care for family members, the development of mechanisms to identify patients who would benefit from palliative care services, and establishment and tracking of performance metrics are critical to achieving high-quality palliative care across a system.

Given limited resources and inadequate reimbursement, the field of palliative medicine has an ethical obligation to evaluate the impact of our services, and to develop high-value (quality/cost) programs based on strong outcome data. Data about the impact of many common palliative care interventions on outcomes remain limited, although notable progress has been made. The early palliative care intervention study at Massachusetts General Hospital (MGH), demonstrating improved quality of life, longer survival, and reduced hospitalization rates is an example of a well-designed and highly impactful evaluation that shows how palliative care both improves quality and reduces cost.[30]

Among the palliative care interventions with the greatest demonstrated efficacy is communication about end-of-life goals and values. Indeed, this was a central element of the MGH palliative care intervention. Advance care planning has now been evaluated in several well-designed trials[31,32] and found to enhance patient receipt of desired care. In addition, patients who report having had end-of-life discussions with their doctors had 36% lower healthcare costs.[33] The combination of improved goal-consistent care and lower costs makes advance care planning a high-value intervention that should be integrated into all healthcare systems. Development of systems within healthcare organizations to identify patients who would benefit from such discussions, prompt clinicians to initiate them, and support best practice in conducting these discussions would support patient control over decisions (autonomy), help clinicians do the right thing for their patients (beneficence), reduce harm (nonmaleficence), and enhance access and probably reduce costs (justice).

Care

How does a healthcare system embody caring? Traditional medical models focus on providing accurate diagnosis and excellent treatment of diseases; patient-centered models emphasize patient and family engagement and empowerment, partnership-building, whole-person care, and respect for patients' needs and values and preferences.[34] Presence, witnessing, solidarity, availability, and responsibility are also core relational elements of caring in the practice of medicine, particularly in the setting of advanced illness,[35] and serve as antidotes to the helplessness, despair, insecurity, uncertainty, and loneliness of the sick person. As Cassell describes, though, healing requires an integration of the diagnosis and treatment model with the caring model. The aim of the care is to restore the well-being of the patient, by restoring the patient's health and allowing the return of the patient's self as a functioning, whole person.[36] Another model for framing this discussion is that of "the ethics of care," which views caring as a practice, embedded in relationships between the caregiver and the care receiver.[37] It is defined as "the meeting of needs of one person by another where face-to-face interaction between carer and cared for is a crucial element of overall activity, and where the need is of such a nature that it cannot possibly be met by the person in need herself."[38] The caregiver's role is viewed as having four key elements: (1) attentiveness, an orientation toward being aware of the other person's need; (2) responsibility, a commitment to take care of that need; (3) competence, the capacity to provide good care; and (4) responsiveness, recognition of the unique perspective and position of the care receiver.[39]

Palliative care has adopted many elements of the healing model described by Cassell. The elements of healing, caring, and patient-centered care, as expressed in the physician-patient relationship, are frequently viewed as the "art" of medicine, rather than as a core and essential element of medical competence; yet this formulation accepts failure in the domain of caring and healing as an inevitable and tolerable feature of medical care. Although medical education has placed more emphasis on professionalism in recent years, the informal, or hidden, curriculum is known to systematically erode the humanistic qualities of students.[40,41] Accepting diagnosis and treatment as sufficient in caring for patients, without equivalent standards for healing, caring and patient-centeredness fails to meet contemporary standards of quality—ensuring systematic adherence to best practices, reducing variability, and focusing on outcomes of value to patients and their families.

One of the innovative features of palliative medicine is its integration of a systematic approach to the provision of whole-person care with attention to the psychological, social, physical, and spiritual elements of the sick person's experience. In general, I would argue that palliative medicine aspires to and very often meets this standard. Yet, this approach still does not adequately permeate the care of patients outside of palliative medicine, leaving major gaps in the experience of many patients and their family members as they live with serious illness.

Even within palliative medicine, it has become increasingly challenging for any one clinician to meet these high aspirations; an interdisciplinary model for the care of patients is viewed as essential. Although it has many advantages, one of the challenges of this approach is that of assuring that there is sufficient personal engagement by at least one clinician to provide the feeling of security, support, clarity, and connection to meet the needs of the patient and the family.

Are there ways to systematize caring? And is systematizing caring an oxymoron? Can we create structures that embed best practices of palliative care into the rest of our clinical care system? Routine identification of patients who are at high-risk of suffering and death can remind and trigger clinicians to address issues such as planning for the future (including end-of-life planning), symptom management, coordination of care, and family support. Regular identification and screening for symptoms and sources of distress for all patients with serious illnesses can make suffering visible, enhancing the likelihood that it will be addressed. Interdisciplinary teams can be deployed to efficiently meet identified patient needs in multiple domains. And a clinician can be designated as the coordinator and overseer of these processes to assure that the team is working together. Metrics, including patient- and family-reported outcomes such as satisfaction with symptom control (patient) and satisfaction with perceived quality of end-of-life care (family) can be generated to evaluate the extent to which these basic standards are met, and can be used to stimulate further improvement in the system.

Conclusions

From an ethical perspective, access, value, and care for patients with serious illness should be an imperative. The care of the most vulnerable tends to highlight issues that are relevant, but perhaps more subtle, throughout the rest of our healthcare system—disparities, dysfunctional cultural norms (such as avoidance of discussion of difficult issues like death), the need for a more comprehensive and coordinated approach to achieving patient well-being and quality of life, failures in communication about patient-centered outcomes, and the value of a secure and close relationship with a physician or other healthcare professional. Although palliative care is improving the care for patients with serious illness, it can also serve as a "Trojan horse," by bringing new practices, attitudes, and values into the house of medicine, and modeling a new approach to the care of all patients.

References

1. Medical Professionalism Project of the ABIM Foundation. ACP-ASIM Foundation and European Federation of Internal Medicine. Medical professionalism in the new millennium: a physician charter. Ann Intern Med 2002;136:243–6.
2. Braddock CH, Snyder L, Neubauer RL, Fischer GS for the American College of Physicians Ethics, Professionalism and Human Rights Committee and the Society of General Internal Medicine Ethics Committee. The patient-centered medical home: an ethical analysis of principles and practice. J Gen Intern Med 2012 [Epub ahead of print. PMID: 22829295].
3. http://reportcard.capc.org/pdf/state-by-state-report-card.pdf (last accessed 10/17/13).
4. Hoyert DL, Xu J. *Deaths: Preliminary Data for 2011*, National Vital Statistics Reports, vol 61 no 6.National Center for Health Statistics, CDC, available online at: http://www.cdc.gov/nchs/data/nvsr/nvsr61/nvsr61_06.pdf (last acessed 10/17/13).
5. Carlson MD, Bradley EH, Du Q, Morrison RS. Geographic access to hospice in the United States. J Palliat Med. 2010 Nov;13(11):1331–8.
6. Walshe C, Todd C, Caress A, Chew-Graham. Patterns of Access to Community Palliative Care Services: A Literature Review. J Pain and Symptom Management 2009;37:884–912.
7. Goldsmith BA, Dietrich J, Du Q, Morrison RS. Variability in Access to Hospital Palliative Care in the United States. J Palliative Medicine 2008;11:1094–102.
8. http://healthaffairs.org/blog/2011/03/30/one-foundations-path-to-expanding-palliative-care-in-californias-public-hospitals/?cat=grantwatch
9. http://www.ahrq.gov/news/nn/nn110409.htm

10. Lupu D. Estimate of current hospice and palliative medicine physician workforce shortage. J Pain Symptom Management 2010;40:899–911.

11. http://reportcard.capc.org/pdf/state-by-state-report-card.pdf (last accessed 10/17/13).

12. Levit L, Smith AL, Benz E, Ferrell B. Ensuring Quality Cancer Care Through the Oncology Workforce. J Oncol Pract. 2010 January;6(1):7–11.

13. Sullivan AM, Lakoma MD, Block SD. The status of medical education in end-of-life care: A national report. J Gen Int Med 2003;18:685–95.

14. Sulmasy DP, Cimino JE, Frishman WH. US medical students perceptions of the adequacy of their schools' curricular attention to care at the end of life: 1998–2008. J Pall Med 2008;11:707–16.

15. Schaefer K, Chittenden E, Periyakoil VJ, Sanchez Reilly S, Sullivan A, Carey E, Morrison L, Block SD. Raising the bar for the care of seriously ill patients: A national survey to define essential palliative care competencies for medical students and residents. Academic Medicine (in press).

16. Douglas C, Murtagh FE, Chambers EJ, Howse M, Ellershaw J. Symptom management for the adult patient dying with advanced chronic kidney disease: a review of the literature and development of evidence-based guidelines by a United Kingdom Expert Consensus Group. Palliat Med. 2009 Mar;23(2):103–10.

17. Sullivan AM, Lakoma M, Billings JA, Block SD, and the PCEP core faculty. A faculty development program to enhance faculty clinical and pedagogical competencies in end-of-life care. Academic Medicine 2005;80:657–68.

18. Sullivan AM, Lakoma MD, Billings JA, Peters AS, Block SD, and the PCEP Core Faculty. Creating enduring change: Demonstrating the long-term impact of a faculty development program in palliative care. J Gen Intern Med. 2006:907–14.

19. http://www.dartmouthatlas.org/data/topic/topic.aspx?cat=18

20. Casarett D, Pickard A, Bailey FA, Ritchie C, Furman C, Rosenfeld K, et al. Do palliative consultations improve patient outcomes? J Am Geriatr Soc. 2008;56(4):593–9.

21. Lienard A, Merckaert I, Libert Y, Delvaux N, Marchal S, Boniver J, et al. Factors that influence cancer patients' anxiety following a medical consultation: impact of a communication skills training programme for physicians. Ann Oncol. 2006;17(9):1450–8.

22. Teno JM, Clarridge BR, Casey V, Welch LC, Wetle T, Shield R, et al. Family perspectives on end-of-life care at the last place of care. JAMA. 2004;291(1):88–93.

23. Wright AA, Zhang B, Ray A, Mack JW, Trice E, Balboni T, et al. Associations between end-of-life discussions, patient mental health, medical care near death, and caregiver bereavement adjustment. JAMA. 2008;300(14):1665–73.

24. Stapleton RD, Engelberg RA, Wenrich MD, Goss CH, Curtis JR. Clinician statements and family satisfaction with family conferences in the intensive care unit. Crit Care Med. 2006;34(6):1679–85.

25. Temel JS, Greer JA, Muzikansky A, Gallagher ER, Admane S, Jackson VA, et al. Early palliative care for patients with metastatic non-small-cell lung cancer. N Engl J Med. 2010;363(8):733–42.

26. Mack JW, Weeks JC, Wright AA, Block SD, Prigerson HG. End-of-life discussions, goal attainment, and distress at the end of life: predictors and outcomes of receipt of care consistent with preferences. J Clin Oncol. 2010;28(7):1203–8.

27. Zhang B, Wright AA, Huskamp HA, Nilsson ME, Maciejewski ML, Earle CC, et al. Healthcare costs in the last week of life: associations with end-of-life conversations. Arch Intern Med. 2009;169(5):480–8.

28. Morrison RS, Penrod JD, Cassel JB, Caust-Ellenbogen M, Litke A, Spragens L, et al. Cost savings associated with US hospital palliative care consultation programs. Arch Intern Med. 2008;168(16):1783–90.

29. Morrison RS, Dietrich J, Ladwig S, Quill T, Sacco J, Tangeman J, et al. Palliative care consultation teams cut hospital costs for Medicaid beneficiaries. Health Aff (Millwood). 2011;30(3):454–63.

30. Temel JS, Greer JA, Muzikansky A, Gallagher ER, Admane S, Jackson VA, Dahlin CM, Blinderman CD, Jacobsen J, Pirl WF, Billings JA, Lynch TJ. Early palliative care for patients with metastatic non-small-cell lung cancer. N Engl J Med. 2010 Aug 19;363(8):733–42.

31. Silveira MJ, Kim SY, Langa KM. Advance directives and outcomes of surrogate decision making before death. N Engl J Med. 2010;362(13):1211–8.

32. Detering KM, Hancock AD, Reade MC, Silvester W. The impact of advance care planning on end of life care in elderly patients: randomized controlled trial. BMJ. 2010;340:c1345.

33. Zhang B, Wright AA, Huskamp HA, Nilsson ME, Maciejewski ML, Earle CC, et al. Healthcare costs in the last week of life: associations with end-of-life conversations. Arch Intern Med. 2009;169(5):480–8.

34. Institute of medicine. Crossing the quality chasm: a new health system for the 21st century. Washington, DC: National Academy Press, 2001.

35. Kleinman A. Caregiver as moral experience. Lancet 2012;380:1550–1.

36. Cassell E. The nature of healing. Oxford: Oxford University Press, 2013. P 83.

37. http://www.iep.utm.edu/care-eth/

38. Tronto, J. Moral Boundaries: A Political Argument for an Ethic of Care. New York, NY: Routledge, 1994.

39. Bubeck, Diemut. Care, Gender and Justice. Oxford: Clarendon Press, 1995.

40. Hafferty FW, Franks R. The hidden curriculum, ethics teaching, and the structure of medical education. Acad Med. 1994 Nov;69(11):861–71.

41. Inui TS. A flag in the wind: educating for professionalism in medicine. Washington, DC: Association of American Medical Colleges, 2003.

SECTION II

Ethical Challenges within Current Systems of Care

4

Emerging Complexities in Pediatric Palliative Care

Renee D. Boss and Nancy Hutton

Pediatric palliative care literally spans the period from before birth to after death. Pediatric palliative care clinicians care for the family whose developing fetus has a life-limiting condition. They care for the toddler in the ICU after near-drowning. They care for the 6-year-old with intractable seizures and feeding intolerance on a ketogenic diet. They care for the 11-year-old with leukemia who wants to attend school despite immunosuppression. And they care for the 18-year-old whose second heart transplant is failing after a lifetime of complications from congenital heart disease. This broad range of pediatric anatomy and physiology, neurological and psychological development, capacity for preferences and decision making, and family preparation for childhood death, result in significant clinical, emotional, and ethical challenges for the pediatric palliative care clinician.

Theory and research in bioethics has traditionally been focused on the adult patient, or at least on the patient who is capable of having values and preferences. Yet the trusted principles of autonomy, justice, beneficence, and nonmaleficence often fall short in pediatric dilemmas, for instance, when considering how to counsel a pregnant adolescent who demands a Cesarean section for her fetus with known anencephaly. This may leave families, clinicians, and ethics consultants struggling to determine what is in the best interests of the young child.

Building on four cases, this chapter will highlight several unique ethical complexities in pediatric palliative care. Underlying many of these challenges is the threat to justice represented by the lack of resources dedicated to pediatric palliative care. The 2003 Institute of Medicine report *"When Children Die: Improving Palliative and End of Life Care for Children and Their Families,"*[1] and the 2000 American Academy of Pediatrics policy statement, *"Palliative Care for Children"*[2] put forward professional standards for providing palliative care alongside disease-directed care for children with life-threatening illnesses, regardless of whether the outcome is cure, living with chronic illness, or death. Yet quality palliative care for infants and children has not been a priority for medical systems, policy makers, and professional societies, including those dedicated to adult palliative care. Because many more adults confront the end of life than do children, financial, administrative, and research support dedicated to palliative care is typically directed at adults. This has limited the expansion of pediatric palliative care services, including hospital-based programs, and inpatient and outpatient hospice services. Of patients with terminal illnesses, more than 40% of adults who die receive hospice services, but only about 10% of children who die receive hospice services.[3-5] Hospice access for infants is most restricted, even though most pediatric deaths occur in infancy.[6] Until access to pediatric hospice and palliative care is more widely available, we cannot discharge our ethical duty to provide quality care to these patients.

Palliative Care before Birth

> Donald and Mirah Brown are pregnant with their first child. Prenatal ultrasound reveals a female fetus with growth restriction and anomalies of the face, hands, and feet. Fetal echocardiogram demonstrates Tetralogy of Fallot. Mirah has an amniocentesis, which reveals a fetal diagnosis of trisomy 18. The obstetrician tells the Browns that most babies born with trisomy 18 die in the first weeks of life, and nearly all die before reaching 1 year old. She recommends pregnancy termination.
>
> The Browns search the Internet, and read how more and more babies with trisomy 18 are receiving medical and surgical interventions like feeding tubes and heart surgery. They meet with a cardiothoracic surgeon, who agrees that surgery is possible. They then meet with a neonatologist who states that his colleagues are unwilling to subject a baby with a "lethal diagnosis" to intensive medical or surgical care; he assures the Browns that compassionate care is the only option.

PERINATAL PALLIATIVE CARE

Approximately half of all children who die do so before 12 months of life; nearly 70% of those infants die in the first month of life.[7] Many infants die from major congenital anomalies or serious genetic syndromes that may be diagnosed prenatally. Perinatal palliative care offers a range of supports for families after the diagnosis of a life-limiting fetal or neonatal condition. Depending on the availability of hospital- and community-based resources, perinatal palliative care team members might include pediatric palliative care clinicians, neonatologists, obstetricians, social workers, child life specialists, psychologists, chaplains, and a variety of pediatric subspecialists. The team can help families set goals about additional prenatal testing, pregnancy termination, or neonatal interventions. Families may need help with developing a palliative care birth plan, supporting their other children, finding alternative birthing classes, or identifying a primary care pediatrician willing to care for a child in home hospice. Diagnostic uncertainty often characterizes decision making, as complete information about the fetal condition is inherently limited during pregnancy. This uncertainty may prompt a decision to "see how the baby does" after birth. This predictably leads to shifting goals that depend on how success and failure are defined after birth. The perinatal palliative care team can provide continuity before and after birth, helping the family consider decisions that could result in neonatal death or chronic disability.

REQUESTS FOR LIFE-PROLONGING INTERVENTIONS AFTER A "LETHAL" FETAL DIAGNOSIS

There are multiple medical, ethical, and legal complexities in caring for a pregnant woman whose fetus is thought to have a life-limiting condition. Depending on the severity of the fetal condition, management options might include pregnancy termination, fetal therapy, delivery at a referral center for neonatal intensive care, or delivery at a community hospital for palliative care only. Evolving professional standards related to several fetal diagnoses call into question the "lethal" nature of those conditions. For example, trisomy 18 was considered nearly uniformly lethal until the last 10 or 15 years. Evolving national practices among neonatologists, geneticists, and cardiologists suggest that more and more clinicians are willing to resuscitate newborns with trisomy 18 and to extend their lives with cardiac surgery and feeding tubes. The American Academy of Pediatrics and American Heart Association have removed trisomy 18 from the list of conditions for which neonatal resuscitation should not be offered in their latest edition of the Textbook of Neonatal Resuscitation.[8] Some of this change in approach reflects data from primarily Japan suggesting that life expectancy can be prolonged in some children with trisomy 18 if they have cardiac surgery—although most of those additional weeks and months of survival occur within the hospital, with a minority surviving to hospital discharge.[9] Shifts in practice which favor increasing interventions for infants with trisomy 18 may also result in delayed integration of palliative care, even though the burdens to infants and families may be substantial.

Many clinicians remain ethically and professionally opposed to medical and surgical interventions aimed at prolonging life for infants with "lethal" conditions like trisomy 18. Serious questions are raised about the obligation that parents can place on the medical profession to provide interventions for children with these conditions. Parents in the United States are automatic surrogate decision makers for their children. As a rule, clinicians can only seek to limit this parental autonomy if they believe that the parents' decisions will harm the child. Clinicians, ethicists, and the legal system are challenged to determine whether a parent's demand to do "everything possible" to extend a child's life causes harm to that child. These questions are even more complicated in the prenatal period, when the fetus is not legally a person. How should an obstetrician respond to a woman's request for Cesarean section with the aim of prolonging life for a fetus with a "lethal" condition, when the Cesarean section poses medical risk to the mother? The growing lack of consensus among the medical profession suggests that the dilemmas in caring for these families will intensify in the coming years.

WHEN PREGNANCY TERMINATION IS PERMISSIBLE, BUT PALLIATIVE CARE ONLY IS NOT

For a pregnant woman and her partner, prenatal testing raises concerns about whether they would want to know about a life-limiting fetal condition, and what their threshold would be for considering pregnancy termination. Currently the option of pregnancy termination is not equally available to all women in the United States. Over the past decade, abortion regulations have become more restrictive, especially for abortions performed later in pregnancy when most prenatal testing results become available. Several states have considered legislation that aims to withhold abnormal prenatal testing results from women who the physician perceives to be likely to consider pregnancy termination. Professional medical organizations have, for the most part, not taken a prominent role in advocating for professional ethical obligations to pregnant women in this area.

Some families do not want to terminate a pregnancy after finding out about a life-limiting fetal diagnosis, but prefer to decline neonatal resuscitation in favor of palliative care alone. Perinatal palliative care clinicians must be aware of legal and ethical distinctions between prenatal and neonatal decision making in this setting. In many areas of the United States, a woman may elect pregnancy termination for any reason up until a defined gestational age. In Maryland in 2012, for example, a woman pregnant with twins could terminate as late as the final trimester the twin whose genetic anomaly is not lethal but causes minor to moderate neurodevelopmental disability. Likewise, a woman whose fetus has a congenital heart disease that is lethal without neonatal surgery, but has a 70% chance of survival with surgery, could terminate that pregnancy. If either woman declines termination on principle, yet believes it is not in her child's best interest to endure the condition, she may not be able to decline neonatal intervention for these nonlethal conditions. Because a fetus is legally not a person, decisions about pregnancy termination do not require consideration of the future child's best interests. From an ethical perspective, some would disagree with this. But once that same fetus is born alive, decisions to withhold life-saving interventions must consider the newborn's best interests. Some clinicians argue that withholding surgery from an infant with a 70% chance of survival is not in that child's best interests. Perinatal palliative care teams should help families in similar situations to understand these shifting thresholds before birth; prenatal ethics consultation may also be helpful in these scenarios.

Palliative Care for Newborns and Infants

Sylvie Crowder is a 23-year-old woman who presents to a hospital in labor; she has received no prenatal care. At delivery the infant appears extremely premature, has no respiratory effort, and a low heart rate; she is intubated with difficulty and receives chest compressions for 10 minutes. Physical exam reveals a birth weight of 540 grams and probable 23 to 24 weeks gestational age. The infant, named Kayla, has a difficult neonatal course, which includes bilateral parenchymal brain hemorrhages with subsequent hydrocephalus requiring a ventriculoperitoneal shunt;

she has ongoing seizures and nearly 100% chance of serious long term neurodevelopmental disability. After 3 months in the neonatal intensive care unit (NICU), she
has not been successfully extubated because of severe chronic lung disease and
cor pulmonale. The pediatric pulmonologist suggests tracheostomy and gastrostomy tube placement. The neonatologist suggests compassionate extubation.

THE EXTREMELY PREMATURE INFANT: URGENT CRISIS

Extremely premature labor is one life-threatening fetal condition that is often unsus-
pected until hours before birth. A neonate is considered "premature" if born before
37 weeks gestation, and is considered "extremely premature" if born between 22
and 28 weeks gestation, the equivalent to the fifth or sixth month of pregnancy.
Survival to hospital discharge is estimated to be 6% for infants born at 22 weeks
gestation, 25% at 23 weeks gestation, and just over 50% at 24 weeks gestation.[8]

Consensus about which extremely premature infants, if any, should receive
resuscitation and intensive care, is elusive despite ongoing medical, ethical, legal,
and societal debate. Consideration of options for neonatal management should
incorporate sound data about predicted morbidity and mortality. Yet because
resuscitation is deliberately forgone for some infants at 22 to 25 weeks gestation,
mortality rates reflect both liveborn infants who did not receive resuscitation and
liveborn infants who were resuscitated unsuccessfully. In addition to prognostic data, professional societies and hospital regulations may define management
options for these infants. Although the American Academy of Pediatrics supports
clinician recommendations of non-resuscitation for the smallest infants, it leaves
room for parents to request interventions even for infants with greater than 90%
chance of death before hospital discharge.[10] Some hospital policies compel resuscitation for any newborn; these policies may not be transparent to families who present to the emergency department with extremely premature labor.

THE EXTREMELY PREMATURE INFANT: CHRONIC DISEASE

Extremely premature infants who are resuscitated experience multiple medical
problems: respiratory distress, intraventricular hemorrhage, recurrent sepsis, necrotizing enterocolitis, and NICU stays in excess of 3 to 6 months. Several models
have described the role for palliative care in promoting infant comfort and supporting families in the NICU.[11-13] Minimizing pain and suffering while maximizing
quality of life are challenging goals, given our incomplete understanding of these
neonatal experiences. Although signs and symptoms of pain are measurable in even
the most premature infant, optimal pain management is unclear. Concerns exist
about adverse effects on the developing brain of pain medications, especially for
premature infants who are likely to receive these medications for protracted periods.
No validated measures of infant suffering or quality of life in the NICU exist.[14]
Ethical considerations about quality of life for premature infants often refer to
future, projected quality of life ("*What will it be like for Jimmie to spend his life in a*

wheelchair?"), with less emphasis placed on current quality of life ("*What is it like for Jimmie that he has not been able to be held for over a month?*").

The acute medical concerns for many premature infants evolve into chronic respiratory, neurological, and growth abnormalities, with future risk of cerebral palsy, mental retardation, blindness, deafness, and behavioral problems. Families and clinicians face new decisions about which ICU interventions that the infant still needs to survive might reasonably be converted to long-term outpatient therapies. Should the infant whose lungs have still not developed enough to breathe without mechanical ventilation be provided with a tracheostomy? Should the child who has liver dysfunction and inability to eat 3 months after a bowel resection from necrotizing enterocolitis be referred for a liver-bowel transplant? Should the infant who has no ability to feed because of intractable seizures following severe brain injury sustained at birth have a surgical gastrostomy?

Some data suggest that patients and families may not perceive the burdens of prematurity-associated morbidities to be as great as they are perceived by clinicians.[15] Others suggest that clinicians without personal experience of disability cannot appropriately counsel families making serious medical decisions based, in part, on predicted disability.[16] Facilitating a conversation between the family and individual(s) with the lived experience of disability can be helpful; many families seek out this information on their own from family support groups and websites.

LONG-TERM DEPENDENCE ON MEDICAL TECHNOLOGY

Since the early 1980s, shifts in healthcare financing have allowed more and more children who are permanently dependent on medical technology to leave the inpatient hospital setting and live at home with their families. It is routine for children dependent on tracheostomy and ventilator, gastrostomy tube, cardiorespiratory monitors, and 24-hour "awake and alert" caregivers to live at home between hospital admissions for intercurrent illness. Insurers can now deny inpatient hospital days because this intensive level of care "should" be provided at home (at less cost to the insurer). The implication is that if the family cannot successfully organize time, physical space, human resources, and medical expertise all while maintaining financial income and caring for other children, then they are failing their child. Perhaps they are even seen by some as "neglectful parents." This "slippery slope" has led to harm for children and parents who are trying to survive in extraordinarily challenging circumstances. When does this well-intended care option cause greater burden than benefit, and when does it cause harm?

As medical professionals, we become desensitized to the shocking experience of a child requiring a tube and machine to breathe. It is part of our routine care. When the child remains intubated for "failure" to wean ventilatory support, we are surprised when parents hesitate to accept tracheostomy. We may wonder—are they giving up? Do they want palliative care "only?" Is that even an "ethically permissible" option for the underlying condition? Don't they know that "kids go home with trachs all the time?" Then, weeks, months, or years later, when the child is repeatedly readmitted to the ICU for tracheitis, respiratory failure, or aspiration pneumonia, we ask, "Why are the parents doing this? Don't they know their child is dying?" It becomes the parents' fault that their child is dependent on a trach and vent, as if we had no role in starting this roller coaster ride.

A key value that varies among parents and clinicians is the value attributed to cognition and awareness of self, others, and one's surroundings, and the ability to interact in some way. Most clinicians can heartily advocate that a child who will think and interact be provided the full array of medical technology and nursing support to permit a life of the fullest potential in the least restrictive environment. There is less consensus about offering the same level of care for children with severe neurological impairment with minimal hope of recovery. How much is too much when parents keep saying, "Do everything"? How can we join with them to assure that their child is treated with respect and dignity? Some parents request all available medical interventions regardless of the medical burden because they believe that each moment of a beating heart is life worth preserving. Many more parents request intensive medical interventions for their neurologically impaired child because they want to give him or her a fair chance to recover to a prior baseline, to be treated like everyone else. They do not seek to cause suffering or prolong dying; they seek fairness and justice.

Palliative Care for Young Children

Austin Dumas is 2 years old. His mother waitresses at night; his father works in construction during the day. Mr. and Mrs. Dumas have argued a lot lately, and she worries that he is going to leave her and Austin. Tonight, at work, she receives a phone call from the police; Austin is in the hospital, she should come right away. At the hospital, a social worker explains that Mr. Dumas told the doctors that he went to check on Austin in his bed and found him blue and not breathing. Austin has some bruises…broken ribs…bleeding…the police question Mr. Dumas and ultimately he is arrested for suspected child abuse. Austin's condition worsens, and the pediatric ICU attending tells Mrs. Dumas that Austin might die, and if he survives will be profoundly disabled. Mrs. Dumas asks if they can end his suffering and turn off the machines. The attending thinks it is reasonable to withdraw life support, but worries that Mrs. Dumas is motivated by anger against her husband, maybe even by her implicit or explicit contribution to Austin's abuse.

WHEN A CHILD'S ILLNESS MAY BE CAUSED BY OTHERS

Approximately half of the young children who can benefit from palliative care have cancer or ongoing complications resulting from premature birth or major congenital anomalies. But many young children who develop life-limiting diseases in the first years of life do so as a result of accidental and nonaccidental trauma, much of which occurs in the child's own home. Rates of fatal and nonfatal drowning are highest among children ages 1 to 4, with most of those events occurring in swimming pools. Injury rates peak in the toddler years, because of falls, poisoning, foreign bodies, and pedestrian injuries. Rates of injury differ significantly by race; for example, young Black children have higher rates of death by fire or homicide than do non–Black children.

Injuries that result from both accidental and nonaccidental trauma often implicate a failure of one or more adults to keep that child safe. Properly securing swimming areas, installing smoke detectors, and using child safety seats in automobiles are proved to decrease the morbidity and mortality associated with childhood injury. Caring for children who are seriously harmed because of a preventable injury raises conflicting priorities and emotions for clinicians. Clinicians may be obligated to notify state child protective services about the injury, which may initiate an investigation of child neglect or abuse. Clinicians may feel blame toward the parents for not protecting the child, yet may feel a duty to support a guilt-ridden and distraught parent. Parents may ask the clinician to withhold from the child the information that the parent could have, or should have, taken steps to prevent the injury.

These conflicts are greatly amplified in cases of intentional child physical and sexual abuse. Child abuse that results in serious injury is most common among infants and young children. Child abuse is usually perpetrated by someone known to the child, most often a parent or other caregiver; the abuse may involve acts of commission or omission. Traumatic brain injury, abdominal organ injury, and bone fractures are common injuries resulting from child maltreatment; these often result in pediatric ICU hospitalization and may be life threatening. Such children who are conscious will have fears above and beyond those typically associated with pain and ICU care. They require significant emotional and psychological support that respects their developmental abilities to remember and understand what happened to them. Young children commonly believe that they did something to deserve the abuse and worry that this "punishment" will recur. They may refuse to discuss what happened, for fear that the perpetrator, usually a parent, will abandon or kill them. Conflicting with their duty to help a child through the psychological sequelae of the abuse, a clinician may feel pressured by child protective services or by legal counsel to either avoid or accelerate the child's discussion of the abuse.

CONFLICTING TIMELINES FOR LEGAL AND MEDICAL DECISIONS

In cases of severe traumatic brain injury and an unconscious child, clinicians may consider withdrawing life support. As with all serious medical decision making in pediatrics, the guiding principle should be what is in the child's best interest. A challenge in cases of suspected child abuse is determining whether the child's parent(s) or caretaker(s) are making biased value judgments about the child's best interest. A mother who was completely unaware of ongoing child abuse by her husband may be partially motivated by a desire for revenge. It may be difficult to separate her motivation to discontinue the child's life support from the reality that this will escalate the criminal charges against her husband to murder. On the other hand, a mother who was aware of the child's abuse by her husband, and who worries that her collusion will result in legal charges against her, may have motivations to keep the child on life support that are not focused on that child's best interests. Palliative care clinicians may struggle to align with families where there are underlying concerns about deception and intent.

What can be most distressing for clinicians in these scenarios is that the "facts" of the abuse are rarely certain at the time when they are considering decisions about withholding or withdrawing particular treatments from the child. Treatment decisions are often desired in days to weeks, whereas legal inquiry can take much longer. As the investigation proceeds, the clinicians often struggle to identify an adult who can reliably engage in deliberations of what is in the child's best interest. The American Academy of Pediatrics recommends that a guardian ad litem be appointed in cases of suspected child abuse in which there is concern that the parent has a conflict of interest, although some courts will not permit this person to make decisions about withdrawing life support.[17] Courts across the United States have been inconsistent in their decisions to override parental wishes in cases of suspected child abuse; in some cases children remain in the ICU and mechanically ventilated for weeks to months during legal deliberation.

Palliative Care for Older Children and Adolescents

Savannah is 17 years old, and has been a patient of the pediatric HIV clinic since she was born. Her mother had acquired immunodeficiency syndrome (AIDS) when she got pregnant with Savannah, took no antiretroviral therapy (ART), and died when Savannah was an infant. Savannah has been in the foster care system since that time. Despite behavioral and learning problems exacerbated by inconsistent caretakers in her life, Savannah's physical health remained good. But as an adolescent, her grief and anger about her mother's absence in her life has made her rebellious against her own human immunodeficiency virus (HIV) treatment, and she has been off of her ART for much of the past 5 years. Now Savannah is hospitalized for the third time in a year, with a CD4 count of 8, chronic diarrhea, and abdominal pain caused by disseminated *Mycobacterium avium* complex (MAC) infection. She says she wants to be healthy ("I don't want to die"), but refuses to take prescribed medications, including her ART, or permit routine abdominal exams.

HELPING OLDER CHILDREN MANAGE CHRONIC DISEASE

Over the past two decades, rates of chronic disease have risen dramatically in the pediatric population. Children are increasingly susceptible to conditions that once primarily affected adults, such as type 2 diabetes or chronic hypertension. Pediatric chronic disease also results from successful management of conditions that were once fatal in childhood, such as cystic fibrosis or congenital heart disease. For many older children and adolescents, serious chronic disease is a burden that demands compliance, consistency, impulse control, and self-regulation—developmental capacities that are often still evolving even in young adulthood.

Models of medical care for children with chronic disease have developed along traditional disease-specific lines, promoting advances in medical and surgical treatments, but inclusion of developmentally appropriate psychosocial care remains inconsistent. Coping with the diagnosis, treatments, hospitalizations, disruption of normal childhood routines, and loss of future dreams is essential to quality of life. When older children and adolescents suffer from a chronic disease that is hereditary or perinatally acquired, such as sickle cell disease or HIV, feelings of blame and anger add to the distress of both the child and the parents. This distress can be prolonged or compounded when families and clinicians avoid opportunities to talk openly and honestly with children about their health condition.

Human immunodeficiency virus is the most recent example of a stigmatizing condition that adults feared disclosing to children. But children and adolescents need to trust their parents and healthcare team; developmentally appropriate truth-telling is the cornerstone of this trust. Parents need compassionate support in planning for diagnosis disclosure. Clinicians should recognize when refusals to include the adolescent in discussions of diagnosis, treatment, and prognosis are potentially harmful. Careful probing regarding parental fears and reassurance that clinicians will not force information on adolescents is necessary for consensus about therapeutic communication. The adolescent's psychological health is particularly at risk when a parent becomes very ill or dies with the same disease that affects the child. Depression, anxiety, and aggressiveness are all increased in children of mothers who are seriously ill with HIV/AIDS, and these risks extend through late adolescence.

ADHERENCE AND CONFLICT

The success of any treatment is dependent on the patient's adherence to recommendations. Adherence decreases during adolescence, setting the stage for conflict between the adolescent and her or his parents and healthcare team. When the treatment is clearly beneficial in the short and long term, such as insulin for type 1 diabetes, then the focus must be on helping the adolescent cope with the practical (self-injection, diet) and emotional (being different than peers) burdens of maintaining optimal glucose control. As the treatment burden increases or the certainty of benefit decreases, the balance in favor of strict adherence becomes more problematic. In the case of Savannah, the prescribed pill burden is high and without anticipated short-term symptom improvement. There may be long-term improvement (if long-term perfect adherence to an intense regimen is maintained), with the best outcome being stable health on lifetime medication; there is no cure. Yet even in this clinical scenario, allowing poor adherence to continue is interpreted as poor medical care. Conflict arises between the patient and everyone else, increasing the adolescent's sense of isolation and hopelessness. For some adolescents, poor adherence leads to disease progression and early death. For others, disease progression and early death are anticipated, although poor adherence may contribute to a more rapid decline. But when does poor adherence become a decision to discontinue treatment? How do we know? And when can we accept this decision?

ADOLESCENTS AND HEALTHCARE DECISION MAKING

Adolescents develop capacity for healthcare decision making in the context of ongoing brain development. Capacity for certain decisions may be present before the age of legal majority and is not guaranteed after, especially when medical or psychiatric illness may impair one's capacity. Clinician assessment is key in determining the adolescent's role in health decisions. The patient needs to be able to (1) communicate a choice, (2) understand the relevant information, (3) appreciate the situation and its consequences, and (4) reason about treatment options.[18] The lived experience of chronic illness generally increases the adolescent's appreciation of the situation and familiarity with the relevant information, and provides prior experience with observing or participating in choices among treatment options. With consistent family and clinician support, adolescents can participate meaningfully in decisions about their care.

Adolescents and young adults who acquired HIV at birth face multiple challenges in decision making. Many have no parents; they are dependent on governmental agencies for guardianship, with no consistent adult support for both the process and outcomes of decisions. Many exhibit evidence of brain dysfunction (executive function, learning, mood) because of HIV or its co-morbidities that can interfere with the development of decisional capacity. With advanced HIV disease, central nervous system complications become more likely, interfering with capacity at a time when concurrent decisions become more complex and less clear. Similar challenges occur with other advanced diseases, such as the altered mental status from hypoxemia in end-stage cystic fibrosis or poor perfusion in congestive heart failure.

The challenge is to respectfully elicit the adolescent's wishes early and often. Clinicians should assess how likely it is that the adolescent can adhere successfully to each option with available supports, and then make a recommendation that optimizes benefit and minimizes burden. Nonadherence that is unresponsive to concerted interdisciplinary efforts can become a terminal condition. When it seems that we should be able to control the disease, if only the patient would follow medical advice, everyone experiences a sense of failure. When this happens, it is especially important to find ways to provide comfort and support for the adolescent during the remainder of his or her life, and for the family members and clinicians who survive them.

WHEN CHRONIC DISEASE BECOMES TERMINAL ILLNESS

Palliative care clinicians have a responsibility to recognize and communicate when the underlying disease is progressing and no treatment can realistically maintain health or prevent death.[19] Prognostication is difficult in many pediatric disorders because of insufficient data regarding long-term outcomes by syndrome or diagnosis; what is available is often out of date, not including newer treatment strategies. When the health conditions are late multisystem complications of static diagnoses (e.g., respiratory failure due to recurrent pneumonia due to recurrent aspiration due to gastrointestinal dysmotility in an adolescent with intellectual disability and cerebral palsy resulting from intraventricular hemorrhage and extreme prematurity), prediction is even more complex. The urge to remain hopeful and positive is likely more intense in pediatric practice than in adult practice—both parents and clinicians hope that this child is the 1 in 20, 1 in 100, 1 in 1,000 who will do well. Communicating a change in prognosis, especially predicting that death may be near, is challenging in and of itself. Parents want honest and complete information, but some report that they have been told their child would die multiple times in the past, and they do not believe this prediction any longer. Parents also seek to protect their children, regardless of age, and may block open and honest discussion between the clinician and the patient, causing conflict and distress. If the standard for open communication is set at the beginning of the clinical relationship, it is more natural to explore a child's understanding of the situation, elicit any questions or concerns, and respond in a trustworthy and balanced manner.

References

1. Institute of Medicine of the National Academies. When Children Die: Improving Palliative and End-of-Life Care for Children and Their Families. Washington, D.C.; 2003.
2. American Academy of Pediatrics. Committee on Bioethics and Committee on Hospital Care. Palliative care for children. *Pediatrics* 2000, **106**: 351–7.
3. National Hospice and Palliative Care Organization. ChiPPS White Paper. A Call for Change: Recommendations to Improve the Care of Children Living with Life-Threatening Conditions; 2001.
4. NHPCO Facts and Figures: Hospice Care in America. National Hospice and Palliative Care Organization. Alexandria, VA; January 2012.
5. Hoyert D, Xu, J. Deaths: Preliminary Data for 2011. National Vital Statistics Reports. Centers for Disease Control, Department of Health and Human Services; 2012. Hyattsville, MD: USA.
6. Feudtner C, Feinstein JA, Satchell M, Zhao H, Kang TI. Shifting place of death among children with complex chronic conditions in the United States, 1989–2003. *JAMA* 2007, **297**: 2725–32.
7. Mathews TJ, Minino AM, Osterman MJ, Strobino DM, Guyer B. Annual summary of vital statistics. *Pediatrics*, 2008, **127**: 146–57.
8. Stoll BJ, Hansen NI, Bell EF, Shankaran S, Laptook AR, Walsh MC, *et al.* Neonatal outcomes of extremely preterm infants from the NICHD Neonatal Research Network. *Pediatrics* 2010, **126**: 443–56.
9. Kaneko Y, Kobayashi J, Achiwa I, Yoda H, Tsuchiya K, Nakajima Y, *et al.* Cardiac surgery in patients with trisomy 18. *Pediatr Cardiol* 2009, **30**: 729–34.
10. Bell EF. Noninitiation or withdrawal of intensive care for high-risk newborns. *Pediatrics* 2007, **119**: 401–3.

11. Truog RD, Meyer EC, Burns JP. Toward interventions to improve end-of-life care in the pediatric intensive care unit. *Crit Care Med* 2006, **34**: S373–9.

12. Nelson JE, Cortez TB, Curtis JR, Lustbader DR, Mosenthal AC, Mulkerin C, *et al.* Integrating Palliative Care in the ICU: The Nurse in a Leading Role. *J Hosp Palliat Nurs* 2010, **13**: 89–94.

13. Catlin A, Carter B. Creation of a neonatal end-of-life palliative care protocol. *J Perinatol* 2002, **22**: 184–95.

14. Boss RD, Kinsman HI, Donohue PK. State-of-the-Art: Health Related Quality of Life in the NICU. *J of Perinatology* 2012, **32(12):** 901–6.

15. Saigal S, Stoskopf BL, Feeny D, Furlong W, Burrows E, Rosenbaum PL, *et al.* Differences in preferences for neonatal outcomes among health care professionals, parents, and adolescents. *JAMA* 1999, **281**: 1991–7.

16. Bach JR. Threats to "informed" advance directives for the severely physically challenged? *Arch Phys Med Rehabil* 2003, **84**: S23–8.

17. American Academy of Pediatrics. Committee on Child Abuse and Neglect and Committee on Bioethics. Foregoing life-sustaining medical treatment in abused children. *Pediatrics* 2000, **106**: 1151–3.

18. Appelbaum PS. Clinical practice. Assessment of patients' competence to consent to treatment. *N Engl J Med* 2007, **357**: 1834–40.

19. National Consensus Project for Quality Palliative Care. Clinical Practice Guidelines for Quality Palliative Care SE. 2009 http://www.nationalconsensusproject.org.

5

Patient-Centered Ethos in an Era of Cost Control: Palliative Care and Healthcare Reform

Emily G. Warner and Diane E. Meier

Health reform in America today is motivated by concerns over both poor quality and high cost. This quotient of quality divided by costs is described in health reform discourse as "value" and the calculus as the "value equation." With healthcare spending increasing at a geometric rate, and access to care blocked for millions by rising insurance premiums and costs of care, the key test for any successful health reform will be whether it can improve value. However, there is frequent public concern that any attempt to rein in costs will result in a reduction in quality and inevitable healthcare rationing—denying desired and beneficial care because of global cost constraints. Modern reforms attempt to undermine this concern by conditioning some payment on the attainment of discrete quality targets, but concerns remain. Unlike many other services, medical care is experienced in exceedingly personal terms. It is borne upon by an individual's religious or spiritual beliefs, deeply held values of bodily integrity, dignity, privacy, and personal autonomy, and the individual's self-concept and what she or he hopes for in life. Consumers are therefore wary of government attempts to define quality, because quality—especially in cases of serious illness—is defined by each patient differently.

Palliative care is a paradigm in which patients participate in the definition of quality through substantial discussions with providers regarding the state of the illness, the costs and benefits of treatment, and the patient's goals of care in light of these factors. And—to the surprise of those who would say that patient autonomy must be sacrificed for cost containment—it has also markedly reduced hospital costs. Palliative care is able to achieve this not by draconian service cuts, but by ferreting out the inefficiency that occurs when treatment is provided that does nothing to advance the patient's goals of care. By allowing patients to participate in the definition of quality, and matching treatment plans to those goals, palliative care is able to increase value through a patient-centered value equation. It is therefore an excellent model for modern health reforms that seek to improve value while maintaining patient autonomy. This chapter describes modern health reforms, paying particular attention to the creation of DRGs in the 1980s and the newer incentive reforms under the Patient Protection and Affordable Care Act of 2010, and discusses them in the context of the patient-centered practice of palliative care.

American Health Reform: Manipulating Incentives to Rectify Inefficiency

THE NEED FOR REFORM

Healthcare in America is exorbitantly expensive. The United States spends a higher percentage of its gross domestic product on healthcare than any other country— at 18%,[1] more than double the median for industrialized nations.[2] Yet for all this spending, Americans do not receive better care. International comparisons rank America low on quality of care in a number of domains, including efficiency, health outcomes, and access.[3] And within the United States, people living in areas that use more health services are not found to have better care. Troublingly, the opposite may be true.[4]

One of the predominant theories of why the American system fails to achieve high quality for its high costs is that its fee-for-service (FFS) system causes substantial inefficiency. This inefficiency is thought to arise from misaligned provider incentives. In the FFS system, each service a healthcare provider performs is billed individually, creating incentives for providers to deliver the highest *quantity* of services possible, without regard for whether such services improve health outcomes.[5] Thus, duplicative services, or services that may have little or no benefit, are frequently provided. Because most healthcare is purchased by third-party insurance, consumers do not perform the balancing function of assessing the benefits of a service—the degree to which they improve quality—in light of their price. And indeed, consumers' perception of quality is skewed by a lack of information about the potential risks and benefits of treatment, and the mistaken assumption that quantity of care is a reasonable proxy for quality. In addition to the perverse incentives regarding quantity of services, the FFS system produces inefficiency by poorly calibrating reimbursements to the value of services. Services that may in fact be very valuable for improving patients' health, such as detailed conversations with patients and families or care coordination among different specialists and providers, are not generally reimbursed, whereas procedures that may not improve a patient's overall health can be reimbursed generously. This results in fractured care delivered by multiple subspecialists that rarely is coordinated to achieve the highest quality care possible for the patient.

These perverse consequences of the FFS system have the worst effect on people with serious illness and multiple chronic conditions. These individuals often see many specialists in many different care settings, and although the work of one specialist may have consequences for several aspects of a patient's well-being, this is not always taken into account. In an elderly patient, for example, a complicated cardiac procedure may restore heart function, but may cause the individual to suffer confusion, worsening dementia, and functional decline. The patient goals that could serve as a touchstone around which the specialists could coordinate care decisions are often never articulated. Without taking into account the patient's overall health, the family structure, caregiver supports available to the patient, and the patient's overall goals of care, excellent specialty services may result in poor quality patient care. In order to strategize the best care possible for patients, providers would need to spend a great deal of uncompensated time speaking with patients and their families and coordinating care with other providers, but this doesn't happen.[6] Thus care is poorly managed and uncoordinated, which can lead to worsened health outcomes, and often leads to unmanaged pain and symptoms, which forces patients to return to emergency departments again and again.

AN EARLY CAPITATION REFORM: DIAGNOSTIC RELATED GROUPS

Many health reforms have sought to undermine the negative effects of the FFS system by utilizing a capitated payment model. In capitated payment systems, a fixed fee is paid to a provider to handle care for a patient in a given setting (or, in more recent reforms, across settings), regardless of the patient's actual use of services. In effect, it puts the provider on a budget, with the hope that this will incentivize a provider to reduce medical waste. One of the capitation reforms of the 1980s that, as discussed later, was important for the efflorescence of palliative care, was the creation of a lump sum payment for inpatient hospital care. In 1982, after seeing the Medicare costs for hospital reimbursements balloon from $5.4 billion in 1970 to $26.4 billion in 1980,[7] Congress passed the Tax Equity and Fiscal Responsibility Act,[8] which included provisions that changed Medicare hospital reimbursements from a FFS system, in which every hospital item was billed separately, to a "prospective payment system."[9] This system provides a lump sum payment to hospitals for each admission. The amount of the payment is based on the patient's Diagnostic Related Group (DRG), which refers to the patient's main diagnosis and various other complexity and comorbidity adjustments. This lump sum payment, itself referred to as a "DRG," creates an incentive for hospitals to provide more efficient care for Medicare patients, because a DRG payment to the hospital will be the same regardless of the length of the patient's admission or intensity of the services provided. However, critics of the DRG program note that, like all capitated programs, it creates an incentive to indiscriminately cut services, even if doing so may reduce quality.[10] These pervasive concerns have led subsequent policy makers to include payment incentives linked to quality of care as well. This is a common feature of the reforms under the Affordable Care Act.

THE AFFORDABLE CARE ACT

In 2008, with nearly 50 million people in the United States without health insurance[11] and healthcare expenses rising relative to GDP at an alarming rate, healthcare became a dominant issue in the presidential election. This provided the political will to enact major reforms. The public sentiment created two calls to action: expand access to healthcare and reduce the cost of healthcare. After heated political debate, Congress passed the Patient Protection and Affordable Care Act,[12] signed into law on March 23, 2010, and the Health Care and Education Reconciliation Act of 2010,[13] signed into law on March 30, 2012. These two statutes are collectively referred to as the Affordable Care Act (ACA). The law contains two main types of reforms: insurance reforms and system reforms aimed at changing provider incentives.

The insurance reforms have taken up the majority of public discourse on the law, owing to both their popularity and their controversy. These reforms included many popular new regulations on health insurance providers, including provisions preventing insurers from denying coverage based on preexisting conditions and provisions requiring insurers to spend a certain percentage of their premiums on care. It also included a controversial provision: the mandate that everyone who meets a certain income threshold must purchase health insurance. This "individual mandate" was designed to balance the perverse incentive, created by the preexisting condition provision, to wait until one got sick before purchasing health insurance. However, some argued that the individual mandate amounted to an unconstitutional intrusion of government into citizens' individual liberty.[14] This mandate has received a great deal of attention, including many lawsuits and a Supreme Court opinion that upheld the mandate as a permissible exercise of Congress' taxing power.[15]

In contrast with the great deal of ink spilled over the insurance reforms, the system reforms have moved forward with relatively little publicity. These provisions received bipartisan support during the healthcare debates and are meant to alter the FFS system to better align provider incentives with efficient, high-quality care. Most of the programs continue to reimburse providers on a partial FFS basis, but they also provide incentives to stay within certain cost targets and to meet quality targets.[16] There are two main incentive programs included under the ACA in this area: hospital reforms and integrated care reforms.

The hospital reforms directly target the weaknesses of the DRG system. Under the DRG, there was some indication that hospital quality was declining. In particular, readmissions were becoming more common, indicating that hospitals were discharging patients too quickly, before the patient was prepared to return home or without adequate home supports.[17] Such readmissions increased revenue for hospitals, because although the fee per admission was fixed, the number of admissions per patient was not. To rectify this, and hopefully to bolster hospital quality generally, the ACA penalizes hospitals for readmissions,[18] and creates a hospital value-based purchasing program (VBP).[19] In this VBP program, most hospitals receive a 2% reduction of their base DRG payments,[20] but will have an opportunity to recoup this loss and more by performing well on certain quality measures. Quality is measured in several domains: clinical processes of care, patient experiences of care, and outcomes of care.[21]

The integrated care reforms seek to improve value not just within one setting, but across settings. One of the challenging aspects of healthcare incentive reform is that better, more efficient care may require cooperation among many different providers, including hospitals and physician groups, and that this might lead to loss of revenue in one setting (hospitals) and more revenue in another (community-based providers). Under FFS or setting-specific capitation plans, each provider is incentivized to maximize its individual revenue and has little investment in the total price of an overall episode of care. Thus, a hospital does not have much incentive to ensure that a patient will not need subsequent hospital visits, and neither does a physician group. Similarly, physicians have no incentive to reduce costs associated with imaging facilities, as this payment stream does not negatively affect the physicians' payment stream. In order to incentivize care that treats patients adequately in the community, minimizes waste, and avoids use of the most expensive and high-risk setting—the hospital—all providers must have an incentive to provide care in the most efficient way possible. In order to achieve this goal, integrated care reforms seek to align provider incentives across settings. The most notable of these programs is the Medicare Shared Savings Program (MSSP),[22] which incentivizes accountable care organizations (ACOs) to provide integrated care across settings, and to be "accountable" for patient outcomes.

Accountable care organizations are single legal entities comprised of many different providers, including hospitals and physicians' groups, who agree to share accountability and risk management for a population—under the MSSP, at least 5,000 people.[23] While participating in the MSSP, an ACO agrees to take responsibility for all healthcare needs of a population—whether patients are receiving care in the community, in the home, or in the hospital. Through the MSSP payment structure, ACOs are paid under the typical FFS arrangement, but they are incentivized to provide efficient care by recouping as profit a portion of any net savings they generate for Medicare—thus the name, Medicare Shared Savings Program. Accountable care organizations only recoup these savings as profit if they are able to meet quality benchmarks at the same time that they are generating savings. Therefore an ACO's overall payment reflects both efficiency and quality—ideally in the form of improved health outcomes for patients. The hope is that ACO leadership will think at a systems level about how to provide a high-quality episode of care at a lower price. This incentive will drive a major shift of healthcare resources out of acute care hospitals (by far the most expensive setting of care), and into the home and community.

Ethical Concerns and a Person-Centered Model of Care

The aspiration guiding the reforms of the ACA, that the dual emphasis on quality and cost will result in higher value healthcare by reducing only those services and procedures that do not contribute to healthcare quality, is apt and achievable: by some estimates, 30% of healthcare spending is waste.[24] However, this discourse of medical waste and the quality measures meant to ensure that needed and beneficial care will not be withheld in service of reducing medical waste does nothing to quell consumer fears that they will lose the autonomy to make healthcare decisions for themselves, because it does nothing to acknowledge what patients value. When asked, patients tend to define quality in functional terms: They hope to be able to walk, to drive, to work, to eat, or to speak with their families. Likewise, the costs they bear come from side effects and opportunity costs of treatment: lost control over their time; inability to travel; inability to engage in activities they find meaningful; days spent in the hospital or a doctor's office, away from their families or the comforts of home; long waits; pain; discomfort; humiliation; embarrassment; and lack of privacy. In order to both calm consumer fears and maintain the integrity of patient autonomy, valuable care must be defined by patients. Thus the challenge for health reform is to create a care paradigm that at once reduces costs and cultivates and honors patient autonomy. This may seem impossible given the current market—that consumers equate quantity with quality and are shielded from the monetary costs of medical services by third-party payers. However, there is substantial evidence that patient autonomy is not antithetical to cost control: the stunning growth of palliative care under the DRG has shown that patients, given the choice and treated with comprehensive, whole-person care, will often need and choose more conservative and less expensive care plans and settings, because this care is actually more valuable for the patient.[25]

Hospital palliative care arose in the 1980s, when some physicians noticed that the FFS care paradigm of reimbursement-driven procedures took the focus off of patients. People with very serious and terminal illnesses were dying painful deaths and receiving medical treatments that subtracted from their quality of life, without first having adequate input as to whether these treatments would help them meet their goals of care. Services that were valuable to patients, such as pain and symptom management and conversations to help navigate increasingly complex treatment options, were not provided, arguably both for want of reimbursement incentives for these services and for lack of professional training in these skills. Initially funded by private foundations, hospital palliative care teams arose to fill in this gap in care, to help patients and families better engage in their treatment options, to counsel and to support, and to treat the individual as a whole. Interdisciplinary palliative care teams—often composed of physicians, social workers, chaplains, and nurses—provide an extra layer of support for patients who are seriously ill and may be receiving treatment from many different specialists.

However, under the FFS system there was no adequate payment mechanism this type of care.[26] In a strictly FFS system, palliative care is not a "profitable" approach to medicine. Often, fewer procedures are performed because patients determine that they prefer less invasive alternatives, and care in a patient's best interests may involve forgoing well-remunerated procedures in order to preserve the patient's quality of life. Time-consuming conversations between chaplains or social workers and patients to determine a patient's values and goals and detailed conversations with physicians and nurses to fully explain a patient's illness and treatment options are compensated at a very low rate, if at all. Conversations with a patient's family—a crucial aspect in care of a seriously ill patient—are not compensated at all if they do not occur "face to face" with the patient. Thus, palliative care teams do not generate substantial revenue in the FFS system—to the contrary, they would reduce revenue in a hospital that was paid on a FFS basis. However, hospitals are not paid on a FFS basis. The imposition of the cost containment reform of DRGs created a financial landscape in which the person-centered practice of palliative care could grow. This is because hospitals, faced with the global budget of DRGs, needed a way to provide care more efficiently, and palliative care does just that.[27]

Although designed to meet patient needs, an epiphenomenon of the palliative care model is that, on average, patients receiving palliative care tend to have shorter hospital admissions and utilize services at a lower intensity. This is a result both of patients choosing less invasive care and of the beneficial effects of pain and symptom management. This lower intensity of services translates to a reduction in costs for hospitals. In a study published in 2009 in the *Archives of Internal Medicine*, Morrison et al.[28] found that by helping patients clarify goals and select treatments that meet those goals, palliative care consultation teams were associated with an average net cost savings of $2,659 per-patient per-admission for patients who were discharged from the hospital alive. For patients who died, this average net cost savings was closer to $7,000 per patient. For a hospital with 300 beds, whose palliative care team serves 500 patients per year, the net savings of a palliative care program is $1.3 million per year. This has added up to significant reduction in costs for hospitals and remains a driving force in the rapid expansion of hospital palliative care. Although hospitals may not see an increase in revenue from interdisciplinary palliative care, they see profit gains from reduced overhead costs. Most important, these cost reductions occur while markedly improving patient satisfaction and sense of autonomy. Indeed, a study of the value of palliative care consultations across multiple settings found that "families of patients who received [a palliative care] consultation were more likely to say that the patient received all the treatment that he or she wanted … and that the patient never received unwanted treatment."[29]

The Need for Palliative Care

Thus a care paradigm that meets the challenge of health reform—to reduce costs and improve quality—while honoring patient autonomy is palliative care. The mechanism by which this genuinely person-centered practice yields cost savings is, in effect, a patient-centered value equation: articulation of the goals of care (quality) and mindful consideration of the costs—both economic and noneconomic—of care. Key practices in palliative care—communicating with patients regarding the realities of the illness and the associated treatment options, taking full assessment of patients' social supports and family situation, and discussing the patient's values and hopes for care at length—allow patients to define "quality" in the context of their unique medical and personal circumstances. Then, treatment plans can be orchestrated that aim to reach these articulated goals while minimizing both economic and noneconomic costs to the patient. This is a goal-directed, person-centered paradigm that will be an essential strategy for providers as they seek to improve quality and reduce costs, and should be a guiding principle for policymakers, as they seek to implement the Affordable Care Act.

The ACA directly addresses palliative care in several of its programs. These include the concurrent care demonstration,[30] which will enable some Medicare beneficiaries to receive hospice care concurrent with curative treatments; a new hospice quality reporting program;[31] changes in the hospice face-to-face recertification requirements;[32] and a concurrent hospice and curative treatment program for children with serious illness.[33] These are all important provisions, but they capture only a small group of Medicare beneficiaries—those in specific communities with clearly terminal illness. They do not apply to people with serious illness for whom prognosis is long or quite uncertain, and are therefore ineligible for hospice. For this large group of seriously and chronically ill beneficiaries who continue to benefit from disease-directed treatment, palliative care can provide enhanced quality at a reduced cost, and will be an important tool for providers under the ACA reforms.

Under the DRG/VBP and MSSP programs, providers must meet quality and cost targets. Hospitals have already begun to utilize palliative care to help deliver care with lower overhead costs, but palliative care will also likely prevent readmissions as patients have fewer crises because of pain and symptoms, and as transitions between settings of care are more coordinated and include more complete information about the individual's care preferences and protocols. Palliative care will likely also enable the hospital to score more highly on quality measures, especially those that relate to patient experience of care. A full 30% of a hospital's quality score will be determined by the patient experience domain.[34] For this measure domain, a random sample of patients discharged from the hospital is surveyed on their perceptions and experience of care. Questions include how well nurses and doctors communicated with patients, how responsive staff was to patients' needs, how well pain was managed, and how clearly hospital providers explained how patients could take care of themselves at home, after discharge from the hospital. These are precisely the special competencies of palliative care, and palliative care teams can help hospitals achieve high scores in these areas.

Under the MSSP, in order for ACOs to meet cost targets, they will have to keep those with serious or chronic illness out of the hospital by providing needed supports in the home and community. Indeed, the demonstration project that tested the principles of ACOs (the Physicians Group Practice Demonstration), indicated that the greatest cost savings came as a result of reduced hospital utilization by those who are dually eligible for Medicaid and Medicare.[35] This population typically has very poor health status and few social supports. Community-based palliative care has been shown to meet this challenge of reducing hospitalizations and costs for the sickest and most vulnerable patients, while improving patient and family satisfaction with the care received. A recent report describing the effects of Kaiser Permanente's home-based palliative care program, which provides interdisciplinary spiritual, social, and medical support to individuals with advanced or terminal illness, described that palliative care led to marked cost reductions for seriously ill individuals—25% lower for those with cancer, 67% lower for those with chronic obstructive pulmonary disease, and 52% lower for people with congestive heart failure. Among patients who received palliative care, 93% said they were very satisfied with their care, compared with 81% of patients who received usual care.[36] This is probably because these individuals were able to receive the interdisciplinary care that they needed, in the setting they preferred—their homes.

Palliative care's person-centered value equation should also serve as a model for policy makers as they implement reforms under the ACA. The successes of palliative care have made clear that costs can be reduced as a consequence of honoring patients' autonomy and values, by paying attention to the *patient's* experience of quality and costs. Thus policies must be implemented that will incentivize providers to fully communicate with patients and their families regarding the realities of the illness and prognosis, the benefits and costs of treatment, and the patient's goals of care; and then to fully communicate these goals of care with the entire healthcare team. There are many opportunities to incentivize this. Under the MSSP and VBP programs, for example, palliative care quality measures should be developed and adopted that effectively measure communication, coordination, and pain and symptom management for the seriously ill. Accordingly, electronic health records must be able to capture this data. Such measurement is crucial, because without it providers are likely to undervalue time-consuming conversations with patients, pain and symptom management, a focus on functional goals, and the importance of effective communication across providers and settings. Defining goals—through a scrupulous process of conversations with patients with an interdisciplinary team— and devising treatment plans to meet those goals were the key to palliative care's success in reducing cost while improving quality. It is also crucial for the health system.

Health reforms have enormous power to transform how healthcare is delivered and how we conceptualize the goals of medicine. Excessive focus on monetary costs and quality measures as defined by payers and providers risks neglecting to correct a source of significant inefficiency in health care: the provision of treatments and services that do not further individual patients' goals for their life and their care. By focusing on individuals' goals and values and on the benefits and burdens of available treatment options, palliative care teams provide higher value care, as defined by the people they are trying to serve. This, in turn, has led to lower monetary costs. In order to further this benefit, providers must focus not on the monetary costs or payer-defined quality, but on the costs and quality as defined by the patient. Policy makers, for their part, should take care to implement reforms that ensure that providers are doing just that. If health reforms fail to take into account person-defined quality and cost, they will likely lose the opportunity to create the most valuable care possible.

Notes

1. World Bank lists 2010 United States expenditures on healthcare as 17.9% of GDP. See http://data.worldbank.org/indicator/SH.XPD.TOTL.ZS.
2. Cathy Schoen et al. *U.S. Health System Performance: A National Scorecard.* 25 Health Aff 457 (Nov. 2006) available at: http://content.healthaffairs.org/content/25/6/w457. abstract?keytype=ref&siteid=healthaff&ijkey=o05rzvque3vQE.
3. Id.
4. See Elliott S. Fisher & John E. Wennburg. Health Care Quality, Geographic Variations, and the Challenge of Supply Sensitive Care. 46.1 Perspectives in Biology and Medicine 69 (2003). Available at: http://muse.jhu.edu/journals/perspectives_in_biology_and_medicine/v046/46.1fisher.html.
5. For a discussion of the limitations of a FFS system, and consideration of the direction for alternative delivery systems, see MedPac's Report to Congress: Reforming the Delivery System. June 2008. Available at: http://www.medpac.gov/documents/Jun08_EntireReport.pdf.
6. As Dr. James Farber explained in an interview with PBS, "You don't get paid to think, to counsel, to coordinate, to plan, to advise, to help guide people through some serious decision making at really critical times in their lives. That's a big failure of the system." Interview with James Farber, Geriatrician, Mt. Sinai Hospital, December 19, 2005. Available at: http://www.pbs.org/wgbh/pages/frontline/livingold/interviews/farber.html.
7. MA Rosenberg & MJ Browne. The Impact of the Inpatient Prospective Payment System and Diagnosis-Related Groups: A Survey of the Literature. North American Actuarial Journal. Vol. 5, No. 4. Pp 84-94. Available at:
8. Pub. L. 97-248. Enacted September 3, http://www.google.com/url?sa=t&rct=j&q=&esrc=s&source=web&cd=2&cad=rja&ved=0CDwQFjAB&url=http%3A%2F%2Fwww.soa.org%2Flibrary%2Fjournals%2Fnorth-american-actuarial-journal%2F2001%2Foctober%2Fnaaj0110_6.pdf&ei=UxHrUOHxA4qW0QHKyYHIBQ&usg=AFQjCNEIL1LuNrBd68IOcuzxOwZacAo8lw&bvm=bv.1355534169,d.dmQ1982.
9. Codified at 42 U.S.C. § 1395ww (d).
10. See Leonard M. Fleck. *DRGs: Justice and the Invisible Rationing of Health Care Resources*, 12 J Med Philos 165 (1987) (arguing that DRG amounts to invisible healthcare rationing) available at: http://jmp.oxfordjournals.org/content/12/2/165. abstract; see e.g. Bill Rumbler, *For Ill, It's Care vs. Cost*, Chicago Sun-Times, Jan. 31, 1986, available at: http://nl.newsbank.com/nl-search/we/Archives?p_product=CSTB&p_theme=cstb&p_action=search&p_maxdocs=200&p_topdoc=1&p_text_direct-0=0EB36CEBD6505BAD&p_field_direct-0=document_id&p_perpage=10&p_sort=YMD_date:D&s_trackval=GooglePM (noting that patients may be released from hospitals too soon because of Medicare payment system).

11. Kaiser Commission on Medicaid and the Uninsured. Covering the Uninsured in 2008: A Detailed Examination of Current Costs and Sources of Payment, and Incremental Costs of Expanding Coverage. August 2008. Available at: http://www.kff.org/uninsured/upload/7809.pdf.

12. Pub. L. 111-148 (124 Stat. 119.)

13. Pub. L. 111-152. (124 Stat. 1029.)

14. See National Federation of Ind't Businesses v. Sebelius, 567 U.S. __, 2012 WL 2427810 (2012).

15. Id.

16. Most of the structural reforms are included under Title III of the law, "Improving the Quality and Efficiency of Health Care."

17. Evidence suggests that the DRG worsened patients' stability at discharge. See http://www.rand.org/pubs/reports/R3930.html.

18. This penalty provides that hospitals will receive a penalty for treatment of patients who, after discharge, are readmitted to the hospital within 30 days for treatment of pneumonia, heart attacks, and/or heart failure. See ACA § 3025.

19. See ACA § 3001. The hospital VBP program builds on the Hospital Inpatient Quality Reporting Program instituted in 2003 as part of the Medicare Prescription Drug, Improvement and Modernization Act.

20. In fiscal year 2013, the percentage will be 1%. This is increased over a period of 4 years, to a maximum percentage of 2% in fiscal year 2017 and beyond. See ACA § 3001.

21. Id. For the initial years of the program, focus will be placed on clinical processes of care measures (e.g., "Surgery Patients on a Beta Blocker Prior to Arrival That Received a Beta Blocker During the Perioperative Period"), and on the patient experience of care. The precise measures are subject to Secretary discretion, and are promulgated as part of the federal rulemaking process each year.

22. PPACA § 3022; 42 U.S.C. §1395jjj.

23. Id.

24. Best Care at Lower Cost: The Path to Continuously Learning Health Care in America. Institute of Medicine. September 2012. Pp 3–9, 3–10. Available at: http://www.iom.edu/Reports/2012/Best-Care-at-Lower-Cost-The-Path-to-Continuously-Learning-Health-Care-in-America.aspx.

25. See Meier, D. E., and J. Brian Cassel. Palliative Care's Positive Outcomes. *Trustee.* March 2011. 2.

26. Physicians can bill for a consultation under Medicare part B, but this consultation is reimbursed at a low rate for the amount of time such a consultation would require for complex patients, and social workers and chaplains—crucial parts of the interdisciplinary team—cannot bill Medicare at all.

27. Morrison et al. 2008. Cost Savings Associated with US Hospital Palliative Care Consultation Programs. *Arch Intern Med. 168*(16):1783–1790.

28. Id.

29. Casarett, D. et al. 2008. Do Palliative Consultations Improve Patient Outcomes? *J Am Geriatr Soc.* 56:596.

30. ACA § 3140.

31. ACA § 3004.

32. ACA § 3132.

33. ACA § 3202.
34. Medicare Program; Hospital Inpatient Value-Based Purchasing Program, 76 FR 26490, 26526 (May 6, 2011).
35. See Carrie H Colla et al. Spending Differences Associated with the Medicare Physician Group Practice Demonstration. *JAMA*. *308*(10):1015–1023. Available at: http://jama.jamanetwork.com/article.aspx?articleid=1357260.
36. In-Home Palliative Care Allows More Patients to Die at Home, Leading to Higher Satisfaction and Lower Acute Care Utilization and Costs. AHRQ innovations exchange. Available at: http://www.innovations.ahrq.gov/content.aspx?id=2366.

6

Palliative Care, Ethics, and Interprofessional Teams

Sally A. Norton, Deborah Waldrop,
and Robert Gramling

Interprofessional teams are a standard for hospice and palliative care services (Meier & Beresford, 2008; National Consensus Project, 2009). One strength of an interprofessional team approach is an explicit use of the varied perspectives that different disciplines bring to patients and families who are facing advanced and/ or end stage illness. The deliberate use of multiple perspectives rounds out the breadth and depth of expertise in developing plans of care for patients and their families. Yet this strength may, at times, be the context for team conflict (Shannon, 1997). The purpose of this chapter is to examine various ethical challenges that manifest among interprofessional palliative care teams and to suggest potential strategies for addressing these challenges. We focus on the roles of social workers, nurses, and physicians because these disciplines are ubiquitous among palliative care programs.

Discipline-Specific Ethical Norms

Nurses, social workers and physicians acculturate to disciplinary norms for ethical practices. Although these norms are generally strongly aligned, they differ subtly in ways that can cause conflict for interprofessional teams. As shown in Table 6.1, the Codes of Ethics for Nursing, Social Work, and Medicine each advocate a primary obligation to the patient or client. However, the disciplinary norms differ with respect to ideal interprofessional collaboration.

In particular, the ANA and NASW standards present nonhierarchical notions of collaboration, while the AMA standards present a hierarchical notion of collaboration. This difference in the "physician as captain of the ship" versus more egalitarian models of team care does not escape members of the interprofessional team. Therefore, although interprofessional collaboration allows for more

TABLE 6.1
Crosswalk of Interprofessional Ethical Principles

	Social Work	Nursing	Medicine
Primary Mission	▫ Enhance human well-being and help meet the basic human needs of all people ▫ Empower people who are vulnerable, oppressed, and living in poverty. ▫ Focus on individual wellbeing in the social context. ▫ Promote the right of self-determination. (*NASW Code of Ethics*)	▫ Respect for dignity, worth, and uniqueness of individuals ▫ To be unrestricted by considerations of social or economic status, personal attributes, or the nature of health problems. (*ANA Code of Ethics Provision 1 and 2*)	▫ Provide competent medical care, with compassion and respect for human dignity and rights. (*AMA Code of Ethics*)
Collaboration	▫ Draw in the perspectives, values, and experiences of the social work profession. ▫ Establish professional and ethical obligations of the interdisciplinary team and its members. (*NASW Code of Ethics 2.03 Interdisciplinary Collaboration*)	▫ Respect all individuals with whom the nurse interacts ▫ Value the distinct contributions of individual/ groups ▫ Work to meet the shared goal of providing quality health services. (*ANA Code of Ethics Provision 1.5*)	▫ Share mutual ethical concern for patients. ▫ Hear nurses' concerns about orders that appear to be erroneous ▫ Explain orders to the nurse involved. ▫ Do not expect or insist that nurses follow orders contrary to standards of good medical and nursing practice... . (*AMA Code of Ethics Collaboration: Opinion 3.02—Nurses*)

Note: Select principles were summarized for comparison.

comprehensive patient care (McLellan, Bateman, & Bailey, 2005), it becomes susceptible to conflicts when role expectations become inflexible (Bateman, Bailey, & McLellan, 2003). As Hewison and Sim (1998) describe, a key barrier to high quality interprofessional collaboration is a dogmatic demarcation of professional members' roles. On the other hand, establishing clarity about the usual roles within a team is essential to efficient team functioning (Bridges, Davidson, Odegard, Maki, & Tomkowiak, 2011; Kipp, Pimlott, & Satzinger, 2007).

Team members who are working together not only share information and knowledge, they also acquire expertise in the role domains of other members of the team (Molleman, Broekhuis, Stoffels, & Jaspers, 2008). Thus, the work of an interprofessional team begins to blur the boundaries of role expertise. Some clinicians respond favorably to the blurring of boundaries and others become defensive of what they perceive to be encroachment on their domains (Molleman, Broekhuis, Stoffels, & Jaspers, 2008). The latter may result in contested realms of expertise and team discord (O'Connor & Fisher, 2011).

Team Cultures Differ

Health care systems are comprised of numerous teams, each having slightly different goals and understandings of best care practices (Hunter, 1996). Therefore, a high functioning palliative care team requires not only an appreciation for multiple disciplinary perspectives within the palliative care (PC) team, but also the need to interact effectively with other teams whose identities, values and norms are dissimilar (Curry et al, 2012). For example, palliative care consult teams that function internally well with an egalitarian model of interprofessional relationships often need to communicate effectively with referring teams that harbor more hierarchical models of relationships.

Understanding the role culture of the groups with whom the PC team interacts is critical for the success of palliative care consultation. The PC team members who are mindful of such cultural rules and norms are better equipped to navigate many of the tensions inherent in multiteam clinical care (Norton et al., 2011). Curry and colleagues (2012) in their work on group dynamics in teams described some of the complexity inherently embedded but not always explicit in an interprofessional group in three ways: (1) Within team—individual-interpersonal view of the group; (2) Team to team—the group to group relationships; (3) Intergroup dynamics—individuals within teams who, in addition, are members of other groups, which all may be encountered by PC teams confronting ethical issues in care delivery.

Case Studies

In the following sections, we describe four clinical scenarios to engage readers more actively in the consideration interprofessional team ethics. Three scenarios involve within team, team to team, or intergroup conflict. The fourth scenario is an exemplar of both intra- and interteam collaboration at its best. Using these scenarios, we highlight key interprofessional issues that can arise in the context of palliative care and suggest strategies that we have found to be effective for addressing them. Our case scenarios represent actual clinical experiences that have been modified sufficiently to preserve the confidentiality of participants.

Identities and Conflict

CASE PRESENTATION

Mrs. Adams is a 60 year-old woman with end-stage metastatic ovarian cancer. The attending oncologist consults palliative care to assist with managing her severe abdominal pain that is "untouched" by anything but opiates. He tells you that some of the nurses are quite distressed about the patient's husband, who they feel is preventing the patient from taking any sedating pain medications. The attending acknowledges that the husband-wife relationship is "complex," but says that the patient is refusing her medications and has the right to do so because she is a competent decision maker.

When you (the palliative care nurse practitioner) and the palliative care attending physician present to the oncology unit for the initial visit, the patient's nurse informs you that the husband is at the bedside and that the patient reports being in pain but is refusing her medications. He explains that the husband is adamantly opposed to any medications that can cause drowsiness or confusion, and that the patient accedes to the husband's wishes. The nurse further states that when the husband goes home at night, Mrs. Adams agrees to take her morphine and appears much more comfortable when she does. The nurse offers that he is a bit less concerned about coercion than some of his colleagues and believes that the husband shows compassion for Mrs. Adams. To minimize conflict, the charge nurse has begun assigning him to Mrs. Adam's care whenever he is on duty. The other nurses voice their frustration that the oncology attending is not addressing the situation and have begun sneaking into the patient's room when the husband steps out in order to offer Mrs. Adams her pain medications. This, in turn, infuriates the husband when he returns. The conflict is escalating between the husband and nursing staff and is also beginning to create unrest among the nursing team.

Thus far, two immediate questions arise:

(1) Is the husband unduly influencing the patient's decision making about pain management?
(2) What is contributing to the differences of opinion among the oncology nursing and physician staff about the husband's behavior?

During the initial visit with Mrs. Adams and her husband, Mrs. Adams looks uncomfortable, confirms that she is in pain, and states that she prefers "to go along with" her husband's wishes regarding avoidance of any sedating pain medications. You ask Mrs. and Mr. Adams about their understanding of her prognosis, and both acknowledge that death is approaching. Neither you nor the palliative care attending observe Mrs. Adams to show any fear of her husband and note that the couple seems to express compassion to one another.

Days pass and Mrs. Adams' condition worsens and her pain levels increase. She continues to refuse both long acting opiates and only will take her "as needed" morphine when her husband leaves for the night. Mrs. Adams confided in the night nurse that her husband has always been very controlling in their relationship and that she was considering leaving him before she became ill.

You notice that men and women members of the nursing and physician oncology teams are becoming more polarized in their opinions. You (a woman) and your attending physician colleague (a man) are both bothered by the situation and discuss whether (and how) to intervene on Mrs. Adams' behalf. You note that you are gravitating more strongly than your physician colleague toward the opinion that Mr. Adams is inhibiting Mrs. Adam's right to self-determination. Given that your opinions are diverging and that the situation is not improving, you both recommend an urgent clinical ethics consult.

As the scenario unfolds, more questions arise that relate to interdisciplinary teamwork:

(1) How is gender and power manifesting within the healthcare teams?
(2) Is a hierarchical model for team roles a relative benefit or burden in this situation?

The next day, Mrs. Adams has become moribund and minimally responsive. Her night-time morphine is beginning to wear off and she is now grimacing and moaning with any movement. Mr. Adams is still hopeful that she will have a few more moments of lucidity and tells the nurses not to give her any pain medications. Before further action can be taken, Mrs. Adams dies. Mr. Adams falls to the floor weeping.

DISCUSSION

We present the scenario with insufficient detail for the reader to determine what the "right" approach would have been for Mrs. Adams' pain control. Indeed, this lack of omniscience is purposeful because this inability to fully know the Adams' decision-making relationship presented confusion and distress for members of the interprofessional teams. Fundamentally, the lenses that focused team members' understanding of this situation appears less dictated by the norms of their specific disciplines per se, but rather by other identities represented by Mr. or Mrs. Adams. The scenario demonstrates several responses to the growing tension, most of which led to forms of avoidance. Avoidance can provide respite for morally distressed and exhausted team members to give them time to reengage in patient care or useful dialogue (e.g., a nurse manager scheduling to provide respite for distressed nurses). Often, however, avoidance can also promote dysfunctional intrapersonal and inter-personal behaviors, miscommunication, fracture of relationships, and delay in time-sensitive decisions. The choice to request an urgent ethics consultation rep-resented shared acknowledgement that this spiraling situation required clinically sensitive and prompt mediation by a trusted and competent source. Unfortunately, the Adams' case represents missed opportunities to mediate a morally distressing situation earlier in her care when it was recognized and when such mediation held the potential to improve Mrs. Adams' clinical care, Mr. Adams' bereavement, and the team's capacity to both function and to respect each others' deep differences of opinion.

 ¤ Decision-making relationships are complex, habitual, and relational. Amid suffering, usual patterns of decision-making relationships can become dysfunctional. Navigating the demands on healthcare professionals to rec-ognize undue coercion requires multiple perspectives and, often, mediation of those important perspectives.

◘ Sociocultural identities (such as those related to gender and power) are important and inextricable aspects of our humanity. Interprofessional teams require time and space to appreciate and discuss differences of perspective that arise in clinical care.

◘ Avoidance, while temporarily providing respite, can delay effective mediation of moral distress in complex situations. Palliative care teams, who are often called to assist in such situations, should remain cognizant of the additional support that clinical ethics consultations can provide in such situations.

Can You "Fix" This?

CASE PRESENTATION

Mary McCormick was a 66 year-old woman with Stage IV lung cancer that had metastasized to her brain. She had been widowed for 25 years and her only daughter, who had experienced a traumatic brain injury, was a resident of the county home. Mrs. McCormick lived in a garage apartment behind her landlady's house. She had an adversarial relationship with her landlady and was estranged from a cousin who was her only other family. Mrs. McCormick had an enduring friendship with Penny Durkin, whom she had known for many years. Penny served as Mary's healthcare proxy and assisted with instrumental activities of daily living (IADL) and groceries. Mary had been treated with chemotherapy but described her experience by saying "my body rejected the chemo." When it was determined that Mary could not tolerate chemotherapy, her oncologist attempted to talk with her about her illness trajectory. Putting her hand up as if to block the words from being spoken, she stated, "I don't want to know." Penny did speak with the oncologist and understood that Mary's prognosis was very short, given her fast-growing small cell lung cancer. Penny also understood that the brain metastases might already have been compromising Mary's cognitive and decisional abilities. The oncologist recommended a hospice referral and Penny was immediately grateful for the offer of help.

During the hospice admission interview, the hospice nurse found that Mrs. McCormick was able to walk but her gait was unsteady. Her pain was not completely controlled and she complained of headaches. The nurse questioned Mary's decision-making abilities. In addition, Mary was incontinent, which she described as "dribbles" for which she wore diapers when she could afford to buy them. Mary had four cats that did not use a litter box. Mrs. McCormick's sofa had been saturated with urine and was infested with maggots. During the admission interview, the nurse expressed her concern that Mary was no longer safe living alone and described the better options for care as the hospice residence or a nursing home. When Mary emphatically said "NO" and took offense, the nurse dropped the subject (for then) and contacted the social worker as soon as she finished the visit to say "I really need you to fix this situation."

Questions:

(1) Can/should people be forced to hear and understand their prognosis especially in light of the fact that it influences decision making?
(2) Can/should Mary continue to make her own decisions?
(3) How/when do you invoke a healthcare proxy when the patient is expressing her wishes clearly but has underlying disease process that may undermine her capacity?
(4) Can/should she be forced to move to a "safer" location for care?
(5) Would a home health aide make it possible for Mary to remain at home?

Mary agreed to let the hospice nurse and social worker make a joint visit. The social worker assessed the home environment and talked with Mary about her very limited resources (social, emotional, and financial). She asked about the healthcare proxy and how Mary wanted Penny to help her make decisions. She learned that Penny had problems that precluded her from doing much more than bringing groceries and doing laundry for Mary. Penny was also caregiving for her mother so she was unable to spend more time with Mary, which meant that there was noone to stay with her when she would become bedbound. The social worker and nurse broached the topic of transferring to another location for care. At this point, Mrs. McCormick stated, "When you keep talking about going to the hospital, I feel that you're trying to shove me in there. I'm not ready to go. I'd rather stay here. I don't want to think about it."

Question:

(1) How do you evaluate the importance of upholding a person's self-determination when his or her choices are in conflict with the patient's best interest?

DISCUSSION

Mary McCormick's resolute determination to remain independent and in her own home until her death clearly emerged in this scenario. Yet, the influence of Mary's declining physical abilities, lack of a readily available caregiver, and the possibility that her decision-making capacity was being compromised by the growth of the brain tumor was becoming central. Balancing Mary's expressed wishes and right to self-determination with her safety and well-being is complex. The team members' individual perspectives seemed to be focused through disciplinary lenses and value systems. Effective interprofessional collaboration in complex situations requires flexible thinking and the ability to think of solutions that are outside of disciplinary "boxes."

◘ This case illustrates the importance of and need for multidisciplinary assessment while underscoring numerous issues that can challenge the team in achieving consensus. If consensus cannot be reached, the issue of whether the team will override the patient's clear wishes because she is unsafe at home becomes a significant dynamic.

◻ Team members may have different personal philosophies about the ethics of Mary remaining at staying home; there is also the likelihood of disciplinary differences in practice standards.

◻ If a consensus cannot be reached with the patient, caregiver, and interprofessional team, the issue of who bears the ethical and legal responsibility if the situation deteriorates (e.g., individual team members, the physician, patient, or caregiver) is central. Assessment of the patient's decisional capacity (and whether it is transient) is a key variable.

◻ If consensus cannot be reached, consultation with an ethics team or protective services for adults may assist in problem solving.

◻ Consideration of the best way to communicate the concerns and recommendation for the patient's relocation could include one of several options: one team member (which one?), a subset (e.g., nurse and social worker), or a conference with the whole team.

Not the "Average" Hospice Patient

CASE PRESENTATION

Charlie Murray was a 70 year-old man who had prostate cancer with bone metastases. He had lived independently until a visiting nurse determined that he was a safety risk. Charlie was described by his sister as the "rogue" in his family. He had a history of alcohol and other drug abuse, and had burned all of his bridges with family members. He had been estranged from his sister Margie until she learned of his terminal diagnosis and admission to the hospice residence. She described their reconciliation as "if not now, when and if not me, who"? Margie described how Charlie's dying trajectory presented challenges for his family and for the hospice team.

Imagine yourself having a loved one who was in an apartment and independent— he took care of all the little old ladies in the building. He even gave them money to help them with their groceries—this was a self-sufficient guy. He had a little bit of dementia going on where he would forget some things but his routine was good. A home health nurse went to his apartment to check on him and took some blood and that's how they found out that the prostate cancer had gone to his bones. On another visit the nurse found that he had burn holes in his shirt from smoking (he was a heavy smoker) and she said he was a safety risk—he was going to burn the place down. Geez, that was tough... he had lived there for years.... She immediately made the decision that he couldn't live alone and made arrangements to move him to the hospice residence. She must have talked with Mark (Charlie's son) who has his power of attorney but I wasn't involved with that part.

By the next day—within 8 hours he was a total zombie. We had a family meeting and the doctor told us that they had given him drugs because he was agitated. It was a total shock to see him like that—he hadn't been agitated and he wasn't on any pain medicine before he came in. We didn't know if he had a breakdown or had finally realized he didn't have to take care of himself anymore and this was a release? He was either getting too many drugs or maybe his condition just progressed rapidly. He was stammering, stumbling, and stuttering. We thought it had to be the mind-altering drugs they were giving him. I couldn't stand seeing him like that.

Question:

1. In patient-centered, family-focused care, how can family wishes be followed when there is a conflict with standard care?

Charlie was also still mobile and when he got out of the chair he wanted to go through doors—he didn't want to be stuck in a bed waiting to die. After a couple months they asked for another family meeting and they wanted us to consider moving because he was an escape risk. The doctor told us that they would continue to medicate him because he was agitated. The nurses seemed frustrated with him because he wasn't bedbound like all the other people. The social worker talked about moving him to a nursing home and said they would send out applications to other places with dementia units. God help him—I was beside myself.

Charlie needed special attention yet they had other patients they had to watch out for—it was a delicate situation for everyone. But by this point I had cleaned out his apartment so he doesn't have anywhere else to go. He wasn't the average hospice patient. In addition to remaining wide awake and active—he had outlived his 6 months. We were between a rock and a hard place—we wanted him to stay, we appreciated the care he was getting but we just wanted them to review how best to serve his medical needs. You can't put a person to sleep because their brain won't work. Charlie didn't fit the hospice model of dying... it was like trying to put a round peg in a square hole and I was so afraid they were going to make him leave.

Questions:

(1) When a patient is estranged from his or her family, is it acceptable for a home healthcare team to take charge of relocation?
(2) How can palliative care teams balance the patient's right for individualized care with the needs of the organization to assure patient safety and remain fiscally viable when the person's dying trajectory involves special needs?
(3) When is it ethical to discharge a "difficult" patient? How should this be handled with patients like Charlie and his family?

DISCUSSION

Charlie Murray's history of the overlay of substance abuse and early stage of dementia in the context of end-stage prostate cancer contributed to behavioral challenges that were difficult for the hospice residence staff to manage. When Charlie's family raised concerns and complaints about the "standard" use of drug protocols to manage his agitation, the team resisted their request for a different approach that they wished would involve more activities to actively engage him rather than expecting he would spend the time in his room and in bed. This scenario raises the question of how interprofessional teams can uphold the individual worth and dignity of patients whose needs do not fall into "normal" or "average" patterns of dying. This case challenges the use of standard protocols and underscores the importance of care being unrestricted by the difficult attributes and characteristics of an illness.

- ◻ The perspectives of all members of the interprofessional team are important to assess the desirability of this patient remaining in the current environment.
- ◻ The perspective of both the residential and hospice teams may be different from the hospice team and may be directed by financial issues.
- ◻ Perspectives about safety and risk may be different from personal and disciplinary perspectives as well between a residential team and visiting team. Developing agreement about the best way to treat this patient has multiple variables and levels of concern (e.g., individual, team, and organization).
- ◻ There is always the potential for differences between patient-family and interprofessional perspectives on good care. Conflict provides both the challenge and opportunity to develop greater understanding of different perspectives and to find the common ground on which the principles of person-centered, family focused care are built.

Going Home

CASE PRESENTATION

A palliative care consultation is called for Mr. Flannigan, a 60-year-old man in the surgical ICU with a completely ischemic bowel. He is awake and alert and ventilator dependent. Married with three adult sons, he and his wife had just finished building their retirement lake home when he became ill. When the palliative care nurse practitioner enters the room, Mr. Flannigan's wife is sitting next to him. She tells you that they know he is dying and that he wants to die in his new home. Mrs. Flannigan states that he would not want to live on a ventilator and wishes to have it withdrawn. Off the ventilator, it is unlikely that he will live longer than a few hours. Although the ICU team understands the Flannigans' wish for him to die at home, his nurse says they are concerned that dying at home is not feasible given his unstable state and ventilator dependence.

(1) Would it be better to have the patient die in the hospital where the teams are certain he can be comfortable or try and discharge him to die at home as he wishes even if the latter comes at a risk?

The first solution discussed is hospital extubation and direct ICU-to-home rapid discharge, but he is unlikely to survive an extubation in the hospital long enough to get him home. Moreover, there is a distinct possibility that he would die in the ambulance on the way home. A second option discussed is to extubate and transfer to the palliative care unit in the hospital. But the sons are upset with the discussion of an in-hospital extubation because that is NOT what their dad wants. The PC team meets separately with Mrs. F. to understand how she is feeling about trying to get her husband home. They discuss some of the risks associated with the plan. She says, "Absolutely—I want him home". The family and Mr. Flannigan are apprised of the risks and still want to try for a home discharge.

After clear and unwavering responses from the Flannigan family, ICU and PC teams agree that it may be feasible for Mr. Flannigan to die at home if he was extubated at home. Though given his deteriorating status, a move had to be made quickly. The two teams, along with the Flannigan family agree to move forward with the transfer. Connected with a shared goal, they move into collaborative problem-solving mode.

(1) What plans need to be in place for a safe discharge and home extubation?
(2) What are some of the organizational and role barriers to the plan?

There is agreement to move forward with developing a discharge plan. The unit social worker calls the hospice and the hospice-hospital liaison. A tentative plan is developed to have the transport nurse extubate the patient in the home with the home hospice nurse present. Medical transport and home hospice teams are called. However, liability concerns are raised about the transfer period. What if the patient dies in transit? Can the transport nurse extubate the patient in the home? The home hospice nurse is concerned about managing breathlessness in a newly extubated patient. Her hospice agency has not participated in a home extubation before.

The nurse practitioner calls a quick conference to address the problems—how could something so simple, wanting to die at home, become so complicated?

(1) Given the major concerns--though not refusal--of the transport and home hospice teams, should the hospital team continue forward?
(2) What contingencies still need to be addressed by the teams?

The teams confer, seeking to identify clinical contingencies. What about medications in transit, pre- and post extubation? Will the patient continue to breathe following extubation? What if the patient asks to go back on the ventilator? They meet with the family. The revised plan is discussed and the family made additions to the plan. A daughter-in-law leaves to get the house ready. The home hospice nurse asks the hospice liaison to bring all the needed medications, out of hospital DNR orders, and extubation orders with her. The PC and ICU physicians connect with the hospice physician to create a detailed discharge order, communication channels, and plans covering contingencies. The transport ambulance arrives and the patient is discharged.

Mr. Flannigan was discharged home from the ICU. The plans go smoothly. The son's wife and friends moved a bed downstairs and placed it by the picture window overlooking the lake. Mr. Flannigan, surrounded by his family, spent time with his family and then said he was ready to be extubated. He died as he wished, surrounded by his family, comfortable, and in his own bed overlooking the lake.

DISCUSSION

This scenario highlights several things that can go well in clinical care. Chief among them was an explicit and shared goal. Note at key points along the way, when the plan appeared to be falling apart, the team champions "huddled" to strategize new options. Communication, availability, shared work, respect for patient self-determination, and a strong patient and family willing to accept risk helped to make this happen. Highlighting and addressing ethical and clinical concerns raised allowed the teams and plan to move from an empathic "no" toward a workable "yes." A clear understanding of and respect for the roles and concerns of coordinating teams helped overcome some of the organizational barriers to discharge, and resulted in a safer and better coordinated plan.

- A conceptually straightforward and important wish (*i.e.,* to go home) often requires complex tasks and responsibilities. Conceptualizing "what is required to do this?" requires the perspectives of all team members. Each member will have intimate knowledge of the particulars relating to their portion of the complex task.
- The team requires trust in their members' capacity to foresee potential threats to the plan and commitment to creative problem solving when unforeseen problems arise. Trust is essential for collaboration within a team. Team members can leverage their relational trust across teams when engaged in complex care in different settings.
- Effective collaboration and coordination require clear and consistent communication. Revisiting shared goals provides a focal point for team members during complex care planning.
- Patients and families are pivotal members of the team. They will ultimately need to assume responsibility for considering whether the risks of the plan are acceptable in relation to the potential benefits.

High Quality Teams

Hoegl and Gemuenden (2001) identified six important facets of teamwork quality: communication, coordination, balance of member contributions, mutual support, effort, and cohesion. Molyneux (2001) described the importance of cooperative and egalitarian styles in creating an atmosphere in which there was flexibility across roles. She found such flexibility required team members to be confident in their own roles and also to have confidence in their team colleagues. She described that early in the formation of a team, the team's new members may follow more traditional roles and hierarchies (physician dominant) but as the team develops and matures, team members tend to think of each other as equal partners and become more flexible about their roles and cross professional boundaries without difficulty.

Perceptions of high quality teamwork have been associated with improved patient outcomes in the critical care setting (Baggs, Norton, Schmitt, & Sellers, 2004; Baggs & Schmitt, 1997; Institute of Medicine, 2001; Thomas, Sexton, Helmreich, 2003). In study findings from hospice and critical care settings, physician team members rated team collaboration higher than members from other disciplines (Baggs & Schmitt, 1997; Casarett, Spence, Haskins, & Teno, 2011; Thomas, Sexton, Helmreich, 2003). In a study of ICU teams, Thomas and colleagues found the majority of physicians (73%) rated collaboration as high or very high compared to only 33% of nurses. Similarly, of the six disciplines reported in hospice settings, Cassaret et al. recently observed that physicians followed by chaplains had the highest total scores of job satisfaction and teamwork and that nurses and social workers total scores ranked at the bottom, fifth and sixth respectively. Interestingly, Baggs and colleagues (1999) found that nurse, but not physician, reports of the degree of collaboration and perceived teamwork significantly predicted mortality and readmission outcomes in the Intensive Care Unit setting.

Palliative Care Team Outcomes

Communication, trusting relationships, commitment to the team, shared philosophies, clear roles, and respect for unique role contributions are characteristics cited for successful palliative care teams (Hunter, 1996; Jünger, Pestinger, Elsner, Krumm & Radbruch, 2007). Much of the research on PC teams has been conducted in the United Kingdom. In a series of metaanalyses, Higginson and colleagues demonstrated that patients receiving care from home and hospital palliative care teams had better outcomes for pain and symptom management (Higginson, Finlay, Goodwin, Hood, Edwards, et al., 2002, 2003). In the United States, Hanson et al. (2005) found the use of PC teams in skilled nursing facilities associated with improved hospice enrollment, advance care planning discussions, and pain assessments.

Resolving Ethical Issues within the Team

Leaders in palliative care continue to champion the interprofessional team approach. Enhancing a team's ability to respond to the intellectually and emotionally challenging work and environment must provide strategies for teams to resolve ethical conflicts. The growing emphasis on team development and interprofessional education is one such avenue. For newly developing or existing teams, Clark et al., (2007) provided a framework for examining ethical issues and challenges that occur in interprofessional teams. Their matrix highlights a systematic examination of ethical challenges and the individual, team, and organizational factors alongside the principles, structures, and processes germane at each level. Such a matrix may allow teams to develop a systematic way to examine and resolve ethical issues arising in interprofessional teams.

Summary

By its nature, the dying process can be emotionally, physically, spiritually and existentially challenging for people and their families. Care at these potentially intense and difficult times can be enhanced by the presence of a palliative care team but team members can also face ethical challenges in the midst of meeting peoples' needs. Interprofessional palliative care teams are strengthened by the triangulation of multiple disciplinary norms, but these differing lenses from which care is perceived can also lead to ethical conflicts. Mutual understanding of others' ethical frames of reference is a fundamental first step toward working as equal partners.

This chapter illuminates some of the common ethical dilemmas that are faced by interprofessional palliative care teams. The case of Mrs. Adams demonstrates how the existence of a hierarchical power differential and gendered perspectives undermines the presence of equal partnerships and detracts from quality of patient care. Mary McCormick's story illustrates conflicting perspectives about autonomy and self-determination in the context of social situations that are seen as unsafe and unpleasant, and making team members uncomfortable. Charlie Murray's dying process highlights the existence of medical paternalism and underscores problems with "template" or standard approaches to managing the dying process which is in actuality, uniquely personal and individual. The case of Mr. Flannigan illustrates how well teams can work together to uphold patient and family wishes while respecting the dignity and worth of individuals even until the very end of life. This exemplary scenario provides hope and inspiration that palliative care teams can make a tremendous difference in peoples' lives. Each of the case scenarios illustrates the facets of teamwork and underscores the importance of communication, cooperation, and collaboration toward the shared goal of working through dilemmas to meet patients' needs.

References

The American Medical Association. (2001). *Code of Ethics*. Available at: http://www.ama-assn.org/ama/pub/physician-resources/medical-ethics/code-medical-ethics.page. Accessed October 31, 2012.

The American Nurses Association. (2001). *Code of Ethics.* Available at: http://www.nursingworld.org/codeofethics. Accessed October 31, 2012.

Baggs, JG, Norton, SA, Schmitt, MH, & Sellers, CR. (2004). The dying patient in the ICU: role of the interdisciplinary team. *Critical Care Clinics* 20(3), 525–40.

Baggs JG, Schmitt MH. (1997). Nurses' and resident physicians' perceptions of the process of collaboration in an MICU. *Research in Nursing and Health* 20(1), 71–80.

Baggs, JG, Schmitt, MH, Mushlin, AI, Mitchell, PH, Eldredge, DH, Oakes, D., & Hutson, AD. (1999). The association between nurse-physician collaboration and patient outcomes in three intensive care units. *Critical Care Medicine* 27, 1992–8.

Bateman, H, Bailey, P, McLellan, H. (2003). Of rocks and safe channels: learning to navigate as an interprofessional team. *Journal of Interprofessional Care* 17(2), 141–50.

Bridges, DR, Davidson, RA, Odegard, PS, Maki, IV, Tomkowiak, J. (2011). Interprofessional collaboration: three best practice models of interprofessional education. *Medical Education Online* April 8, 16. Available at: http://www.ncbi.nlm.nih.gov/pmc/articles/PMC3081249/

Casarett, DJ, Spence, C, Haskins, M, Teno, J. (2011). One big happy family? Interdisciplinary variation in job satisfaction among hospice providers. *Journal of Palliative Medicine* 14(8), 913–7.

Clark, PG, Cott, C, Drinka, T. (2007). Theory and practice in interprofessional ethics: a framework for understanding ethical issues in health care teams. *Journal of Interprofessional Care* 21(6), 591–603.

Committee on Quality of Health Care in America, Institute of Medicine. Crossing the quality chasm: a new health system for the 21st century. Washington, DC: National Academy Press; 2001.

Curry, LA., O'Cathain, A, Clark, VLP., Aroni, R, Fetters, M, Berg, D. (2012). The role of group dynamics in mixed methods health sciences research teams. *Journal of Mixed Methods Research* 6(1), 5–20.

Hanson LC, Reynolds K, Henderson M, Pickard CG. (2005). A quality improvement intervention to increase palliative care in nursing homes. *Journal of Palliative Medicine* 8, 576–83.

Hewison, A, Julius, S. (1998). Managing interprofessional working: using codes of ethics as a foundation. *Journal of Interprofessional Care* 12(3), 309–21.

Higginson IJ, Finlay IG, Goodwin DM, Hood K, Edwards AG, Douglas, HR, Norman, CE (2002) Do hospital-based palliative teams improve care for patients or families at the end of life? *Journal of Pain and Symptom Management* 23, 96–106.

Higginson IJ, Finlay IG, Goodwin DM, Hood K, Edwards AG, et al. (2003). Is there evidence that palliative care teams alter end-of-life experiences of patients and their caregivers? *Journal of Pain and Symptom Management* 25, 150–68.

Hoegl, M, Gemuenden, HG. (2001). Teamwork quality and the success of innovative projects: a theoretical concept and empirical evidence. *Organization Science* 12, 435–49.

Hunter, DJ (1996). The changing roles of health care personnel in health and health care management. *Social Science & Medicine* 43, 799–808.

Jünger, S., Pestinger, M., Elsner, F., Krumm, N., Radbruch, L. (2007). Criteria for successful multiprofessional cooperation in palliative care teams. *Palliative Medicine* 21(4), 347–54.

Kipp, J, Pimlott, JF, Satzinger, F. (2007). Universities preparing health professionals for the 21st century: can something new come out of the traditional establishment? *Journal of Interprofessional Care* 21(6), 633–44.

McLellan, H, Bateman, H, Bailey, P. (2005). The place of 360 degree appraisal within a team approach to professional development. *Journal of Interprofessional Care* 19(2), 137–48.

Meier, DE, Beresford, L. (2008). The palliative care team. *Journal of Palliative Medicine* 11(5), 677–81.

Molleman, E, Broekhuis, M, Stoffels, R, Jaspers, F. (2008). How health care complexity leads to cooperation and affects the autonomy of health care professionals. *Health Care Annals* 16, 329–41.

Molyneux, J. (2001). Interprofessional teamworking: what makes teams work well? *Journal of Interprofessional Care* 15(1), 29–35.

National Association of Social Workers. (2008). *Code of Ethics*. Available at: http://www.socialworkers.org/pubs/code/default.asp. Accessed October 31, 2012.

National Consensus Project for Quality Palliative Care. (2009). *Clinical practice guidelines for quality palliative care*, 2nd ed. Available at: http://www.nationalconsensusproject.org/guideline.pdf. Accessed October 12, 2012.

Norton, SA, Powers, BA, Schmitt, MH, Metzger, M, Fairbanks, E, Deluca, J, Quill, TE. (2011). Navigating tensions: integrating palliative care consultation services into an academic medical center setting. *Journal of Pain and Symptom Management* 42(5), 680–90.

O'Connor, M., Fisher, C. (2011). Exploring the dynamics of interdisciplinary palliative care teams in providing psychosocial care: "everybody thinks that everybody can do it and they can't." *Journal of Palliative Medicine* 14(2), 191–6.

Shannon, SE. (1997). The roots of interdisciplinary conflict around ethical issues. *Critical Care Nursing Clinics of North America* 9(1), 13–28.

Thomas EJ, Sexton JB, Helmreich RL. (2003). Discrepant attitudes about teamwork among critical care nurses and physicians. *Critical Care Medicine* 31(3), 956–9.

Addressing Dimensions of Suffering

7

Pain Relief and Palliative Care

Nathan Cherny

Severe pain, which can undermine quality of life and cause incapacitating distress to patients and their accompanying family members, is a common consequence of advanced cancer and of other advanced incurable illnesses. Patients have a right to the adequate relief of their pain, and indeed a strong case has been made for having this recognized as a basic human right. This right is derived from principles of respect for persons, beneficence, nonmaleficence, and justice. Substantial obligations and duties derive from this claim that are relevant to individual health care providers (such as the professional staff attending to patients), the institutions in which they work, and the authorities responsible for public health policy in the provision and allocation of healthcare resources. This chapter explores these ethical domains and issues through a longitudinal case history of Michael, a 68-year-old man suffering from pain caused by metastatic colon cancer beginning from a pain crisis, through his ambulatory management and ultimately to his end of life care, which necessitated the use of sedation to manage otherwise refractory pain.

Michael: A Cry for Help

CASE PRESENTATION

Michael was a 68-year-old Russian immigrant with a 2-year history of metastatic cancer of the colon. At presentation he had a metastasis in the left iliac crest that was initially treated with palliative radiotherapy and chemotherapy. Now, after 2 years of chemotherapy and biological treatments his disease is refractory to systemic therapies. Six weeks ago he reported to the palliative care nurse that he developed severe incapacitating pain in the right hip that was not responding to his usual doses of oxycodone. His wife reported that he was crying uncontrollably and was unable to walk. Compounding the situation was the fact that he lived on the third floor of an apartment building with no elevator and that, in this situation, he would be unable to walk down the stairs to get the hospital.

The hospital incorporates an integrated oncology and palliative medicine service with a proactive telephone follow-up program for patients considered to be at high risk of pain or other complications, to promote early identification of poorly controlled symptoms before they became catastrophic. Additionally, the service provides 24/7 telephone backup for palliative care emergencies. The palliative care nurse case manager recognized this was an emergency situation. Based on her familiarity with the logistical difficulties of Michael's housing situation (84 steps to the road), she arranged for an ambulance to transport him to the emergency room for urgent evaluation and treatment. The emergency room staff was notified in advance of his arrival and was prepared to respond to this as high priority, emergency situation.

Rights and Duties in the Relief of Pain

Severe pain, which can undermine quality of life and cause incapacitating distress to patients and their accompanying family members, is a common consequence of advanced cancer (1-3), and of other advanced incurable illnesses (4, 5). Among cancer patients, the most common causes of severe pain are bone metastases, metastases that compress adjacent neural structures, visceral pain from tumors involving internal organs, and headaches caused by either tumors involving the brain or meninges of the surrounding skull (6, 7). In addition to pains caused by the tumor, many patients suffer from severe and persistent iatrogenic pains related either to previous surgical procedures or as a long-term consequence of chemotherapy treatments (7, 8). Finally, some patients will suffer from acute pain syndromes related either to an acute complications (such as a pathological fracture or a hemorrhaging tumor) or as a side effect of some aspect of their treatment (9, 10).

Irrespective of the cause, patients have a right to the adequate relief of their pain, and indeed a strong case has been made for having this recognized as a basic human right (11-14). This right is derived from principles of respect for persons, beneficence, nonmaleficence, and justice.

There are substantial obligations and duties that derive from this claim that pertain to individual healthcare providers (such as the professional staff attending to patients), the institutions in which they work, and the authorities responsible for public health policy in the provision and allocation of healthcare resources (11-14).

At the macro level, the authorities responsible for public health policy have an obligation to provide adequate infrastructure for the relief of pain including adequate availability and accessibility to the medications and other resources (such as imaging modalities and radiotherapy facilities) that are necessary for the evaluation and management of pain (13, 15). These obligations are confounded by parallel obligations to reduce and to control the diversion and abuse of prescription pain medications, and to prevent the development of drug dependency disorders. These duel obligations require a delicate balance to ensure that patients' pain relief needs are met while simultaneously providing safeguards against drug diversion, abuse, and the risk of addiction. These are not trivial considerations and on an international scale, many governments and healthcare systems fail to meet these basic obligations. Indeed the problem of excessive regulatory restrictions (over-regulation, and therefore inadequate access) is endemic outside of the economically developed Western world. This makes it near impossible for many palliative care patients in such settings to achieve relief pain, thereby undermining their quality of life. Furthermore, regarding the provision of available and accessible therapeutic drugs for the relief of pain, recent surveys have demonstrated that many countries do not provide adequate medications that are on the essential drug lists of the World Health Organization or the International Association for hospice and palliative care. Even when the medications are theoretically available on formulary they are often expensive, not actually available in pharmacies, and/or provision is hampered by a host of regulations that make it profoundly difficult for patients to either receive the prescription or to have it dispensed in an adequate quantity to provide relief for more than just a small number of days.

This problem of overregulation has been highlighted by The Open Society Institute International Palliative Care Initiative (http://www.soros.org/initiatives/health/focus/access/about), the International Observatory on End of Life Care (http://www.eolc-observatory.net), The International Narcotics Control Board (16-19), The World Health Organization (20, 21), the Council of Europe (22), and Human Right Watch (23).

Institutional, national, organizational, and departmental commitments are needed to make the relief of pain a high clinical priority. This ought to be reflected in international and national healthcare policy, and in legally binding definitions of good practice. This priority also ought to be reflected in the development of a staffing infrastructure that is adequately skilled and resourced to be able to respond effectively in a timely manner and to follow up and adjust as necessary with the capacity and commitment (24-27).

Finally, individual clinicians have a host of duties connected with the right to adequate pain relief: to ensure that they are adequately skilled in the relief of pain, to assess pain and its severity, to provide care in a timely manner (recognizing also that unrelieved pain in a patient with incurable disease is a medical emergency), and to provide care safely and with follow-up and ensure that there is an appropriate balance between adequate relief without excessive adverse effects, including addiction and misuse. Increasingly, physicians are expected to identify persons at risk of addiction or abuse for special considerations in treatment planning and follow-up (28, 29). Failure to recognize, or to act upon, any one of these duties can have profound consequences for individual patients and their families (30-33).

In the Emergency Room

CASE PRESENTATION CONTINUED

As soon as Michael presented to the emergency room, an intravenous line was inserted and, after evaluation of the pain severity (which he reported to be "intolerable"), a dose of intravenous morphine was calculated based on the knowledge of his preexisting background analgesic requirements. Because he had previously been taking 300 mcg per hour of transdermal fentanyl, which is approximately equivalent to 200-300 milligrams of parenteral morphine per day, he was given 30 mg IV morphine on an as-needed basis, to be titrated against pain relief and drowsiness. After a total of 60 mg of intravenous morphine, a careful physical examination was performed that indicated severe pain with movement of the right hip and an inability to bear weight. Neurological examination was normal. The provisional diagnosis of a pathological fracture involving the right hip was made, and emergency imaging with a CT scan was undertaken. The CT scan demonstrated a lytic lesion involving the anterior column of the acetabulum with the destruction of the acetabular cortex. The situation was reviewed by an oncologic orthopedist who did not feel that surgical intervention was indicated. Michael was admitted to the inpatient oncology service for pain stabilization.

Scope of Duties in Assessment

The evaluation of palliative care patients with pain requires assessment of the severity and consequences of the pain and of the clinical context in which it is occurring. Evaluation of pain severity is critical for prioritization of clinical attention. Mild to moderate pain may not warrant acute diversion of resources or clinical attention from other tasks; in contrast, severe or overwhelming pain should be viewed as a medical emergency that requires appropriate prioritization.

In most cases the identification of the specific underlying mechanism is also important, because there are many potential causes of cancer pain. Some causes have particular consequences both in terms of potential risk (such as risk of pathological fracture, or damage to vital organ structures such as spinal cord compression, or bowel perforation) and in terms of the need for specific treatment approaches (such as the fixation of the pathological fracture, decompression of the spinal cord, and the medical or surgical management of bowel obstruction).

The other critical aspect of assessment, one that is often overlooked, is the context of the pain problem in relation to the trajectory of the patient's illness and the prevailing goals of care (34-37). The prevailing goals of care may be summarized by the relative priority of optimizing duration of survival, optimizing physical and psychological functioning, and optimizing comfort. When relevant goals include optimizing survival and function, this has profound implications for the selection of relevant therapeutic modalities and also for the degree of intensity with which patients are monitored for adverse effects of analgesic therapy that may adversely affect these goals (38). In contrast to patients with far advanced illness for whom the only relevant goal of care is the provision of comfort, relatively well-functioning patients at an earlier stage of disease progression require adequate pain relief without compromising consciousness and the ability to interact.

Even in countries with all of the best resources available to address pain, cancer pain is often inadequately relieved because of substandard assessment (39, 40). When treating clinicians fail to appreciate the severity of the patient's pain they will often prescribe analgesics that are inappropriately weak for the prevailing circumstances (39, 40). This phenomenon has been demonstrated in repeated studies over a span of almost two decades (40-45).

An additional level of complexity is added when cancer survivors have persistent pains that are often more closely related to side effects of treatment than to their previous cancer(s). In this situation, particularly among persons with a history of tobacco or alcohol abuse or preexisting psychiatric disorder, patients with ongoing pain may also be at risk of analgesic drug dependency or abuse (46, 47). Indeed, evaluation of abuse risk and the setting of clear goals of care and the monitoring strategy for both therapeutic efficacy and abuse-related behaviors may be required in the management of strong chronic pain problems among cancer survivors (46).

CASE PRESENTATION CONTINUED

In this case, Michael had bone metastases in the right acetabulum that were limiting his ability to walk and which were also associated with a risk of pathological fracture. His prevailing goals of care were equally to simultaneously optimize comfort and physical functioning as well as to live as long as is possible. Additionally, he wanted to be able to return to his home. Based on these considerations, efforts were made to find an effective therapeutic strategy that could be easily administered in the home and would minimize the need for transport to medical facilities (given that this could only be done with ambulance assistance because of his third-floor walk-up residence).

On the Oncology and Palliative Care Ward

CASE PRESENTATION CONTINUED

Michael's pain was much better alleviated by the addition of steroids and oral methadone. A trial of methadone was selected because it was a cheap, long-acting medication that could be easily administered by mouth, it potentially addressed both somatic and neuropathic components of his pain, and it would not require high-intensity nursing care or invasive, potentially painful methods of administration. Within 24 hours his pain intensity was dramatically reduced. On the second day of treatment he became drowsy and somewhat confused. Regular methadone was discontinued and was subsequently administered on an "as needed" basis only and at a reduced dose; these changes restored his mental clarity and alertness. Michael was mobilized with the assistance of a rehabilitative physiotherapist who evaluated his ability to walk with a walking frame and to manage a small number of stairs without risk of falling. Radiotherapy to the affected bone was arranged to reduce his analgesic requirement and to lower his risk of pathological fracture. Prior to his discharge home by ambulance directly up to his third floor apartment, he was sent for a single fraction dose of radiotherapy. He was only discharged after appropriate checks of the home care infrastructure, including access to the bathroom and availability of home-based pain and palliative care services.

Ethical Considerations and Therapeutic Planning

The management of pain for palliative care patients is a collaborative endeavor between the patient and the professional healthcare providers. Successful outcomes are predicated on a common understanding of the aims of analgesic therapy, the potential risks and side effects of therapy, and other potential consequences. Although pain relief is generally possible, it is rarely complete; indeed, manageable pain is often the best that can be reasonably expected. All of the opioid analgesics that are appropriate for the management of strong pain have the potential for side effects: Some like constipation are almost inevitable unless preventative steps are taken; others such as nausea and vomiting, drowsiness, myoclonus, or confusion may be either idiosyncratic or dose related (48, 49). For some patients, the potential side effects of opioids may be prohibitive, and they may prefer a therapeutic strategy that does not include opioid medications (48, 49). More often than not, however, patients accept these risks as long as the therapeutic plan includes close monitoring for the development of side effects and a commitment to review of the therapeutic strategy if side effects occur.

All patients who are started on opioid analgesics for strong pain should have a management plan that incorporates follow-up and even the possibility of out-of-hours reporting of any substantial adverse effects, in particular of drowsiness or confusion. Drowsiness may be the first warning sign of a central depressant effect of opioids, which, if ignored, may culminate in catastrophic respiratory depression and possibly even death. Patients do not necessarily require inpatient admission to start opioid therapy; initiation can be achieved as an out-patient as long as there is a strong line of communication both to evaluate the relief of pain and to monitor for the development of side effects. This approach requires telephone access to a responsible clinician who is able to respond effectively to the development of significant adverse effects.

The level of risk of medication overdose is higher with methadone than with other opioid analgesics because of the distinctive characteristic of a very long, variable, dose-dependent half-life, and consequent dose accumulation during the titration phase (31). Obligations of precaution and stewardship would suggest that methadone should only be initiated by physicians with substantial experience in its use, and with provision for close and regular monitoring at least over the first week until steady-state levels are likely to be achieved.

In addition to issues of efficacy and potential for adverse effects, other relevant considerations in the selection of analgesic medications include actual availability and affordability. Some medications, despite being listed on formulary, are not readily available in the community. Furthermore, some formulations are expensive and may not be affordable if they are not covered by insurance plans or if there are high copayments. The clinician's role of stewardship of scarce resources is essential in these determinations (50).

Achieving Michael's goal of being able to return home required an approach of intensive collaborative care involving physicians, nurses, social workers, physiotherapists, occupational therapist, and a community care team. Ethical discharge planning requires an evaluation of the home care resources, augmentation of resources when needed, and a careful evaluation of the patient's ability to manage safely in a home environment (51, 52). Failure to ensure these steps can have catastrophic consequences for patients or for their family caregivers. Sadly, inadequate discharge planning is commonplace, and many patients are discharged to home care situations without previously checking if the patient is safe from falling or can access personal hygiene facilities in the home. To ensure Michael's ongoing safe care and the coping of his family caregivers, a communication network was established among his home palliative care providers, his oncologist, and the hospital based palliative care service.

Pain Relief at the End of Life

CASE PRESENTATION CONTINUED

Michael was cared for at home over the ensuing 2 months. His condition gradually deteriorated and he became bedbound. His wife and daughter attended to his nursing care with substantial support of visiting nurses and palliative care physician. With time, his pain became increasingly difficult to control, and the combination of intense nursing needs, inadequate home care supports, and poorly controlled symptoms made ongoing home care too difficult. All parties agreed that Michael ought to be admitted to an inpatient setting for pain relief and end-of-life care.

When Michael was admitted he was weak, jaundiced from advanced liver metastases, and in the severe distress from the left-sided lumbosacral plexopathy caused by nerve compression from the tumor mass arising from his left hemi pelvis. Initial attempts to stabilize his pain without making him more drowsy were unsuccessful and, after an interdisciplinary meeting including input from a consulting anesthesia pain specialist, it was concluded that this was a situation of refractory pain at the end-of-life and that Michael would be unlikely to achieve adequate relief without some level of sedation.

At this point, Michael was confused, agitated, and distressed. He was unable to participate in any sort of meaningful discussion about treatment options. His wife and daughter related that he had previously discussed his fears about dying in pain with a home-care palliative care physician who had promised that "everything would be done" to ensure that he would "die in comfort." They pleaded that his request be respected. At the conclusion of this discussion it was agreed that Midazolam (a strong sedative medication) would be added to his analgesic medications, and that the dose would be adjusted until Michael appeared comfortable. Additionally, they agreed that because the only relevant goal of care for Michael was to ensure that he was comfortable, other noncritical medications interventions were discontinued, including measurements of blood pressure, temperature and pulse oximetry.

Michael's agitation was controlled after two small doses of midazolam. This situation was maintained with an ongoing infusion at a dose of 0.5mg/hr of midazolam alongside his continued maintenance infusion of opioids. Provision was made to give him extra boluses of both medications if needed. He never needed them, and he remained comfortable but sleepy until his death a day later.

Ethical Considerations Regarding the Use of Sedation as an Option for Patients with Refractory Pain at the End of Life

Sedation in the context of palliative medicine is the monitored use of medications intended to induce a state of decreased or absent awareness (unconsciousness) to relieve the burden of otherwise intractable suffering. The aim is to provide adequate relief of distress in a manner that is ethically acceptable to the patient, family, and healthcare providers. It is most commonly used to manage situations of severe refractory distress caused by agitated delirium, dyspnea, pain, and/or convulsions in patients at the end of life. In this chapter, I will focus on the use of sedation to help manage otherwise intractable pain. There will be a broader discussion of risks and benefits of the use of various forms of palliative sedation for additional clinical indications and situations in Chapter 14.

The decision making and application of this therapeutic option is predicated on careful patient evaluation that incorporates assessment of current goals of care in a manner that is consistent with ethical professionalism and good clinical practice. Because all medical treatments involve risks and benefits, each potential option must be evaluated for its potential to achieve the goals of care (53). The potential risks of such treatment must be proportionate to the gravity of the clinical indication. As with any other high-risk clinical procedure, clinician considerations are guided by an understanding of the patient's goals of care and must be within accepted medical guidelines of beneficence and nonmaleficence. The risks of hastening death with usual pain management are very low, especially if doses are adjusted carefully and systematically. But when doses of opioid analgesics are escalated rapidly and/or strong sedatives are added to help a patient escape otherwise intractable suffering, these risks are increased substantially. Finally, the ultimate decision to act on these considerations depends on informed consent, an advance directive or, in the absence of these, substituted judgment of authorized surrogate decision makers based on evidence regarding the relevant preferences of the patient. When nothing is known about the patient's preferences, the decision should be based on the best interests of the patient.

Despite the potential for shortening life, this approach of providing sedation for intractable pain or other severe suffering has been endorsed as acceptable normative practice by legal precedent (54). In the 1957 English case of *R v. Adams,* Justice Devin wrote in his judgment that "If the first purpose of medicine, the restoration of health, can no longer be achieved, there is still much for a doctor to do, and he is entitled to do all that is proper and necessary to relieve pain and suffering, even if the measures he takes may incidentally shorten life." He justified this approach by rejecting the notion that this is a special defense; rather, he endorsed the pragmatic perspective that "The cause of death is the illness or the injury, and the proper medical treatment that is administered and that has an incidental effect on determining the exact moment of death is not the cause in any sensible use of the term "(55). This approach was lent further support by a decision of the Supreme Court of the United States when it rejected a constitutional right that encompasses assisted suicide but endorsed the use of sedation as an extreme form of palliative care in the management of refractory symptoms at the end of life (56).

However, the use of sedation has the potential for harm. Indeed, there are many ways in which the care of patients can be undermined by the abusive, injudicious, or unskilled use of sedation.

ABUSE OF PALLIATIVE SEDATION

The most common abuse of sedation occurs when clinicians sedate patients approaching the end of life with the primary goal of hastening the patient's death (57-64). This has been called "slow euthanasia." Indeed, some physicians administer very high doses of opioid analgesic medication out of proportion to the patient's pain, ostensibly to relieve symptoms, but with a covert intention to hasten death. In extreme situations, this might include the deliberate use of deep sedation in patients who have no refractory symptoms, or more subtly in the deliberate use of opioid analgesic doses that far exceed that which is necessary to provide adequate comfort. Excess doses of opioids can compromise physiological functions such as spontaneous respiration and hemodynamic stability. These duplicitous practices represent an unacceptable, and often illegal, deviation from normative ethical clinical practice.

INJUDICIOUS USE OF PALLIATIVE SEDATION

Injudicious palliative sedation occurs when sedation is applied with the intent of relieving symptoms but in clinical circumstances that are not appropriate. In this situation, sedation is applied with the intent of relieving distress and is carefully titrated to effect, but the indication is inadequate to justify such a radical intervention. The following are representative examples of injudicious use:

(1) Instances of inadequate patient assessment in which potentially reversible causes of pain or other distress are overlooked (58, 65)

(2) Situations in which, before resorting to sedation, there is a failure to engage clinicians expert in relief of pain despite their availability (58, 66)

(3) The case of an overwhelmed physician resorting to sedation because he or she is fatigued and frustrated by the care of a complex symptomatic patient (67)

(4) Situations in which the demand for sedation is generated by the patient's family based on their own needs rather than the patient's otherwise intractable symptoms (67)

INJUDICIOUS WITHHOLDING OF PALLIATIVE SEDATION

Injudicious withholding of sedation in the management of refractory distress occurs when clinicians defer the use of sedation excessively while persisting with other therapeutic options that do not provide adequate relief. Given the subjectivity of refractoriness and the profound interindividual variability of responsiveness to palliative interventions for pain or other symptoms, these assessments are often very difficult to make. Clinicians should be aware of the potential for a "counter phobic determination to treat" whereby anxiety about having to deal with all of the difficult discussions about sedation and end of life care leads to avoidant behaviors and futile therapeutic trials, ultimately resulting in increased patient distress or reservations based on exaggerated concerns about hastening death.

SUBSTANDARD CLINICAL PRACTICE OF PALLIATIVE SEDATION

This occurs in situations in which sedation is used for an appropriate indication but without the appropriate attention to one or more processes essential to good clinical care. Examples of substandard clinical practices include:

(1) Inadequate consultation with the patient (if possible), family members, or other staff members to ensure understanding of the indication for the intervention, the goals of the care plan, the anticipated outcomes, and the potential risks

(2) Inadequate monitoring of symptom distress or adequacy of relief

(3) Inadequate assessment of psychological, spiritual or social factors that may be contributing to the patient's pain (67)

(4) Inadequate monitoring of physiological parameters that may indicate risk of drug overdose (when clinically relevant)

(5) Hasty dose escalation of sedative medications without titration to effect and use of minimal effective doses

(6) Use of inappropriate medications to achieve sedation (i.e., opioids) (68, 69)

(7) Inadequate care of the patient's family (67)

(8) Inadequate attention to the emotional and spiritual well being of distressed staff members (67, 70)

Some authors argue that although sedation in the relief of uncontrolled symptoms may be justifiable, the concurrent discontinuation of nutrition and hydration may constitute "slow euthanasia," because this act does not contribute to patient comfort and almost certainly hastens death by starvation and dehydration (71-74). In response, however, it is important to assert that the discontinuation of hydration and nutrition is **not** an essential element to the administration of sedation in the management of refractory symptoms (75) and there are no data to support the assertion that it is "typical" (76). In this context, artificial hydration and nutrition should be considered a separate decision that warrants joint, informed decision making with the patient and/or his surrogates if he is incapable of decision-making at that point.

Euthanasia refers to the deliberate termination of the life of a patient by active intervention, at the request of the patient in the setting of otherwise uncontrolled suffering. Sedation in the management of refractory pain is distinct from euthanasia insofar as: (1) The intent of the intervention is to provide pain relief, not to end the life of the suffering patient; (2) the intervention is proportionate to the severity of the pain and the prevailing goals of care; and (3) most importantly, unlike euthanasia or assisted suicide, the death of the patient is not a criteria for the success of the treatment.

Final Thoughts

Procedural guidelines for pain management in general and for sedation at the end of life can provide a framework for decision making and implementation to best promote and protect the interests of patients, their families and the healthcare providers administering care. Sound procedural guidelines, such as checklists, can reduce the risk of adverse outcomes in medicine (77, 78). Guidelines have been, and may be, be developed at a national, local, or institutional level. An excellent framework for the development of guidelines to regulate the practice were published by The European Association of Palliative Care (38).

References

1. Goudas LC, Bloch R, Gialeli-Goudas M, Lau J, Carr DB. The epidemiology of cancer pain. *Cancer Inves.* 2005;23(2):182–90.

2. van den Beuken-van Everdingen M, de Rijke J, Kessels A, Schouten H, van Kleef M, Patijn J. Prevalence of pain in patients with cancer: a systematic review of the past 40 years. *Ann Oncol.* 2007;18:1437–49.

3. Marcus DA. Epidemiology of cancer pain. *Curr Pain Headache Rep.* 2011;15(4):231-4

4. Solano JP, Gomes B, Higginson IJ. A comparison of symptom prevalence in far advanced cancer, aids, heart disease, chronic obstructive pulmonary disease and renal disease. *J Pain Symptom Manage.* 2006;31(1):58–69.

5. Ostgathe C, Alt-Epping B, Golla H, Gaertner J, Lindena G, Radbruch L, et al. Non-cancer patients in specialized palliative care in Germany: what are the problems? *Palliat Med.* 2011;25(2):148–52.

6. Chang VT, Janjan N, Jain S, Chau C. Update in cancer pain syndromes. *J Palliat Med.* 2006;9(6):1414–34.

7. Caraceni A, Portenoy RK. An international survey of cancer pain characteristics and syndromes. IASP Task Force on Cancer Pain. International Association for the Study of Pain. *Pain.* 1999;82(3):263–74.

8. Chapman S. Chronic pain syndromes in cancer survivors. *Nurs Stand.* 2011; 25(21):35–41.

9. Stull DM, Hollis LS, Gregory RE, Sheidler VR, Grossman SA. Pain in a comprehensive cancer center: more frequently due to treatment than underlying tumor (Meeting abstract). *Proc Annu Meet Am Soc Clin Oncol.* 1996;15:abstract 1717.

10. Jain PN, Chatterjee A. Development of acute pain service in an Indian cancer hospital. *J Pain Palliat Care Pharmacotherapy.* 2010;24(2):129–35.

11. International Pain Summit of the International Association for the Study of Pain. Declaration of Montreal: declaration that access to pain management is a fundamental human right. *J Pain Palliat Care Pharmacother.* 2011;25(1):29–31.

12. Lohman D, Schleifer R, Amon JJ. Access to pain treatment as a human right. *BMC Med.* 2010;8:8.

13. Brennan F, Carr DB, Cousins M. Pain management: a fundamental human right. *Anesth Analg.* 2007;105(1):205–21.

14. Cousins MJ, Brennan F, Carr DB. Pain relief: a universal human right. *Pain.* 2004;112(1–2):1–4.

15. Rich BA, Dubois M. Pain, ethics, and public policy. *Pain Med.* 2011;12(9):1295–6.

16. International Narcotics Control Board. *Demand for and supply of opiates for medical and scientific needs.*: Vienna, Austria: United Nations, 1989.

17. International Narcotics Control Board. *Availability of opiates for medical needs*: Report of the International Narcotics Control Board for 1995. Vienna Austria: United Nations. 1995.

18. International Narcotics Control Board. *Freedom from pain and suffering.* Report of the International Narcotic Control Board for 1999. Vienna, Austria: United Nations, 1999.

19. International Narcotics Control Board. Report 2004; available at http://www.incb.org/documents/Publications/AnnualReports/AR2004/AR_04_English.pdf (last accessed 10/23/13).

20. World Health Organisation. *Achieving balance in national opioids control policy: guidelines for assessment.* Geneva: World Health Organisation, 2000.

21. World Health Organization. Access to Controlled Medications Programme. Geneva: World Health Organisation, 2007.

22. Council of Europe. Recommendation Rec(2003)24 of the Committee of Ministers to member states on the organisation of palliative care and explanatory memorandum. Available from https://wcd.coe.int/ViewDoc.jsp?id=85719 (last accessed 10/23/13)

23. Human Rights Watch. *"Please, do not make us suffer any more..."* Access to pain treatment as a human right. NY: Human Rights Watch, 2009.

24. Ferrell BR, Dean GE, Grant M, Coluzzi P. An institutional commitment to pain management. *J Clin Oncol.* 1995;13(9):2158–65.

25. Glickman SW, Boulding W, Staelin R, Mulgund J, Roe MT, Lytle BL, et al. A framework for quality improvement: an analysis of factors responsible for improvement at hospitals participating in the Can Rapid Risk Stratification of Unstable Angina Patients Suppress Adverse Outcomes with Early Implementation of the ACC/AHA Guidelines (CRUSADE) quality improvement initiative. *Am Heart J.* 2007;154(6):1206–20.

26. Tarzian AJ, Hoffmann DE. Barriers to managing pain in the nursing home: findings from a statewide survey. *J Am Med Dir Assoc.* 2005;6(3 Suppl):S13–9.

27. Ryan M, Ambrosio DA, Gebhard C, Kowalski J. Pain management: an organizational commitment. *Pain Manag Nurs.* 2000;1(2):34–9.

28. Sloan PA. Opioid risk management: understanding FDA mandated risk evaluation and mitigation strategies (REMS). *J Opioid Manag.* 2009;5(3):131–3.

29. Lipman AG. The Food and Drug Administration opioid Risk Evaluation and Mitigation Strategy. *J Pain Palliat Care Pharmacother.* 2009;23(3):219–21.

30. Starrels JL, Becker WC, Weiner MG, Li X, Heo M, Turner BJ. Low use of opioid risk reduction strategies in primary care even for high risk patients with chronic pain. *J Gen Intern Med.* 2011;26(9):958–64.

31. Vital signs: risk for overdose from methadone used for pain relief—United States, 1999–2010. *MMWR Morb Mortal Wkly Rep.* 2012;61(26):493–7.

32. Grant KJ, Baca CT. Methadone deaths in pain and addiction populations. *J Gen Intern Med.* 2010;25(9):898; author reply 9.

33. Manchikanti KN, Manchikanti L, Damron KS, Pampati V, Fellows B. Increasing deaths from opioid analgesics in the United States: an evaluation in an interventional pain management practice. *J Opioid Manag.* 2008;4(5):271–83.

34. Kumar G, Markert RJ, Patel R. Assessment of hospice patients' goals of care at the end of life. *Am J Hosp Palliat Care.* 2011;28(1):31–4.

35. Haberle TH, Shinkunas LA, Erekson ZD, Kaldjian LC. Goals of care among hospitalized patients: a validation study. *Am J Hosp Palliat Care.* 2011;28(5):335–41.

36. Kaldjian LC, Curtis AE, Shinkunas LA, Cannon KT. Goals of care toward the end of life: a structured literature review. *Am J Hosp Palliat Care.* 2008;25(6):501–11.

37. Duggleby W, Berry P. Transitions and shifting goals of care for palliative patients and their families. *Clin J Oncol Nurs.* 2005;9(4):425–8.

38. Cherny NI, Radbruch L. European Association for Palliative Care (EAPC) recommended framework for the use of sedation in palliative care. *Palliat Med.* 2009;23(7):581–93.

39. Breivik H, Cherny N, Collett B, de Conno F, Filbet M, Foubert AJ, et al. Cancer-related pain: a pan-European survey of prevalence, treatment, and patient attitudes. *Ann Oncol.* 2009;20(8):1420–33.

40. Fisch MJ, Lee JW, Weiss M, Wagner LI, Chang VT, Cella D, et al. Prospective, observational study of pain and analgesic prescribing in medical oncology outpatients with breast, colorectal, lung, or prostate cancer. *J Clin Oncol.* 2012;30(16):1980–8.

41. Wu HS, Natavio T, Davis JE, Yarandi HN. Pain in outpatients treated for breast cancer: prevalence, pharmacological treatment, and impact on quality of life. *Cancer Nurs.* 2012;36(3):229–35.

42. Moskovitz BL, Benson CJ, Patel AA, Chow W, Mody SH, McCarberg BH, et al. Analgesic treatment for moderate-to-severe acute pain in the United States: patients'

perspectives in the Physicians Partnering Against Pain (P3) survey. *J Opioid Manag.* 2011;7(4):277–86.

43. Foley KM. How well is cancer pain treated? *Palliat Med.* 2011;25(5):398–401.

44. Cohen MZ, Musgrave CF, Munsell MF, Mendoza TR, Gips M. The cancer pain experience of Israeli and American patients 65 years and older. *J Pain Symptom Manage.* 2005;30(3):254–63.

45. Von Roenn JH, Cleeland CS, Gonin R, Hatfield AK, Pandya KJ. Physician attitudes and practice in cancer pain management. A survey from the Eastern Cooperative Oncology Group. *Ann Intern Med.* 1993;119(2):121–6.

46. Koyyalagunta D, Burton AW, Toro MP, Driver L, Novy DM. Opioid abuse in cancer pain: report of two cases and presentation of an algorithm of multidisciplinary care. *Pain Physician.* 2011;14(4):E361–71.

47. Starr TD, Rogak LJ, Passik SD. Substance abuse in cancer pain. *Curr Pain Headache Rep.* 2010;14(4):268–75.

48. Berde C, Nurko S. Opioid side effects—mechanism-based therapy. *NEJM.* 2008; 358(22):2400–2.

49. Cherny N, Ripamonti C, Pereira J, Davis C, Fallon M, McQuay H, et al. Strategies to manage the adverse effects of oral morphine: an evidence-based report. *J Clin Oncol.* 2001;19(9):2542–54.

50. Minogue B. The two fundamental duties of the physician. *Acad Med.* 2000;75(5):431–42.

51. Benzar E, Hansen L, Kneitel AW, Fromme EK. Discharge planning for palliative care patients: a qualitative analysis. *J Palliat Med.* 2011;14(1):65–9.

52. Mor V, Besdine RW. Policy options to improve discharge planning and reduce rehospitalization. *JAMA.* 2011;305(3):302–3.

53. Pauker SG, Kassirer JP. The threshold approach to clinical decision-making. *NEJM.* 1980;302(20):1109–17.

54. Gevers S. Terminal sedation: a legal approach. *Eur J Health Law.* 2003;10(4): 359–67.

55. Devlin P. *Easing the passing.* London: Bodley Head, 1985.

56. Burt RA. The Supreme Court speaks—not assisted suicide but a constitutional right to palliative care. *NEJM.* 1997;337(17):1234–6.

57. Levy MH, Cohen SD. Sedation for the relief of refractory symptoms in the imminently dying: a fine intentional line. *Semin Oncol.* 2005;32(2):237–46.

58. Hasselaar JG, Reuzel RP, van den Muijsenbergh ME, Koopmans RT, Leget CJ, Crul BJ, et al. Dealing with delicate issues in continuous deep sedation. Varying practices among Dutch medical specialists, general practitioners, and nursing home physicians. *Arch Intern Med.* 2008;168(5):537–43.

59. Kuhse H, Singer P, Baume P, Clark M, Rickard M. End-of-life decisions in Australian medical practice. *Med J Aust.* 1997;166(4):191–6.

60. Stevens CA, Hassan R. Management of death, dying and euthanasia: attitudes and practices of medical practitioners in South Australia. *Arch Intern Med.* 1994;154(5):575–84.

61. Willems DL, Daniels ER, van der Wal G, van der Maas PJ, Emanuel EJ. Attitudes and practices concerning the end of life: a comparison between physicians from the United States and from The Netherlands [In Process Citation]. *Arch Intern Med.* 2000;160(1):63–8.

62. Meier DE, Emmons CA, Wallenstein S, Quill T, Morrison RS, Cassel CK. A national survey of physician-assisted suicide and euthanasia in the United States [see comments]. *NEJM*. 1998;338(17):1193–201.

63. Douglas CD, Kerridge IH, Rainbird KJ, McPhee JR, Hancock L, Spigelman AD. The intention to hasten death: a survey of attitudes and practices of surgeons in Australia. *Med J Aust*. 2001;175(10):511–5.

64. Rietjens JA, van der Heide A, Vrakking AM, Onwuteaka-Philipsen BD, van der Maas PJ, van der Wal G. Physician reports of terminal sedation without hydration or nutrition for patients nearing death in the Netherlands. *Ann Intern Med*. 2004;141(3):178–85.

65. Fainsinger RL, De Moissac D, Mancini I, Oneschuk D. Sedation for delirium and other symptoms in terminally ill patients in Edmonton. *J Palliat Care*. 2000;16(2):5–10.

66. Murray SA, Boyd K, Byock I. Continuous deep sedation in patients nearing death. *BMJ*. 2008;336(7648):781–2.

67. Higgins PC, Altilio T. Palliative sedation: an essential place for clinical excellence. *J Soc Work End Life Palliat Care*. 2007;3(4):3–30.

68. Reuzel RP, Hasselaar GJ, Vissers KC, van der Wilt GJ, Groenewoud JM, Crul BJ. Inappropriateness of using opioids for end-stage palliative sedation: a Dutch study. *Palliat Med*. 2008;22(5):641–6.

69. Hasselaar JG, Reuzel RP, Verhagen SC, de Graeff A, Vissers KC, Crul BJ. Improving prescription in palliative sedation: compliance with dutch guidelines. *Arch Intern Med*. 2007;167(11):1166–71.

70. Rietjens JA, Hauser J, van der Heide A, Emanuel L. Having a difficult time leaving: experiences and attitudes of nurses with palliative sedation. *Palliat Med*. 2007;21(7):643–9.

71. Craig GM. On withholding artificial hydration and nutrition from terminally ill sedated patients. The debate continues [published erratum appears in J Med Ethics 1996 Dec;22(6):361]. *J Med Ethics*. 1996;22(3):147–53.

72. Craig GM. On withholding nutrition and hydration in the terminally ill: has palliative medicine gone too far? [see comments]. *J Med Ethics*. 1994;20(3):139–43; discussion 44–5.

73. Craig G. Is sedation without hydration or nourishment in terminal care lawful? *Med Leg J*. 1994;62(Pt 4):198–201.

74. Orentlicher D. The Supreme Court and physician-assisted suicide—rejecting assisted suicide but embracing euthanasia. *NEJM*. 1997;337(17):1236–9.

75. Hahn MP. Review of palliative sedation and its distinction from euthanasia and lethal injection. *J Pain Palliat Care Pharmacother*. 2012;26(1):30–9.

76. Sulmasy DP, Ury WA, Ahronheim JC, Siegler M, Kass L, Lantos J, et al. Palliative treatment of last resort and assisted suicide. *Ann Intern Med*. 2000;133(7):562–3.

77. Haynes AB, Weiser TG, Berry WR, Lipsitz SR, Breizat AH, Dellinger EP, et al. A surgical safety checklist to reduce morbidity and mortality in a global population. *NEJM*. 2009;360(5):491–9.

78. Hoffman GM, Nowakowski R, Troshynski TJ, Berens RJ, Weisman SJ. Risk reduction in pediatric procedural sedation by application of an American Academy of Pediatrics/American Society of Anesthesiologists process model. *Pediatrics*. 2002;109(2):236–43.

8

Management of Dyspnea

Thomas W. LeBlanc, David C. Currow,
Jane L. Phillips, and Amy P. Abernethy

Dyspnea is among the most prevalent, variable, and difficult to manage symptoms arising in hospice/palliative care clinical practice; its complexity introduces a host of ethical issues. Ambiguity in the clinical presentation of dyspnea is apparent in the American Thoracic Society's definition of this symptom as "a subjective experience of breathing discomfort that consists of qualitatively distinct sensations that vary in intensity" [1]. Dyspnea can occur as an acute episode, as a chronic experience resulting from clearly identified precipitating factor(s), or as an "acute-on-chronic" phenomenon, in which the patient suffers a worsening, with or without a trigger, of the ongoing symptom [2, 3].

Often termed "shortness of breath" or "breathlessness," dyspnea is commonly experienced by patients with advanced disease. Prevalence ranges from 56% among patients with severe chronic obstructive pulmonary disease (COPD) [4] to 90% among those near the end of life [5], typically increasing significantly in severity between 3 months and 1 month before death [6]. Half of patients reporting dyspnea at the end of life rate their symptom as severe, [7] although many of these patients have no apparent cardiorespiratory disease. Despite its prevalence, dyspnea remains under-recognized and under-treated. To combat these tendencies, the American College of Chest Physicians' consensus statement on dyspnea affirms that clinicians have an ethical obligation to recognize, assess, and treat dyspnea [8].

Impact of Dyspnea

The particularly subjective nature of dyspnea makes its clinical management challenging, and contributes to the problems of under-recognition and under-treatment. Studies have consistently found physiological factors such as airway resistance, respiratory flow rate, static lung volume, and arterial blood gas to be minimally correlated with patients' reports of dyspnea [9, 10]. Instead, the interactions of physiological, psychological, social, and environmental factors, often exacerbated by secondary physiological and behavioral changes that the dyspnea itself induces, create the patient's composite experience of this symptom [11]. Thus, the patient's perception largely determines the way in which dyspnea manifests and its reported nature and severity, with patients' descriptions of dyspnea varying based on multiple factors such as the individual's underlying disease, ethnic/racial background, previous experiences, and emotional state.

The impact of dyspnea on patients and their caregivers is far-reaching [12]. Historically, the literature has described a host of changes in the patient's experience associated with dyspnea, including: poor concentration, anorexia, memory loss, sweating, "smothering," tiredness and fatigue, depression, anxiety, and panic [13-16]. Studies such as the National Emphysema Treatment Trial, which enrolled 1,621 patients with severe COPD, have found strong correlations between higher dyspnea scores and poorer quality of life [17, 18]. Decreased functionality resulting from dyspnea can lead to disturbance of social relationships and social isolation, especially when the patient relies on therapeutic oxygen for symptomatic relief [19]. To fully capture the patient's experience of this disabling, distressing experience, theorists have proposed a construct, "total dyspnea," which encompasses four domains of symptom-related suffering—physical, psychological, interpersonal, and existential [20].

Dyspnea exacts a toll on the caregiver as well [12]. Studies have reported increases in stress, depression, and physical illness, and decreases in quality of life among family caregivers. Among caregivers of patients who are not recipients of hospice/palliative care services, there is a broad association between caregiving and increased mortality [21]. The breadth of effects on the caregiver has given rise to the aggregate term, "caregiver burden" [22], defined as "a multidimensional response to physical, psychological, emotional, social, and financial stressors associated with the caregiving experience" [23]. These issues may continue through the period of bereavement, well after the actual caregiving has ceased.

Complexity and Challenge of Dyspnea Management

To relieve dyspnea, intervention first targets any potentially modifiable anatomical and pathological causes of the symptom, provided the intervention remains consistent with the patient's goals of care. As underlying etiologies are treated, clinicians must also encompass symptom relief either alone or in conjunction with disease-targeted approaches. Definitive studies support regular, low-dose, sustained-release opioids, preferably in oral formulation, as the standard first-line pharmacological treatment [24-29]; parenteral administration is also effective and safe.

Despite the preponderance and clarity of evidence supporting opioids for dyspnea management, its use is constrained by pervasive misperceptions and misgivings. Many healthcare providers have concerns about the potential for respiratory depression, or the risks of confusion or drowsiness associated with the use of opioids. Many are not familiar with the demonstrated benefits of regular low-dose opioids for dyspnea relief; some feel that opioids should not be necessary to manage breathlessness, or that doing so is only appropriate in the terminal stages of a life-limiting illness (last hours of life). Among patients and their families, unease surrounds the stigma of using an opioid, fear of addiction, fear of hastening or even causing death, and misconceptions about prior experience ("They killed grandma with morphine."). Healthcare administrators and systems may hesitate to condone opioid use for newly emerging purposes, such as for dyspnea management; opioids are controlled substances, a designation which these individuals may associate with potential theft, misuse, and abuse [30].

Although the supporting evidence is less definitive, alternatives and adjuncts to opioids for dyspnea management have been studied. Emerging data may in the future support a role for anxiolytics (benzodiazepines, selective serotonin reuptake inhibitors [SSRIs]) [31] and inhaled furosemide [32-39] as helpful adjunctive pharmacological options. Supplemental oxygen is one of the interventions most frequently requested by patients and used in the hospital setting to relieve dyspnea [40, 41]. The benefits of oxygen therapy for COPD patients, in terms of survival, dyspnea, and quality of life, are well established [42-44]. However, although oxygen is often prescribed to alleviate dyspnea in people who are not hypoxemic, it may be no more effective than less burdensome approaches (e.g., a small, hand-held, battery-operated fan blowing across the face to stimulate receptors in the nasopharynx that relieve breathlessness); if oxygen is prescribed, then the impact on dyspnea should be monitored and the intervention discontinued if there is no improvement after 3 days [45]. It should be noted that oxygen therapy poses significant burdens on patients and families, sometimes resulting in social isolation [19]. Nonpharmacological options warranting consideration include walking aids, and breathing training; future data may also support the use of pulmonary rehabilitation and may show benefit from acupuncture [46].

Palliative Dyspnea Management: Potentially an Ethical Quagmire

Grounded by the injunction typically attributed to Hippocrates, "First do no harm," medical practice is often an exercise in ethical judgment. Over the ensuing centuries, physicians have sought to apply overarching bioethical principles—autonomy, nonmaleficence, beneficence, and justice—in their clinical practice. In hospice/palliative care, the potential proximity of death and patients' vulnerability amplify the ethical dimension of many clinical decisions, among them, how to best manage dyspnea. When suffering, such as that caused by breathlessness is involved, the physician can no longer consider the omission to treat as an ethically acceptable option; the principle of beneficence mandates intervention to manage the patient's symptom to the best of current abilities and evidence. This attention to symptoms, however problematic they might be, requires assessment, knowledge about evidence-based strategies, consultation with experts as appropriate, assurance that patient and caregiver concerns are heard, and conscientious consideration of ethical concerns. The following cases provide examples of ethical issues that frequently arise in the management of dyspnea for patients with advanced disease.

Palliative Dyspnea Management: An Ideal Scenario

CASE PRESENTATION

Mrs. White, a 78-year-old woman with advanced lung cancer, was admitted to the hospital from the oncology clinic for management of severe dyspnea and general weakness. Chest imaging shows progression of her cancer despite ongoing chemotherapy; her oncologist says there are no remaining disease-modifying treatment options. Overnight the admitting hospitalist began empiric treatment for pneumonia with intravenous antibiotics and nebulized bronchodilators. Despite having normal oxygen saturation, Mrs. White continued to report considerable discomfort. The hospital's palliative care specialist was called to see her, and recommended initiating treatment with oral morphine solution, starting with 2.5 mg by mouth every 4 hours and regular docusate with sennosides. Within a few hours, Mrs. White felt much more comfortable, reporting that her breathlessness had decreased significantly. To amend her care plan in the context of her goals of care, a hospice/palliative care meeting was convened that afternoon, involving the patient, Mr. White (her husband), her oncologist, the palliative care specialist, a palliative care nurse, and a clinical social worker. The clinical team was alert to signs of emotional and existential (spiritual) distress in addition to the more obvious physical markers of tachypnea, and logistical considerations. To maintain a focus on comfort and quality of life after discharge, Mrs. White was referred for home hospice services, and it was agreed that her medication regimen would include oral long-acting morphine tablets to provide more consistent dyspnea relief throughout the day, with as-needed oral morphine solution for acute exacerbations of breathlessness. The hospice interdisciplinary care team worked together to create a plan for nonpharmacological interventions as well, including the use of a battery-operated hand-held fan to help the sensation of dyspnea, occupational therapy consultation for helpful assistive devices, support from the chaplain, and a visiting hospice volunteer to provide periodic respite for her husband.

CASE DISCUSSION

Mrs. White's care highlights many aspects of "best practice" in dyspnea management for patients with advanced, life-limiting illness. The hospital-based treatment team recognized dyspnea as an important symptom to address, one that impacted her quality of life as well as presenting a potential direct health concern to her and her husband. Her dyspnea persisted despite normal oxygen saturation; rather than considering the symptom conquered, and the patient's continued perceptions of dyspnea to be residing "in her head," the hospital staff understood the importance of this complex symptom—despite its subjectivity—and called the palliative care specialist for further assistance.

Ethical care of the patient with dyspnea begins with an honoring of the symptom as reported by the patient, as recommended by the American College of Chest Physicians [8]. Because the experience of breathlessness oftentimes does not correlate, or aligns only loosely, with physiological measures, many people with serious progressive disease are at risk of under-treatment for their dyspnea; this risk can be compounded in patients who have multiple co-morbid symptoms, and/or who hold back on naming this concern out of a desire not to be viewed as "complaining." Under-treatment of dyspnea, a violation of the principle of beneficence (discussed in the following), can also have roots in physician tendencies. Physicians may interpret the ethical injunction, "First do no harm," as a mandate to refrain from intervening when the symptom is poorly described or when they perceive the risk as being only a rare, although catastrophic, harm.

Given the prevalence of dyspnea in the palliative care population, physicians should directly query each patient about its presence and, if present, its nature and severity. In order to accurately understand the patient's experience of dyspnea—the target of intervention in palliative care's symptom-focused approach—depiction of the symptom must go beyond objective assessments, such as pulmonary function tests and 6-minute walk tests, and to include the patient's direct report of the symptom either through verbal account or through use of a robust instrument that collects patient-reported outcomes. Several clinical tools, many of them well recognized, such as the Edmonton Symptom Assessment Scale, incorporate numerical ratings of dyspnea into an overall symptom inventory; these have been comprehensively reviewed [47]. Often, however, a more holistic characterization of dyspnea is needed to understand and address all four biopsychosocial domains; clinicians may find greater utility in an instrument such as the Cancer Dyspnea Scale [48, 49], a 12-item multidimensional dyspnea scale for patients with cancer designed to capture the patient's experience of the symptom. Many clinicians will continue to opt for a simple verbal report; to the extent possible, standardization of the assessment will improve the quality of information obtained and will allow for more consistent monitoring of patients' dyspnea over time and across the population. It is important to ask the patient about his or her symptom experience using the same wording and the same kind of scale (e.g., 0–10 numerical rating scale) each time. This attention to the patient and his or her symptom experience initiates the process of ethical management of dyspnea in palliative care, and sets the stage for decisions about the timing of intervention.

Ethical Sensibilities Related to Timing

Timing is of paramount importance in palliative care, and, although not strictly an ethical consideration, it can feel to the practitioner like an ethically laden and sensitive decision. Early integration of palliative care with usual medical care has been shown to significantly improve not only traditional palliative care outcomes such as symptom control and mood, but also survival in patients with metastatic non–small cell lung cancer [50]. Clinicians, however, may hesitate to seek an early specialist palliative care consultation for symptom management for fear that this act may signal to the patient and/or caregivers that the prognosis has worsened, that there is no longer any hope for recovery, or that he or she has "given up" on the patient. Referral to palliative care should be viewed, instead, as the initiation of active effort to optimize the patient's function and comfort, while minimizing dependency.

In the case of Mrs. White, early initiation of opioids for refractory dyspnea might have improved this patient's comfort across the duration of her advanced illness. Hers, like most referrals to hospice or palliative care services, came late in the trajectory of care and she, like the majority of patients admitted to hospice or palliative care, likely missed out on much of the benefit that this service can offer to patients and their families. Best supportive care would have included an earlier referral to palliative care, when Mrs. White was an outpatient, for aggressive symptom management alongside active cancer treatment; the palliative care team would have followed Mrs. White across her transitions in care, adjusting dyspnea management in step with changes in the patient's symptom experiences and overall health status, aligned with her goals of care and the psychosocial needs of the patient and her family. With this approach, Mrs. White might have avoided the hospitalization described.

Balancing Positive and Negative Effects of Symptom Management

CASE PRESENTATION CONTINUED

Mrs. White has been home for 6 weeks, receiving care from a local hospice agency along with loving support from her husband and friends. She enjoys the hospice nurse's weekly visits. Her breathlessness continues to be a focus of care. At times, she experiences a crescendoing cycle in which anxiety worsens her breathlessness that, in turn, worsens her anxiety; dyspnea management therefore includes both regular and as-needed benzodiazepines in addition to her prescribed opioids. Mr. White has expressed concerns that this combination of medications makes his wife very drowsy and forgetful, and in response, the nurse has placed a fan in the room, positioning it so that the air blows gently across Mrs. White's face. She also ordered an oxygen concentrator for the couple to try. Although these measures help reduce Mrs. White's symptoms somewhat, she still requires continued medications to be comfortable.

Mr. White, himself showing evidence of considerable distress related to his wife's breathlessness and treatment effects, is torn between wanting his wife to be more awake and alert, and wanting her to be comfortable. Knowing that she has advanced disease, he wants to spend as much "quality time" with her as possible.

CASE DISCUSSION

Mrs. White's care, as her disease progresses, illustrates the difficult balancing of effects that is a classic, and ethically challenging, aspect of palliative care. It is not always possible to achieve effective symptom management (positive effects) without also inducing unwanted side effects (negative effects). Additional complexity is introduced when those effects impact individuals within the care system, such as the patient and family members, differently. Here, for example, Mrs. White bears the burden of the symptom itself and stands to benefit most from its positive effect (relief of dyspnea) and may prefer being sleepy than experiencing severe shortness of breath, whereas Mr. White is most negatively impacted by the somnolence and the associated increasing caregiving demands. Data suggest that where possible most patients value preserved cognition more highly than symptom control [51].

If the dose of opioids and sedatives that are required pose a significant risk of knowingly but unintentionally hastening death, then the "rule of double effect" might be invoked. This term is used to refer to ethically complex cases in which a desired positive result cannot be achieved without also knowingly risking a negative result. In classical bioethics, the action in question (to achieve the positive result) is ethically permissible only if four conditions are met:

(1) The action, itself, is either ethically good or ethically neutral;
(2) The negative result can be foreseen, but not intended;
(3) The negative result is not the means for achieving the positive result; and
(4) The positive result is proportionate to the negative result. (The negative result can only be permitted when there is a "proportionately grave" reason for it.) [52]

Using sedation to help a patient escape otherwise intractable dyspnea would not in itself warrant the application of double effect reasoning (the sedation was indeed intended to help the patient escape suffering); it is only when that sedation knowingly risks hastening death that such reasoning might be invoked.

The palliative care physician's basic mandate is to assess and manage, to the best of current knowledge and capacity, symptoms that are causing distress or discomfort. Tension arises, however, between the principles of beneficence ("doing good") and nonmaleficence ("doing no harm"). In the case of dyspnea management using opioids and benzodiazepines, the method known to best reduce suffering (beneficence) also may incur a negative effect, somnolence, with accompanying emotional suffering on the part of the caregiver or patient. In more extreme cases it might even hasten death. To act most beneficently, the physician cannot always entirely avoid maleficence; in such cases, the two ethical principles—beneficence and nonmaleficence—are, in a sense, competing. The framework of classical ethics is thus somewhat limiting and problematic, but we utilize it here to help illustrate the different sources of conflict and their interaction. Of course, for patients who willing and able to participate in decision making, involving the patient in these discussions can make the process much less murky.

The "art" of clinical practice at times implies the application of wisdom to a clinical decision fraught with ethical ambiguity. Side effects such as sedation, confusion, and even respiratory depression (discussed in the following)—although known possibilities—are never the intended outcome of palliative care (nonmaleficence), but rather, may be unintended consequences of using an effective dose of medication to provide comfort and symptom reduction (beneficence) while generating side effects (maleficence). Nonetheless, it is incumbent upon the palliative care clinician to attend to the undesirable effects of the symptom management plan. Support for family members is thus integral to hospice/palliative care practice and includes discussion with relevant individuals, such as Mr. White, to listen to their concerns and distress, discuss treatment options, review the goals of care, and address caregiver needs in their own right as far as possible. As the patient's disease progresses, discussions with family members and other caregivers should seek to normalize the dying process, through conversations that are not vague and general, but specific, informative, supportive, and open in format to allow individuals to ask questions, express concerns, and review information.

The Challenge of Opioids: Resistance among Physicians

CASE PRESENTATION

Mr. Brown has had repeated hospitalizations over the last 6 months. At 62 years old, he is hospitalized now for an acute exacerbation of his end-stage heart failure. His dyspnea, which has persisted despite aggressive diuresis and optimization of his heart failure regimen, causes him to be largely bedbound. Even attempts to brush his teeth or get dressed induce an alarming level of discomfort. Mr. Brown's physician hesitates to prescribe an opioid for fear of respiratory depression, given his overall tenuous condition. His 34-year-old son, a bachelor and local businessman, visits daily. Visibly distressed, he demands action to relieve the suffering associated with his father's shortness of breath. The son's distress may be contributing to the father's apparent anxiety, which seems to exacerbate his dyspnea.

CASE DISCUSSION

At times, it is the physician him- or herself who stands as the barrier to appropriate use of opioids for dyspnea, and thus to optimal symptom management. Individual clinicians can bring biases to patient care that they acquired during medical education. Often, these biases stem from instruction about the danger of opioids when used injudiciously, or from the physician's own experience, for example, the observation of opioid-naïve patients who receive large parenteral doses in the postoperative or trauma settings, and who then experience considerable side effects. Alternatively, clinicians may lack knowledge about the substantial benefits to be gained by prescribing regular low-dose opioids for symptom relief. Fear of respiratory depression has inhibited many physicians' use of opioids to successfully manage dyspnea in palliative care. Their concern is that, although relieving dyspnea, opioids might decrease the patient's respiratory rate, resulting in dangerous change in other respiratory parameters, including reduced arterial oxygen saturation and increased partial pressure of carbon dioxide. This belief has been refuted, provided the opioid is properly titrated [29, 53, 54]. Only under unusual circumstances (discussed in the following) is the risk of respiratory depression sufficient to influence the decision about whether or not to prescribe regular, low-dose, systemic opioids for palliative management of dyspnea.

Education is essential to ensure that clinicians themselves, out of ethical concerns not supported by evidence, do not stand between the patient and best care. One could argue that it is an ethical responsibility of all clinicians who serve seriously ill patients to educate themselves and their colleagues about best, evidence-based, palliative symptom management. Continuing medical education (CME) and periodic specialty board re-certification examinations offer formal vehicles for disseminating this information, but the onus remains on the individual clinician to regularly update him- or herself on the latest evidence, current best practices, clinical guidelines, and standards of care. When palliative care specialists face misperceptions among referring colleagues, peer-to-peer education may facilitate effective patient care. An open, nonconfrontational, and informative discussion between the palliative care specialist and, for example, Mr. Brown's referring cardiologist, may help build support among the patient's clinical team for the best, evidence-based, treatment option—use of opioids to optimally manage his dyspnea. In an institution in which a palliative care specialist repeatedly encounters misunderstandings and/ or resistance to the palliative use of opioids, he or she may consider offering an in-service to educate relevant colleagues.

The Challenge of Opioids: Resistance among Patients and Family Members

CASE PRESENTATION CONTINUED

The palliative care specialist and Mr. Brown's referring cardiologist discuss the latter's concerns about respiratory depression. With newfound confidence grounded in the evidence base, the cardiologist recommends initiating a low dose of oral morphine to help alleviate Mr. Brown's dyspnea. Mr. Brown's son, however, is outraged at this suggestion; his highly emotional reaction draws its charge from recent experience with his mother's death from colon cancer, which metastasized to the bone. "Momma was on hospice, and they just doped her up with morphine. Toward the end, she was totally out of it. I don't want that for Dad." Mr. Brown, too, expresses concern and allies with his son in language that, likewise, is emphatic. "People get addicted to that stuff. I don't want anything to do with it."

CASE DISCUSSION

Not uncommonly, patients and families harbor a fear or mistrust of opioids and many other medications, based either on their own experience with the medication or on hearsay. Even some physicians remain wary of opioids, due not only to concerns about potential adverse effects including addiction, but also to worries about possible legal repercussions. The evidence, however, shows that fears regarding opioid use and addiction in this clinical setting are unjustified, and concerns are often exaggerated [55]. In the setting of life-limiting illness, the incidence of addiction is low and is generally negligible in people who have not had a substance abuse problem; this concern should not limit the appropriate use of opioids to effectively manage dyspnea [8]. Potential for life-threatening side effects is quite low as well when the medication is prescribed and taken properly [53, 54].

When the palliative care clinician encounters ethically couched resistance to opioids among patients and/or family members, and when these views seem to be based on misperception, misinformation, or lack of information, the clinician must educate all relevant individuals in a way that is both respectful and professional. Communication is the core function in this mission, and should involve face-to-face discussion in which the clinician:

(1) Listens to and legitimizes the patient's/family's experience and concern
(2) Presents the pertinent evidence in a manner that the patient and family members present can understand, checking to ensure that they actually do understand (e.g., by stopping regularly to allow them to ask questions, or asking them to repeat their understanding)
(3) Discusses the fact that virtually every treatment has some measure of risk or undesirable effect, in addition to its desired benefits, and that these risks and benefits must be weighed against one another and constantly reviewed
(4) Places the question at hand in the overarching context of the patient's goals of care
(5) Moderates a process of genuine shared decision making that is oriented by the patient's goals and desires

Whenever initiating a new treatment, including opioids for dyspnea, the clinician should explain to the patient and caregiver(s) that the patient will be closely monitored for the treatment's benefit and potential side effects, and that the course of treatment will be immediately adjusted on request and as warranted by the patient's response. A time-limited trial is recommended to evaluate whether or not the specific treatment is effective for the individual patient [56, 57].

When a patient and/or family express a strong aversion to the concept of opioid treatment, the physician must explore the sentiments and probe for underlying reasoning. Often biases against opioids stem from misconceptions about a prior experience; in the case of Mr. Brown, learning about what happened to "Momma" will help explain the fears, advance the conversation, and potentially help to dispel the misperception. It is likely, for example, that education about the intense pain associated with bone metastases could help the son understand why, perhaps, high doses of opioids represented the kindest, and most preferable, treatment path for his mother despite their unfortunate sedating effects, or that the somnolence was likely a result of the dying process itself rather than solely an adverse effect of medication. Some people think the opioid caused the death of their loved one, relaying stories such as, "the nurse gave her a dose of liquid morphine under her tongue, and then she breathed her last breath." Here the clinician can explain that death was occurring anyway, and that a low dose of an opioid did not cause the death, but made the process of dying more comfortable. This explanation can be given with confidence: When people are on regular medications there will always be a last dose.

When Agreement Cannot Be Reached

At times, even with the best of explanations, the patient and/or family members will remain fixed in their resolve not to accept an evidence-based treatment option, such as opioid therapy, which the physicians deems to be best aligned with the patient's goals of care. The physician finds him- or herself caught in a clash between the imperative to respect the patient's desires on the one hand, and the ethical mandates to practice beneficence, and to avoid maleficence, on the other. In the case of Mr. Brown, the action required of the physician in order to help the suffering patient entails prescribing the opioid so as not to perpetuate (by act of omission) unnecessary dyspnea. The patient and family oppose this treatment plan. The physician's ethical duty in such a situation is confusing at best, and can be exceptionally distressing to him or her.

Ethically, patients who have decision-making capacity may refuse even clearly beneficial treatments—provided that they demonstrate a sound understanding of the risks, benefits, and alternatives to the treatment they are declining, and the likely result of not accepting it. The physician has fulfilled his or her ethical responsibility by fully informing the patient and making sure that he or she understands well the treatment options, their risks, benefits, and other implications. With respect to opioid use for dyspnea, although a difficult ethical conundrum lurks, most patients do accept an opioid prescription once their physician has engaged them in a clear discussion about the actual risks and benefits, a discussion based on the evidence indicating the benefits significantly outweigh the risks.

Decision Making in the Context of Genuine Clinical Uncertainty

CASE PRESENTATION

At age 34, Mr. Black has cystic fibrosis which was first diagnosed when he was an infant. Following lung transplantation, he has suffered chronic rejection interspersed with acute episodes of infection and other complications. His lung function is poor. He requires nightly support with BiPAP, which effectively serves as a less-invasive version of a ventilator; without it, he develops progressive CO_2 retention, resulting in somno-lence and confusion, and which would otherwise lead to his death. He knows that he will likely die in the coming months, and has decided not to be maintained full-time on a ventilator, yet he struggles with dyspnea every day. The BiPAP helps but requires him to wear a large facemask, which limits his interactions with family and friends, and makes it difficult to eat. His dyspnea borders on unbearable; he is desperate for relief. His quality of life is poor. He has unbearable nausea whenever opioids are prescribed. The pulmonary team is hesitant to prescribe benzodiazepines because of concerns about making his hypercapnia (elevated pCO_2 in his blood) worse and hastening death.

CASE DISCUSSION

Although, as discussed, fears about medication-induced respiratory depression (and hence CO_2 retention) and harm are generally unfounded for the majority of pallia-tive care patients, there are cases in which respiratory depression is a serious and legitimate concern. Mr. Black is one such patient; in his case, benzodiazepines—although likely helping to control the dyspnea—may indeed cause potentially dangerous clinical parameters. Mr. Black's tenuous lung function already causes hypercapnia; if benzodiazepines were to even slightly impair his respiratory rate or function, the result could be a worsening of his hypercapnia, leading to CO_2 narco-sis and even possibly death. His treating physician must consider this potential sce-nario, and simultaneously recognize the fact that the patient describes his symptom as "unbearable," that he is clearly suffering with significant and uninterrupted and largely untreated dyspnea.

Mr. Black has made clear the priority he places on his quality of life. He does not want a ventilator, although it might help alleviate his breathlessness, because he feels it would destroy his quality of life. He has stated that even the BiPAP has an unacceptable impact on his quality of life; for this reason, he does not wish to use it during the day.

Clinical options for Mr. Black are limited. The palliative care team has already tried other strategies for managing dyspnea. Mr. Black's situation presents a par-ticularly stark example of the ethical challenges of "double effect." Here, according to classical bioethics, the conditions are met to justify the use of opioids, despite reasonable expectation that they may worsen the patient's clinical condition. The intended effect of opioid prescription for Mr. Black is to reduce his suffering through relief of dyspnea; for a patient who is in the late stage of a terminal illness, whose suffering is intense, and who does not wish to pursue more aggressive, potentially life-prolonging, strategies such as mechanical ventilation, relief of symptoms and suffering is the topmost clinical priority. Both the patient and the healthcare team can foresee that the addition of opioids and/or benzodiazepines might hasten his death, but it is not their intention to do so. Even the lowest effective benzodiazepine dose that could improve his dyspnea might still potentially result in hypercapnia and CO_2 narcosis, followed by death.

In cases such as that of Mr. Black, the clinician's only option is to explain the risk of palliative treatment in full to the patient, and to allow him to make an informed treatment decision based on his acceptance or rejection of the risk. Psychosocial care, alternative therapies such as acupuncture, and other nonpharmacological interventions that may minimize dyspnea while preserving respiratory function should be considered. These may have collateral benefits such as reduction in negative emotional states or greater sense of peace and quietude, but are generally insufficient to relieve dyspnea when used in isolation. Close monitoring of benefits and harms is a crucial part of any care that is administered. Finally, whenever there is an open clinical trial of a novel dyspnea management strategy that does not increase the risk of respiratory failure and that offers the opportunity to explore a new solution, this option should be presented to the patient.

CASE PRESENTATION CONTINUED

Mr. Black and his physician had an open, honest discussion about the risks and benefits of adding an opioid to his medication regimen to treat his severe, persistent dyspnea. The patient expressed understanding about the possibility that such medication might hasten his death, and decided that the risk was worth taking because his primary goal was to improve the quality of his life, regardless of its duration. Given the risks they decided to proceed cautiously, with a very low dose of oral morphine solution (1 mg every 4 hours, as needed). After 2 days of gentle dose escalation, Mr. Black's dyspnea was significantly improved without any apparent untoward effects. He did well on this regimen for 1 week, but his dyspnea again worsened, requiring higher dosages of opioids. Despite dose escalation he remained very uncomfortable, in respiratory distress. Given his symptom burden and the amount of hands-on caregiving required, he was transferred to the local inpatient hospice house. Even subcutaneously infused higher-dose opioids did not result in adequate improvement of his dyspnea, so the palliative care team started a subcutaneous benzodiazepine infusion in order to induce sedation, as a way of maintaining his comfort. He died 5 days later, surrounded by family and friends.

CASE DISCUSSION

It is sometimes impossible to achieve symptom relief while maintaining alertness and preserving a patient's mental faculties. Despite initial concerns about respiratory depression and hastening death, Mr. Black did quite well with low doses of opioids, but as his dyspnea worsened it became more difficult to control with oral opioids. In such cases of so-called "terminal dyspnea," it is sometimes necessary to deliver higher doses of opioid via intravenous or subcutaneous methods, often at the expense of alertness and ability to interact with family. Patients in these situations often have just hours or days left to live, so it is of paramount importance to aggressively aim treatments at providing comfort and peace during their last days. Consistent with the philosophy of palliative care, treatments like this strive to maximize comfort and quality of life, rather than life prolongation. As such, potential concerns about oversedation, hypercapnia, or impairment of oral nutrition and hydration are not justifications for withholding these kinds of aggressive, comfort-directed treatments. In this case, even a higher dose of a subcutaneously infused opioid was ineffective. The addition of a benzodiazepine was thus deemed necessary, with the intent of inducing some sedation so as to achieve comfort for the patient and family in those last days of life. Sometimes called "terminal sedation," this technique is somewhat controversial, yet in clinical practice it is sometimes the only way to achieve comfort for patients with terminal dyspnea or other significant symptoms in their last hours or days.

Summary

Hospice and palliative care practice is increasingly recognized as integral to best clinical practice. Specialist palliative care consultation is now considered standard of care in certain settings, such as in patients with advanced solid tumors [58]. Typically, palliative care patients present with complex clinical characteristics including a heavy symptom burden. Dyspnea, one of the most prevalent symptoms encountered in palliative care, and one that is highly subjective and variable in nature, raises a number of ethical challenges. These challenges arise in the complex scenarios typical of palliative care, with the waters further muddied by factors such as discomfort on the part of clinicians, patient, and families; misunderstandings related to genuine versus perceived risks; and the necessity of compromise between symptom relief and treatment side effects. With any intervention targeting dyspnea in hospice/palliative care, it can also be difficult to discern whether changes in patient status (such as somnolence or confusion) are the result of the treatment, or are natural aspects of advanced disease or the dying process itself, or both.

In general, an ethical approach to dyspnea management in palliative care will rest upon integrity, transparency, and empathic communication. The practice of integrity entails the clinician's explicit commitment to serve in the patient's best interests, and to honor the patient's desires and informed preferences, while providing the highest quality medical care. Transparency can be achieved when the clinician:

(1) Openly acknowledges the ethical issues, concerns, and ambiguities arising in the specific patient's care

(2) Expresses these ethical parameters to individuals involved in decision making for that patient, including relevant colleagues, the palliative care team, and the patient/family unit

(3) Once a treatment plan has been determined, clearly articulates how the ethical issues are being resolved, and why they are being resolved in this particular way

Communication, throughout the process of palliative care and within that care, throughout the palliative management of dyspnea, involves, above all else, meaningful and respectful conversations and recognition of the emotionally charged nature of these scenarios. It is in face-to-face discourse, grounded in scientific information but tempered with compassion, that understanding, trust, and shared commitment to the patient's goals and well-being are cemented.

If, despite the implementation of integrity, transparency, and communication, differences or conflicts persist regarding the best treatment option to control the patient's dyspnea, modern bioethical principles stipulate that the ethical path for the clinician is to defer to the patient's autonomy, provided that decisions made by the patient (or surrogates, as appropriate) are fully informed. Ultimately, each patient has the authority to choose his or her care, and thus his or her experiences of symptoms and of treatment side effects, in the remaining portion of his or her life.

References

1. Parshall, M.B., et al., *An official American Thoracic Society statement: update on the mechanisms, assessment, and management of dyspnea.* Am J Respir Crit Care Med, 2012. **185**(4): p. 435–52.
2. Simon, S.T., et al., *Episodic and continuous breathlessness: a new categorization of breathlessness.* J Pain Symptom Manage, 2013. **45**(6): p. 1019-29.
3. Simon, S.T., et al., *Episodic breathlessness in patients with advanced disease: a systematic review.* J Pain Symptom Manage, 2013. **45**(3): p. 561–78.
4. Claessens, M.T., et al., *Dying with lung cancer or chronic obstructive pulmonary disease: insights from SUPPORT. Study to Understand Prognoses and Preferences for Outcomes and Risks of Treatments.* J Am Geriatr Soc, 2000. **48**(5 Suppl): p. S146–53.
5. Currow, D.C., et al., *Do the trajectories of dyspnea differ in prevalence and intensity by diagnosis at the end of life? A consecutive cohort study.* J Pain Symptom Manage, 2010. **39**(4): p. 680–90.
6. Elmqvist, M.A., et al., *Health-related quality of life during the last three months of life in patients with advanced cancer.* Support Care Cancer, 2009. **17**(2): p. 191–8.
7. Kutner, J.S., C.T. Kassner, and D.E. Nowels, *Symptom burden at the end of life: hospice providers' perceptions.* J Pain Symptom Manage, 2001. **21**(6): p. 473–80.
8. Mahler, D.A., et al., *American College of Chest Physicians consensus statement on the management of dyspnea in patients with advanced lung or heart disease.* Chest, 2010. **137**(3): p. 674–91.

9. Dudley, D.L., C.J. Martin, and T.H. Holmes, *Dyspnea: psychologic and physiologic observations.* J Psychosom Res, 1968. **11**(4): p. 325–39.

10. McFadden, E.R., Jr., R. Kiser, and W.J. DeGroot, *Acute bronchial asthma. Relations between clinical and physiologic manifestations.* N Engl J Med, 1973. **288**(5): p. 221–5.

11. *Dyspnea. Mechanisms, assessment, and management: a consensus statement. American Thoracic Society.* Am J Respir Crit Care Med, 1999. **159**(1): p. 321–40.

12. Gysels, M.H. and I.J. Higginson, *Caring for a person in advanced illness and suffering from breathlessness at home: threats and resources.* Palliat Support Care, 2009. **7**(2): p. 153–62.

13. Janson-Bjerklie, S., V.K. Carrieri, and M. Hudes, *The sensations of pulmonary dyspnea.* Nurs Res, 1986. **35**(3): p. 154–9.

14. Dudley, D.L., et al., *Psychosocial concomitants to rehabilitation in chronic obstructive pulmonary disease. Part I. Psychosocial and psychological considerations.* Chest, 1980. **77**(3): p. 413–20.

15. Moody, L., K. McCormick, and A. Williams, *Disease and symptom severity, functional status, and quality of life in chronic bronchitis and emphysema (CBE).* J Behav Med, 1990. **13**(3): p. 297–306.

16. Bernhard, J. and P.A. Ganz, *Psychosocial issues in lung cancer patients (Part 2).* Chest, 1991. **99**(2): p. 480–5.

17. Smith, E.L., et al., *Dyspnea, anxiety, body consciousness, and quality of life in patients with lung cancer.* J Pain Symptom Manage, 2001. **21**(4): p. 323–9.

18. Moy, M.L., et al., *Multivariate models of determinants of health-related quality of life in severe chronic obstructive pulmonary disease.* J Rehabil Res Dev, 2009. **46**(5): p. 643–54.

19. Leidy, N.K. and G.A. Traver, *Adjustment and social behaviour in older adults with chronic obstructive pulmonary disease: the family's perspective.* J Adv Nurs, 1996. **23**(2): p. 252–9.

20. Abernethy, A.P. and J.L. Wheeler, *Total dyspnoea.* Curr Opin Support Palliat Care, 2008. **2**(2): p. 110–3.

21. Christakis, N.A. and T.J. Iwashyna, *The health impact of health care on families: a matched cohort study of hospice use by decedents and mortality outcomes in surviving, widowed spouses.* Soc Sci Med, 2003. **57**(3): p. 465–75.

22. Schulz, R., et al., *Predictors of complicated grief among dementia caregivers: a prospective study of bereavement.* Am J Geriatr Psychiatry, 2006. **14**(8): p. 650–8.

23. Kasuya, R.T., P. Polgar-Bailey, and R. Takeuchi, *Caregiver burden and burnout. A guide for primary care physicians.* Postgrad Med, 2000. **108**(7): p. 119–23.

24. Jennings, A.L., et al., *A systematic review of the use of opioids in the management of dyspnoea.* Thorax, 2002. **57**(11): p. 939–44.

25. Ben-Aharon, I., et al., *Interventions for alleviating cancer-related dyspnea: a systematic review.* J Clin Oncol, 2008. **26**(14): p. 2396–404.

26. Viola, R., et al., *The management of dyspnea in cancer patients: a systematic review.* Support Care Cancer, 2008. **16**(4): p. 329–37.

27. Abernethy, A.P., et al., *Randomised, double blind, placebo controlled crossover trial of sustained release morphine for the management of refractory dyspnoea.* BMJ, 2003. **327**(7414): p. 523–8.

28. Allard, P., et al., *How effective are supplementary doses of opioids for dyspnea in terminally ill cancer patients? A randomized continuous sequential clinical trial.* J Pain Symptom Manage, 1999. **17**(4): p. 256–65.

29. Currow, D.C., et al., *Once-daily opioids for chronic dyspnea: a dose increment and phar-macovigilance study.* J Pain Symptom Manage, 2011. **42**(3): p. 388–99.

30. Gott, M., et al., *The effect of the Shipman murders on clinician attitudes to prescrib-ing opiates for dyspnoea in end-stage chronic obstructive pulmonary disease in England.* Progress in Palliative Care, 2010. **18**(2): p. 79–84.

31. Navigante, A.H., M.A. Castro, and L.C. Cerchietti, *Morphine versus midazolam as upfront therapy to control dyspnea perception in cancer patients while its underlying cause is sought or treated.* J Pain Symptom Manage, 2010. **39**(5): p. 820–30.

32. Wilcock, A., et al., *Randomised, placebo controlled trial of nebulised furosemide for breathlessness in patients with cancer.* Thorax, 2008. **63**(10): p. 872–5.

33. Kohara, H., et al., *Effect of nebulized furosemide in terminally ill cancer patients with dyspnea.* J Pain Symptom Manage, 2003. **26**(4): p. 962–7.

34. Ong, K.C., et al., *Effects of inhaled furosemide on exertional dyspnea in chronic obstruc-tive pulmonary disease.* Am J Respir Crit Care Med, 2004. **169**(9): p. 1028–33.

35. Nishino, T., et al., *Inhaled furosemide greatly alleviates the sensation of experimentally induced dyspnea.* Am J Respir Crit Care Med, 2000. **161**(6): p. 1963–7.

36. Jensen, D., et al., *Mechanisms of dyspnoea relief and improved exercise endurance after furosemide inhalation in COPD.* Thorax, 2008. **63**(7): p. 606–13.

37. Stone, P., et al., *Re: nebulized furosemide for dyspnea in terminal cancer patients.* J Pain Symptom Manage, 2002. **24**(3): p. 274–5; author reply 275–6.

38. Shimoyama, N. and M. Shimoyama, *Nebulized furosemide as a novel treatment for dyspnea in terminal cancer patients.* J Pain Symptom Manage, 2002. **23**(1): p. 73–6.

39. Stone, P., A. Kurowska, and A. Tookman, *Nebulized frusemide for dyspnoea.* Palliat Med, 1994. **8**(3): p. 258.

40. Roberts, C.M., *Short burst oxygen therapy for relief of breathlessness in COPD.* Thorax, 2004. **59**(8): p. 638–40.

41. Escalante, C.P., et al., *Dyspnea in cancer patients. Etiology, resource utilization, and survival-implications in a managed care world.* Cancer, 1996. **78**(6): p. 1314–9.

42. *Continuous or nocturnal oxygen therapy in hypoxemic chronic obstructive lung dis-ease: a clinical trial. Nocturnal Oxygen Therapy Trial Group.* Ann Intern Med, 1980. **93**(3): p. 391–8.

43. *Long term domiciliary oxygen therapy in chronic hypoxic cor pulmonale complicating chronic bronchitis and emphysema. Report of the Medical Research Council Working Party.* Lancet, 1981. **1**(8222): p. 681–6.

44. Eaton, T., et al., *Long-term oxygen therapy improves health-related quality of life.* Respir Med, 2004. **98**(4): p. 285–93.

45. Abernethy, A.P., et al., *Effect of palliative oxygen versus room air in relief of breathless-ness in patients with refractory dyspnoea: a double-blind, randomised controlled trial.* Lancet, 2010. **376**(9743): p. 784–93.

46. Buckholz, G.T. and C.F. von Gunten, *Nonpharmacological management of dyspnea.* Curr Opin Support Palliat Care, 2009. **3**(2): p. 98–102.

47. Dorman, S., A. Byrne, and A. Edwards, *Which measurement scales should we use to measure breathlessness in palliative care? A systematic review.* Palliat Med, 2007. **21**(3): p. 177–91.

48. Tanaka, K., et al., *Development and validation of the Cancer Dyspnoea Scale: a multi-dimensional, brief, self-rating scale.* Br J Cancer, 2000. **82**(4): p. 800–5.

49. Uronis, H.E., et al., *Assessment of the Psychometric Properties of an English Version of the Cancer Dyspnea Scale in People With Advanced Lung Cancer.* J Pain Symptom Manage, 2012. **44**(5): 741–9.

50. Temel, J.S., et al., *Early palliative care for patients with metastatic non-small-cell lung cancer.* N Engl J Med, 2010. **363**(8): p. 733–42.

51. Steinhauser, K.E., et al., *Factors considered important at the end of life by patients, family, physicians, and other care providers.* JAMA, 2000. **284**(19): p. 2476–82.

52. Quill, T.E., R. Dresser, and D.W. Brock, *The rule of double effect—a critique of its role in end-of-life decision making.* N Engl J Med, 1997. **337**(24): p. 1768–71.

53. Clemens, K.E., I. Quednau, and E. Klaschik, *Is there a higher risk of respiratory depression in opioid-naive palliative care patients during symptomatic therapy of dyspnea with strong opioids?* J Palliat Med, 2008. **11**(2): p. 204–16.

54. Clemens, K.E. and E. Klaschik, *Symptomatic therapy of dyspnea with strong opioids and its effect on ventilation in palliative care patients.* J Pain Symptom Manage, 2007. **33**(4): p. 473–81.

55. Minozzi, S., L. Amato, and M. Davoli, *Development of dependence following treatment with opioid analgesics for pain relief: a systematic review.* Addiction, 2012.

56. Abernethy, A.P. and D.C. Currow, *Time-limited trials.* JAMA, 2012. **307**(1): p. 33–4; author reply 34.

57. Currow, D.C. and A.P. Abernethy, *The ultimate personalised medicine.* Int J Clin Pract, 2012. **66**(9): p. 824–6.

58. Smith, T.J., et al., *American Society of Clinical Oncology provisional clinical opinion: the integration of palliative care into standard oncology care.* J Clin Oncol, 2012. **30**(8): p. 880–7.

9

Diagnosis and Treatment of Delirium

Maxine de la Cruz and Eduardo Bruera

Delirium is a prevalent neuropsychiatric condition in patients with severe illness such as advanced cancer. It also occurs in 15% to 50% of elderly patients admitted to the hospital [1]. A vast majority of patients at the end of life are also reported to have delirium. Delirium is a source of significant suffering and distress to patients and their families, as well as in healthcare professionals taking care of such patients. It prevents meaningful interaction between the patient and his or her family, particularly at the end of life [2]. A diagnosis of delirium also impacts a patient's ability to make sound decisions because such fluctuations in cognition compromise the patient's ability to understand complex medical issues. The development of delirium has also been shown to be associated with increased mortality, greater morbidity, persistent functional decline, and increased rate of institutionalization, particularly in the frail elderly population. It is often misdiagnosed or underdiagnosed, causing potential conflicts in several clinical situations [3, 4]. The presence of delirium likewise raises several clinical and ethical concerns regarding the treatment approach and appropriate treatment strategies, goals of care, and participation in clinical trials.

In this chapter we will discuss delirium in palliative care settings and outline the different clinical scenarios that pose ethical dilemmas to clinicians who are confronted with patients who develop delirium.

Overview of Delirium

Delirium is a complication that is frequently observed in severely ill patients and at the end of life. It is an acute disorder of cognition and attention, and is characterized by diminished level of consciousness, inability to focus and sustain attention, developing over a short period of time, often with a fluctuating course. It is important to note that delirium is often caused by an underlying medical condition, and is potentially reversible. However, in about 50% of cases, delirium persists despite appropriate medical management aimed at correcting underlying conditions [5]. Delirium can likewise develop in the last hours to days of life. About 80% of patients who were determined to be "actively dying" experienced terminal delirium [6].

Delirium is generally believed to be multifactorial in etiology. Inouye et al. describe the interaction between predisposing or vulnerability factors and precipitating or incident factors. The more significant the predisposing factors, the higher the risk of developing delirium when exposed to precipitating factors. Individuals with baseline cognitive impairment, poor functional status, presence of underlying neurological disease, advanced age as well as increased severity of illness and high burden of co-morbidity are at increased risk of developing delirium. Precipitating factors include medications, intercurrent illness, surgery, sleep deprivation, and certain environmental conditions [7].

Delirium is acknowledged to occur frequently, but is most commonly misdiagnosed and underdiagnosed [8-10]. Frequently cited reasons for this include the under-utilization of assessment tools to facilitate in the diagnosis by the medical team and poor understanding of the course of the disease and its implications. Delirium may be difficult to diagnose by the untrained eye because of the fluctuating nature of the symptoms and its intensity, inability to accurately assess cognition, absence of psychomotor agitation, and presence of underlying cognitive impairment that may mask other symptoms of delirium. Screening tools frequently used include: the Confusion Assessment Method, the Memorial Delirium Assessment Scale, and the Delirium Rating Scale [11].

From a psychomotor point of view, delirium can be classified as hypoactive, hyperactive, or mixed. Patients with hypoactive type of delirium are often misdiagnosed as having depression or dementia and receive treatment less frequently that those with agitated (associated with hypervigilant level of consciousness) or mixed type [12-14].

Untreated delirium causes significant psychological distress to patients, their families, and the healthcare professionals involved. Treatment includes correction of suspected underlying pathology, and use of nonpharmacological as well as pharmacological interventions to control the symptoms. Nonpharmacological therapies include orientation and emotional support, orientation techniques, provision for a safe and quiet environment, and avoidance of physical restraints and noxious environmental stimuli. There are no evidenced-based pharmacological guidelines for delirium, but neuroleptics such as haloperidol are considered by most specialists as the first line of treatment. The use of other antipsychotics such as chlorpromazine, olanzapine, risperidone, and quetiapine has also been shown to be effective in controlling symptoms [15, 16]. Benzodiazepines are generally not used, especially in the elderly, because they cause worsening of delirium. They are useful, however, in patients whose delirium is caused by alcohol withdrawal.

Ethical Dilemmas in Patients with Delirium

NATURAL PROCESS VERSUS REVERSIBILITY

One of the challenges in the management of delirium is finding a balance between aggressive investigation and treatment of the delirium episode versus recognition that the episode is part of the dying process and that further aggressive measures may result in more harm for the patient and his or her family. Several studies have shown that about half of diagnosed delirium cases are reversible, particularly those related to opioid neurotoxicity, dehydration, metabolic abnormalities. However, a significant number of patients do not show improvement in symptoms despite efforts to treat the underlying cause. Delirium is less likely to resolve in patients with underlying dementia, or delirium related to hypoxic or metabolic encephalopathy, or disseminated intravascular coagulopathy. A study by Bruera et al., which showed delirium reversibility to be 49% and an 88% occurrence rate for terminal delirium, illustrates the complexity of the decision regarding how to proceed with delirium management [5]. It is generally recommended that a search for reversible cause is made, with appropriate symptom management and family education concurrently in place. Conversations with the family should focus on assuring them that the potential cause will be sought for and treated. But at the same time, they should be cautioned that sometimes despite the clinician's best efforts, the patient's previous cognitive and psychological functioning may not return to baseline.

PATIENT DISTRESS WITH THE DELIRIUM EPISODE

Hypoactive delirium is more often missed and under-treated compared with the hyperactive and mixed subtypes. Patients who have hypoactive type delirium do not exhibit agitation or restlessness seen in hyperactive or mixed types. Most often, these patients are sluggish or lethargic. It may be that in such cases, clinicians do not perceive patients to be in distress because of the absence of agitation, or there is a lack of appreciation with the distress that caregivers experience witnessing such episodes. In recent years, however, several investigators have reported that the majority of patients who recovered from their delirium episode recalled their experience and were quite distressed by it. Delirium recall was not associated with any particular form of delirium. In a study by Schofield et al., 19 elderly patients who recovered from their delirium episode reported that they remember experiences of perceptual disturbance including delusions and hallucinations that ranged from pleasant to frightening [17]. Other investigators reported that patients cited presence of hallucinations as major stressors, along with extreme anxiety while being aware of their confusional state. Breitbart et al. reported in their study of 101 patients that 54% recalled their delirium experience. Further analysis showed that recall was associated with less severe episodes and better performance status, and was negatively associated with impairment in consciousness, disorientation, and short-term memory impairment, as well as age and the presence of baseline cognitive impairment.

A majority of patients, particularly those who had delusions and perceptual disturbances, reported severe distress [18]. A study of 99 cancer patients indicated that 80% of patients recalled their delirium episode and that there was no association with delirium subtype. For those who recovered from delirium, higher level of distress was associated with psychomotor agitation [19]. These findings suggest that delirium needs to be treated despite the absence of obvious psychomotor agitation. And with this information, clinicians may be more inclined to treat delirium.

Delirium in a Patient with Dementia

CASE PRESENTATION

A 90-year-old nursing home resident with Alzheimer's dementia for 7 years was brought in to the emergency room for failure to thrive. Her records indicate that she had a rapid decline in her oral intake over the last week. She is able to feed herself, but requires assistance with all of her other activities of daily living. She is verbal, but utters only a few words. The patient is confused, but does not appear to be in any distress and she is unable to give details of her history. Laboratory and imaging studies show that she has a urinary tract infection. She was admitted to the hospital and started on intravenous antibiotics and subsequently discharged back to the nursing home.

DISCUSSION

This patient is at very high risk of developing delirium, given her underlying dementia, poor functional status, and overall frailty. From the history, the patient appears to have hypoactive delirium. The diagnosis is often missed, particularly in patients with underlying dementia. Patients with this delirium subtype often do not get treated with antipsychotics because of the absence of psychomotor agitation. However, as shown in the delirium recall studies, patients with hypoactive delirium will also benefit with pharmacotherapy along with nonpharmacological interventions. Less sedating antipsychotics, given at low doses would be appropriate for this frail geriatric patient. Treatment of possible underlying etiology would require discussion of overall treatment goals. If reversibility is unlikely and quality of life is severely compromised, symptomatic treatment of the delirium to alleviate suffering may be the most judicious intervention.

FAMILY AND CAREGIVER DISTRESS

Delirium causes significant emotional distress for families and caregivers, as well as members of the healthcare team. Families are often troubled by signs that the patient is suffering from perceptual disturbances, fluctuating cognition and emotional liability, delusions and paranoia, and psychomotor agitation that often accompany delirium.

Interviews conducted with 37 caregivers showed that caregivers were distressed when patients develop delirium, and most attribute this to the pain medication [20]. Misinformation regarding delirium has also been shown to result in conflicts with family and the healthcare team. Often, delirious patients have high symptom expression and families may perceive that the healthcare team is not effectively managing symptoms if they are not properly educated and given support to understand that this cognitive dysfunction is often not reversible. Caregivers reported more severe emotional distress in patients with hyperactive delirium and severe debility. It often helps to advise families about how to respond to patients who are delirious. Behavioral interventions that include redirection, use of nonconfrontational statements, compassion and empathy, and reassurance can be used to improve interaction with patients who have delirium.

Hospital staff may likewise report distress in caring for patients with delirium. It is also more common in patients with more severe delirium and those who have delusions and perceptual disturbances. In one study, however, investigators found that despite high distress reported in patients and families, nurses and other medical staff reported their distress level to be minimal. Investigators conclude that this may have something to do with level of staff experience [21]. This may be true in units in which nurses and medical staff are trained to care for patients who have delirium.

Overexpression of Symptoms as a Source of Conflict

CASE PRESENTATION

AB is a 20-year-old woman with metastatic breast cancer. The patient was admitted to the hospital because of severe pain in the hip. She reports that she has had increasing pain over the last week, and on average she has been taking six to eight breakthrough opioids per day with minimal to moderate relief. She was started on a continuous infusion of hydromorphone with a nurse bolus every hour for breakthrough pain. The following day, the patient was noted to be drowsy, but was still complaining that pain is not well controlled. She had been requiring breakthrough medications almost every hour. The family voiced their frustration that pain was not being managed effectively; the nurse caring for her has likewise expressed concern that the patient is suffering. Review of her blood work showed that she had hypercalcemia. The attending physician informs the family that she thinks the patient has delirium.

DISCUSSION

Studies have shown that there is an over-expression of pain and other symptoms in patients with delirium. A case report by Delgado et al. describes patients with delirium who report high symptom burden on the Edmonton Symptom Assessment Scale (ESAS); that treatment of the underlying medical etiology of the delirium, opioid rotation, and hydration improved the delirium episode and the overall symptom burden [30]. When families and healthcare providers are not aware that there is underlying delirium, and that patients are overexpressing their symptoms as a consequence of disinhibition, conflicts may arise. There may be a tendency to overtreat pain with more opioids, potentially worsening the situation, or families may feel that healthcare providers are not doing their best in ensuring improvement of the patient's symptoms. Educating families is a cornerstone in the management of delirium. It not only prepares the families emotionally for the difficulty of seeing the patient act very differently from baseline, it also helps them understand the complexity of management.

Response to a Patient's Unrealistic Requests

CASE PRESENTATION

KR is a 71-year-old man with pancreatic cancer with metastasis to the liver. He was brought to the emergency room for worsening confusion and jaundice. His wife reports that the patient has been having difficulty sleeping at night and sometimes does not respond appropriately to questions over the last 3 weeks. There is no history of hallucinations. Jaundice was noted about 1 week before the emergency room visit. The patient was alert and was able to hold conversation for short periods. He was easily distracted and incoherent at times. The patient repeatedly verbalized that he wanted to go home and was angry at his family when they declined his request. This caused a lot of distress among his family members. Workup revealed intrahepatic biliary duct dilatation and progression of the hepatic mass. A stent was placed along with scheduled haloperidol.

DISCUSSION

It is often difficult when patients make unreasonable requests and families and healthcare providers do not recognize that there is generalized brain dysfunction. There may be feelings of guilt on the part of the family when they do not comply with patient's wishes. It must be made clear that when patients have delirium, sound judgment may be compromised to varied degrees, depending on the severity of delirium. Therefore, they cannot be relied upon to make complex decisions about their care. It is important to remember that a confrontational and argumentative stance would not be helpful in such cases. Redirection can help decrease agitation.

HYDRATION AS TREATMENT FOR DELIRIUM

Advancement in medical science sometimes creates new ethical dilemmas and re-evaluation of how we compassionately practice medicine. Although it has been shown that forcing nutrition in advanced cancer patients results in harm, the role of hydration is more controversial and requires more evidence for its resolution. Hydration is categorized as a medical procedure, which should be evaluated with respect to its potential benefits and burdens for the patient. Continuation of hydration therefore should depend on the informed decision of the patient or surrogates based on appropriate medical input regarding pathophysiology of dehydration, effects on patient's quality of life, and the natural course of the dying process. There is a paucity of research regarding hydration at the end of life, yet there are strong and differing views on the matter. Those arguing against the use of hydration at the end of life cite that dehydration is a natural consequence of the dying process and that providing hydration would in some cases prolong the dying process. Other experts argue that hydration at the end of life will not prolong dying or alter the course of the disease, but promote overall well-being. Critical to this argument is the issue of delirium and medication that is common in dying patients. Bruera et al. demonstrated that careful hydration decreased the incidence of delirium in patients admitted to the palliative care unit. The burdens of increased urine output may be overcome by the risk of adverse drug effects secondary to the body's failure to clear toxic drug metabolites. Hydration has likewise been shown to improve other symptoms common in the palliative care patient, such as sedation, myoclonus, and a trend toward reduction in hallucinations in those with delirium [22]. In sum, hydration may be useful in selected cases such as in those patients with opioid-induced neurotoxicity, delirium as a consequence of dehydration, or patients with hypercalcemia. The decision to implement hydration must be individualized and consistent with the goals of care of the patient.

Hydration at the End of Life

CASE PRESENTATION

TM is a 40-year-old woman with metastatic ovarian cancer. She was admitted to the hospital for intractable pain and nausea. She was found to have malignant small bowel obstruction. The patient was a poor surgical candidate and the decision was made to focus on controlling symptoms followed by discharge home with hospice care. After a week, the patient developed delirium believed to be secondary to opioids and dehydration.

DISCUSSION

Hydration at the end of life is a controversial topic that warrants further research and review of current evidence. In this patient, gentle hydration may improve symptoms of delirium along with initiation of antipsychotics and opioid rotation. There is minimal risk to the patient, and it is relatively easy to deliver. Given the absence of clear evidence-based guidelines, each case should be individualized depending on perceived balance of benefits and burdens in light of the patient's medical condition, values, and preferences.

Determination of Decision-Making Capacity

The principle of respect for autonomy is an important ethical principle that requires clinicians to obtain the competent patient's consent or agreement before proceeding with any medical intervention deemed beneficial. Autonomy implies that patients have the appropriate information necessary to make sound decisions for their care and are free from undue influence. A precondition for patient autonomy is decision-making capacity, which in general pertains to a person's ability to understand factual information, use it, and subsequently communicate a decision to others. Patients with delirium are generally regarded as having compromised autonomy. In patients in whom the predominant symptom is psychomotor agitation and perceptual disturbance, the loss of capacity is clearly evident. However, patients with hypoactive delirium, who may appear alert and responding appropriately, may lead clinicians to believe falsely that they have capacity if no standard testing is employed. Fluctuating cognition makes it difficult for clinicians to assess autonomy and clinical decision capacity, but clinicians must always try to involve patients to the degree that is appropriate in discussions about their care.

Avoiding unwanted aggressive treatment that may be harmful or nonbeneficial is a concern shared by patients, families, and healthcare providers. Because patients with delirium may lose decision-making capacity, advance directives may be helpful in assuring that treatment decisions are consistent with their preferences and values. Advance directives could range from assigning a surrogate decision maker, to general statements about the patient's values and preferences, decisions not to attempt resuscitation, artificial hydration, feeding, and withdrawal of aggressive treatment. In a study by Detering et al., bereaved members of the family of patients with an advance directive were found to have significantly less stress, anxiety, and depression. The presence of advance directives may relieve the family from the burden of having to decide treatment options [23]. Thus, encouraging patients to have this legal document prepared is an important step in carrying out patients' preferences of treatment,

TABLE 9.1
Risk factors for delirium

Risk Factors for Delirium in Surgical Patients
Advanced age
Existing cognitive impairment
Existing functional impairment
History of CVA/TIA/CNS disorder
History of alcohol abuse
Metabolic abnormalities: albumin, sodium, potassium, and glucose
Diabetes
Type and complexity of surgery

Risk Factors for Delirium in Medical Patients
Vision impairment
Severe illness
Cognitive impairment
BUN/crea ratio ≥18
Precipitating factors
Use of physical restraints
Three new medications during hospitalization
Use of bladder catheter
Any iatrogenic event

particularly at the end of life. One concern, however, is that most often advance directives are worded vaguely and are too simplistic. Patients should be encouraged to address values and goals such as "to prolong life and preserve cognition" versus "minimizing suffering or avoid unacceptable functional status." Clinicians should evaluate decisions in the light of the best interest of the patient, working with families to have a clearer sense of patient's goals, preferences, and values.

TREATMENT VERSUS SEDATION

Palliative sedation (PS) is commonly employed in patients whose delirium is refractory to conventional treatments with antipsychotics and other nonpharmacological therapies. Several studies have shown that delirium is a common symptom for which palliative sedation is started [24, 25]. In a study by Carceni, delirium was present in 31% of patients who underwent palliative sedation [26]. A systematic review by Mercadante et al. reported that delirium was a common problem requiring palliative sedation in advanced cancer patients followed in the home setting [27].

Intractable Delirium

CASE PRESENTATION

CT is a 60-year-old man with metastatic non–small cell lung diagnosed less than a year ago. The patient has progressive disease despite several courses of chemotherapy. A few days after his last chemotherapy, he developed fever and dyspnea. He was neutropenic with chest x-ray showing pleural effusion and possibly pneumonia on top of his extensive lung involvement. He was initiated on antibiotics, steroids, high flow concentrated oxygen, and continuous opioid infusion. On the third hospital day, the patient continued to complain of dyspnea and pain and was very anxious and restless. The family, advocating for the patient, constantly asked the nurse for more pain medications. A diagnosis of delirium was made. Opioid rotation was done and scheduled haloperidol was added to his regimen. Worsening agitation prompted the team to start him on chlorpromazine and eventually initiate the palliative sedation protocol. The family and nursing staff were very distressed seeing the patient suffering.

DISCUSSION

This case illustrates what we commonly encounter in our practice. When delirium is diagnosed, efforts to diagnose and treat the underlying medical etiology concurrent with treating the distressing symptoms that often accompany the syndrome are the initial steps. Conversations with the family regarding the etiology, the symptoms, and what can be expected foster understanding of the syndrome and prepares families to deal with a worsening clinical picture. When treatment options have been exhausted and it is becoming clear that the patient is approaching the end of life, then discussions with the family should change from trying to reverse the condition to reducing the suffering as much as possible. This may be accomplished through palliative sedation (see chapter 14 for a more extensive discussion of this topic). It should be explained that the intent of the sedation is to control distressing symptoms and alleviate suffering. The distress can also be experienced by families and health professionals caring for the patient. As shown in multiple studies, distress is particularly high in those patients with psychomotor agitation. The distress expressed is in part related to the imminent loss of a loved one. Families need psychosocial support during this difficult experience.

RESEARCH PARTICIPATION OF PATIENTS WITH DELIRIUM

Delirium poses serious concern with regard to the inclusion of patients in clinical research. On the one hand, laws in place to protect vulnerable research subjects are also on the other hand depriving such groups from representation in clinical trials. Although a surrogate decision maker can be used in certain in situations, it is often difficult to obtain surrogate consent for participation in research. Previous studies have shown that when consent is sought from surrogates, almost half decline to participate despite minimal risk to the patient [28]. This is a critical barrier to further our understanding of delirium and its treatment through research.

Missed delirium is a significant issue in patients participating in research. It has been reported that delirium is missed in a significant number of patients with advanced disease. In a study of Bruera et al., they reported that of 67 patients who were recruited to participate in research and signed a consent form, 19% were found to have a Mini Mental State Exam Score of 24/30 or less [29]. This raises the question of the validity of the informed consent in such patients. This poses a challenge for researchers to evaluate cognition in populations with a risk for cognitive impairment or delirium to ensure that appropriate patients are included in the study.

Conclusion

Delirium is a common neuropsychiatric symptom in older patients and those at the end of life. It is an atypical presentation of illness in frail older patients, and is also present in a significant proportion of patients who are near death. It is often under-reported and underdiagnosed despite its prevalence. It causes severe distress in patients, family members, and medical staff. Screening patients at risk for developing delirium is desirable. Delirium presents with several ethical dilemmas, which require careful assessment and intervention. A good understanding of delirium is imperative in judicious medical management. In patients with delirium, carefully working with the family through education and interdisciplinary support to alleviate distress cannot be overemphasized.

References

1. Fong, T.G., S.R. Tulebaev, and S.K. Inouye, *Delirium in elderly adults: diagnosis, prevention and treatment.* Nat Rev Neurol, 2009. **5**(4): p. 210–20.
2. Breitbart, W. and Y. Alici, *Agitation and delirium at the end of life: "We couldn't manage him."* JAMA, 2008. **300**(24): p. 2898–910, E1.
3. Inouye, S.K., *Delirium in older persons.* N Engl J Med, 2006. *354*(11): p. 1157–65.
4. Inouye, S.K., et al., *Does delirium contribute to poor hospital outcomes? A three-site epidemiologic study.* J Gen Intern Med, 1998. **13**(4): p. 234–42.
5. Lawlor, P.G., et al., *Occurrence, causes, and outcome of delirium in patients with advanced cancer: a prospective study.* Arch Intern Med, 2000. **160**(6): p. 786–94.
6. Centeno, C., A. Sanz, and E. Bruera, *Delirium in advanced cancer patients.* Palliat Med, 2004. **18**(3): p. 184–94.
7. Inouye, S.K., *Predisposing and precipitating factors for delirium in hospitalized older patients.* Dement Geriatr Cogn Disord, 1999. **10**(5): p. 393–400.
8. Inouye, S.K., *The recognition of delirium.* Hosp Pract (Off Ed), 1991. **26**(4A): p. 61–2.
9. Lawlor, P.G. and E.D. Bruera, *Delirium in patients with advanced cancer.* Hematol Oncol Clin North Am, 2002. **16**(3): p. 701–14.
10. Fang, C.K., et al., *Prevalence, detection and treatment of delirium in terminal cancer inpatients: a prospective survey.* Jpn J Clin Oncol, 2008. **38**(1): p. 56–63.
11. Breitbart, W., et al., *The Memorial Delirium Assessment Scale.* J Pain Symptom Manage, 1997. **13**(3): p. 128–37.
12. Breitbart, W., *Psycho-oncology: depression, anxiety, delirium.* Semin Oncol, 1994. **21**(6): p. 754–69.
13. Fick, D.M., J.V. Agostini, and S.K. Inouye, *Delirium superimposed on dementia: a systematic review.* J Am Geriatr Soc, 2002. **50**(10): p. 1723–32.
14. Stagno, D., C. Gibson, and W. Breitbart, *The delirium subtypes: a review of prevalence, phenomenology, pathophysiology, and treatment response.* Palliat Support Care, 2004. **2**(2): p. 171–9.
15. Boettger, S. and W. Breitbart, *Atypical antipsychotics in the management of delirium: a review of the empirical literature.* Palliat Support Care, 2005. **3**(3): p. 227–37.
16. Breitbart, W., et al., *A double-blind trial of haloperidol, chlorpromazine, and lorazepam in the treatment of delirium in hospitalized AIDS patients.* Am J Psychiatry, 1996. **153**(2): p. 231–7.
17. Schofield, I., *A small exploratory study of the reaction of older people to an episode of delirium.* J Adv Nurs, 1997. **25**(5): p. 942–52.
18. Breitbart, W., C. Gibson, and A. Tremblay, *The delirium experience: delirium recall and delirium-related distress in hospitalized patients with cancer, their spouses/caregivers, and their nurses.* Psychosomatics, 2002. **43**(3): p. 183–94.
19. Bruera, E., et al., *Impact of delirium and recall on the level of distress in patients with advanced cancer and their family caregivers.* Cancer, 2009. **115**(9): p. 2004–12.
20. Cohen, M.Z., et al., *Delirium in advanced cancer leading to distress in patients and family caregivers.* J Palliat Care, 2009. **25**(3): p. 164–71.
21. Inouye, S.K., et al., *Nurses' recognition of delirium and its symptoms: comparison of nurse and researcher ratings.* Arch Intern Med, 2001. **161**(20): p. 2467–73.
22. Bruera, E., et al., *Effects of parenteral hydration in terminally ill cancer patients: a preliminary study.* J Clin Oncol, 2005. **23**(10): p. 2366–71.

23. Detering, K.M., et al., *The impact of advance care planning on end of life care in elderly patients: randomised controlled trial.* BMJ, 2010. **340**: p. c1345.

24. Alonso-Babarro, A., et al., *At-home palliative sedation for end-of-life cancer patients.* Palliat Med, 2010. **24**(5): p. 486–92.

25. Elsayem, A., et al., *Use of palliative sedation for intractable symptoms in the palliative care unit of a comprehensive cancer center.* Support Care Cancer, 2009. **17**(1): p. 53–9.

26. Caraceni, A., et al., *Palliative sedation at the end of life at a tertiary cancer center.* Support Care Cancer, 2012. **20**(6): p. 1299–307.

27. Mercadante, S., et al., *Palliative sedation in advanced cancer patients followed at home: a retrospective analysis.* J Pain Symptom Manage, 2012. **43**(6): p. 1126–30.

28. Mason, S., et al., *Brief report on the experience of using proxy consent for incapacitated adults.* J Med Ethics, 2006. **32**(1): p. 61–2.

29. Bruera, E., et al., *Cognitive failure in cancer patients in clinical trials.* Lancet, 1993. **341**(8839): p. 247–8.

30. Delgado-Guay, M.O., S. Yennurajalingam, and E. Bruera, *Delirium with severe symptom expression related to hypercalcemia in a patient with advanced cancer: an interdisciplinary approach to treatment.* J Pain Symptom Manage, 2008. **36**(4): p. 442–9.

10

Psychosocial and Psychiatric Suffering

Yesne Alici, Kanan Modhwadia,
and William S. Breitbart

Suffering is a universal and unavoidable part of human existence. Viktor Frankl (1959) described three existential facts of life, or what he called the "tragic triad"; that in life we must all inevitably encounter "suffering," "death," and "existential guilt" (Frankl, 1959). Karl Jaspers (1955) defined suffering as "any encounter with a limitation" and death, or the finiteness of life as intimately confronted by a terminally ill patient, as the ultimate limitation (Jaspers, 1955). Eric Cassel (1982) defined suffering as a "loss of personhood" (Cassel, 1982). This concept of suffering as a loss of personhood is often related to such issues as loss of dignity (Chochinov, 2002) and loss of meaning (Breitbart et al., 2004).

Over the last two decades, our research group at Memorial Sloan-Kettering Cancer Center has focused on expanding the concept of what it means to provide adequate palliative care. Our goal has been to expand the concept of adequate palliative care beyond a focus on pain and physical symptom control (absolutely essential goals) to include psychiatric, psychosocial, existential, and spiritual domains of care (Breitbart and Chochinov, 2009). We have attempted to do this through our writing and teaching, but primarily through our focus of psychiatric palliative care research. Our research has been conducted within a laboratory headed by Dr. Breitbart, formally called the Psychotherapy, Psychopharmacology and Symptom Control Laboratory. Unofficially, we called it the Laboratory of Despair. "Despair" may be an even more informative term than "suffering" for the goals of psychiatric, psychosocial, and existential palliative care. We defined "despair" not merely as a "loss of hope," but rather as a "loss of essence of what makes one human." This is perhaps what Eric Cassel (1982) meant by loss of personhood. Human beings, as opposed to all other animals, have certain unique characteristics. Human beings are aware of their existence (and their mortality), and as such experience "Awe and Dread" (Kierkegard, Hong, and Hong, 1983). Human beings are "meaning-making" creatures, and as such are responsible to create lives of meaning and purpose (Yalom, 1980). Only human beings are capable of transformation, posttraumatic growth, and even transcendence in response to loss and limitations.

Finally, "connection and connectedness" is essential to human survival and is at the essence of the human experience. When cancer illness or other life-threatening or degenerative illness robs human beings of these unique and "essential" aspects of what it means to be human, then we experience a sense of loss of meaning and a loss of what is the spirit or "essence " of what makes us human.

Despair is caused by many consequences of advanced cancer and life-threatening illness. As death approaches, it is common for patients with terminal illness to experience an exacerbation in the number and severity of their physical and psychosocial symptoms and stressors. Although these stressors can include increased physical symptom burden (e.g., pain, dyspnea), physical debilitation, loss of independence, and even loss of bowel and bladder control, a significant contribution to "despair" comes from psychosocial, psychiatric, and existential sources. In our "Laboratory of Despair" we have studied the assessment and management of psychiatric disorders in the palliative care settings (e.g., anxiety, depression, delirium) that contribute to "despair." We have also examined "meta-diagnostic" sources of despair, including hopelessness, loss of meaning, loss of dignity, demoralization, loss of spiritual well-being, and the results of despair that include a desire for hastened death as well as suicidal ideation.

Palliative care practitioners, along with their mental health colleagues, have always had the sense of responsibility and desire to intervene with these psychiatric, psychosocial, and existential sources of suffering and despair. Fortunately, the clinical science of psychiatric palliative care has advanced to a point where effective methods of assessment and intervention are now available.

In this chapter we will provide an overview of the main sources of psychiatric and psychosocial suffering encountered in palliative care settings, including assessment and management recommendations that would benefit clinicians caring for the terminally ill patients and their families.

Psychiatric Disorders

ANXIETY

Anxiety is a common source of suffering in palliative care settings, and can range from situational anxiety to intolerable anxiety. Often patients are faced with new information or discussion centered around the unknown of their medical illness, which can lead to anxiety. This may be because of fear of dying, fear of medical treatment, fear of anticipated pain, or side effects of medications. Understanding and recognizing anxiety by the physician will allow the patient to be alleviated from the suffering caused by anxiety.

The prevalence of anxiety in palliative care settings has been reported to range from 13% to 28% depending on the population studied and the assessment method used (Derogatis et al., 1983a; Wilson et al., 2007a; Roth and Massie, 2009; Kolva et al., 2011). The Canadian National Palliative Care Survey (Wilson et al.,

2007) found a prevalence of 13.1% anxiety disorders and 20.7% for depressive disorders with frequent comorbidity of depression and anxiety disorders in patients receiving palliative care. Patients with depression and anxiety reported more physical symptoms and worsened quality of life.

Diagnosis of anxiety in palliative care population can be challenging, as these patients at times may endorse this in somatic forms (Roth and Massie, 2009). Somatization of anxiety can take the form of unexplained worsening pain, insomnia, loss of appetite, or increased nausea and vomiting. Indecisiveness or inability to make decisions, which can also be caused by poor concentration, recurrent unpleasant thoughts about cancer, fear of death, and dependency on others are the most common nonsomatic (cognitive or psychological) anxiety symptoms in this population.

The gold standard for diagnosis of anxiety symptoms in palliative care settings is the clinical interview given the complexities in diagnosis caused by physical debilitation and the effects of cancer, cancer treatments, or other supportive medications that present a challenge in assessment of anxiety. Clinical scales are available such as Brief Symptom Inventory (Derogatis and Melisaratos, 1983b), the Hospital Anxiety and Depression Scale (Zigmond and Snaith, 1983), the Rotterdam Symptoms Checklist (De Haes et al., 1990), and the Distress Thermometer (Roth et al., 1998) may be useful in conjunction with the clinician's assessment.

Previous anxiety disorder can be exacerbated in the medically ill, especially panic disorder and posttraumatic stress disorder, from several medical procedures, intensive care unit (ICU) stays or entering magnetic resonance imaging (MRI) machines. Uncontrolled pain, akathisia (inner state of restlessness secondary to medication side effects), or confusional states may present as anxiety. Assessment for suicidality is also important in advanced cancer patients presenting with anxiety particularly in the presence of physical distress such as pain, fatigue, and nausea (Roth and Massie, 2009).

Treatment of anxiety disorders involves psychotherapy, medication management, and treating underlying etiologies such as decreasing medications that exacerbate anxiety symptoms (e.g., glucocorticosteroids, metoclopramide).

Psychotherapy in cancer patients with anxiety may take on a supportive approach focusing on support, and a nurturing role, which can help contain the anxiety patients feel regarding medical settings or death anxiety. This therapy focuses on helping patients' psychological suffering and physical comfort. Patients who are also depressed or delirious may not benefit from psychotherapy unless underlying delirium and depression are managed first. A patient's anxiety can also develop from unknown treatment procedures, prognosis, or expected side effects from treatments received. This population would benefit from candid communication by the physician regarding what to expect when undergoing various treatments and side effects. Relaxation techniques such as mindfulness can help patients in pain and those who are overwhelmed by anxiety. Behavioral interventions, progressive muscle relaxation, and hypnosis have been proved effective in advanced cancer patients with anxiety symptoms (Holland et al., 1991; Roth and Massie, 2009). Cognitive psychotherapy interventions help patients identify their negative thoughts, rehearse impending stressful events, approach the fear of death, and restructure one's expectations for life in palliative care settings (Moorey et al., 1998).

Psychopharmacological management for anxiety in the palliative care population may be a challenge given the medication route, doses, and drug-drug interactions, or its effectiveness in alleviating anxiety in patients (Levin and Alici, 2010). Shorter half-life benzodiazepines can be used to control anxiety and may be beneficial in palliative care patients because they also potentially reduce nausea and vomiting. Excessive use of benzodiazepines may increase the risk of delirium in this population; therefore, it is important to be cautious when using in elderly patients, patients on other central nervous system (CNS) depressant medications, or those with impaired hepatic function, or reduced pulmonary function. Low dose of non-sedating antipsychotics such as haloperidol and atypical antipsychotics such as olanzapine or quetiapine have often been used to reduce anxiety. Selective serotonin reuptake inhibitors can also be used as long-term management; however, given 3 to 4 weeks to obtain symptomatic relief, they may not be suitable for a patient who is suffering at the present time with anxiety (Levin and Alici, 2010).

Relieving anxiety symptoms through use of pharmacological options and/or nonpharmacological interventions is essential to minimize suffering in palliative care settings.

DELIRIUM

Delirium is the most common neuropsychiatric syndrome seen in palliative care settings. Up to 80% of patients with terminal illness develop delirium near death (Breitbart and Alici, 2008). In the palliative care setting, delirium is often the harbinger of impending death. It is distressing for patients, families, and health care professionals.

The *Diagnostic and Statistical Manual of Mental Disorders*, Fourth Edition, Text Revision (DSM-IV-TR, 2000) diagnostic criteria define delirium as a syndrome composed of disturbances of consciousness, attention (i.e., arousal), and cognition, with abrupt onset and fluctuating course, and require that the disturbance be etiologically related to medical causes.

Delirium is classified according to three clinical subtypes, based on either motor or arousal disturbances: hypoactive, hyperactive, and mixed. The *hypoactive* (hypoalert, hypoaroused) subtype is characterized by psychomotor retardation, lethargy, sedation, and reduced awareness of surroundings (Stagno et al., 2004; Spiller and Keen, 2006; Meagher et al., 2007). Hypoactive delirium is often mistaken for depression and is difficult to differentiate from sedation caused by opioids, or obtundation in the last days of life (Stagno et al., 2004). The *hyperactive* (hyperalert, hyperaroused) subtype is more commonly characterized by restlessness, agitation, hypervigilance, hallucinations, and delusions. In the palliative care setting, hypoactive delirium is most common. Hypoactive delirium has generally been found to occur with hypoxia, metabolic disturbances, and anticholinergic medications (Spiller and Keen, 2006; Kiely et al., 2007). Hyperactive delirium is correlated with alcohol and drug withdrawal, drug intoxication, or medication adverse effects (Spiller and Keen, 2006; Kiely et al., 2007; Meagher et al., 2007).

Clinically, the diagnostic gold standard is the clinician's assessment using the *DSM-IV-TR* criteria (American Psychiatric Association, 2000) for delirium. Several delirium screening and evaluation tools have been developed, including the Delirium Rating Scale-Revised 98 (Trzepacz, 1999), Confusion Assessment Method (Inouye et al., 1990), and Memorial Delirium Assessment Scale (Breitbart et al., 1997). In the medically ill, delirium can interfere significantly with the recognition and control of symptoms such as pain.

Delirium causes distress in patients, family members, clinicians, and staff. In a study of 101 terminally ill cancer patients, Breitbart et al. (2002) found that 54% of patients recalled their delirium experience after recovering from the episode. The more severe the episode, the less likely the patient was to recall it, but the presence of hallucinations and delusions made delirium more likely to be recalled and to be reported as distressing. Of note, patients with hypoactive delirium were just as distressed as patients with hyperactive delirium. DiMartini et al. (2007) reported posttraumatic stress disorder in patients who experienced hallucinations and delusions during delirium. These findings highlight the significance of distress and suffering caused by both hypoactive and hyperactive subtypes of delirium and the importance of treating the causes and controlling the symptoms of delirium in both subtypes.

In a study of caregiver distress related to delirium, Breitbart et al. (2002) found that family caregivers and nurses rated their distress to be high. Two-thirds of 300 bereaved Japanese families who participated in a survey (Morita et al., 2004) reported that delirium in their family members was highly distressing. Symptoms that caused the most distress included agitation and cognitive impairment. Caregivers of delirious terminally ill patients have been shown in one study to be 12 times more likely to develop an anxiety disorder than caregivers of nondelirious patients (Buss et al., 2007).

In the medical setting, the diagnostic workup typically includes an assessment of potentially reversible causes. However, when confronted with delirium in the terminally ill or dying patient, the clinician must take an individualized and judicious approach to such testing, consistent with the goals of care.

In the last days of life, the ideal goal of delirium management is a patient who is comfortable, not in pain, awake, alert, calm, cognitively intact, and able to communicate coherently with family and staff. Treatment of the symptoms of delirium (by using both pharmacological and nonpharmacological interventions) should be initiated before, or in concert with, a diagnostic assessment of possible etiologies. When delirium is a consequence of the dying process, the goal of care may shift to providing comfort, minimizing suffering through the judicious use of sedatives, even at the expense of alertness (Breitbart and Alici, 2008).

Nonpharmacological and supportive therapies play an essential role in the treatment and prevention of delirium. Assessment and modification of key clinical factors that may precipitate delirium for persons at risk for delirium, including cognitive impairment or disorientation, dehydration, constipation, hypoxia, infection, immobility or limited mobility, several medications, pain, poor nutrition, sensory impairment, and sleep disturbance, constitute the main components of nonpharmacological intervention trials. Although a study by Gagnon et al. (2012) conducted in terminally ill cancer patients demonstrated no benefit in prevention of delirium, several studies among hospitalized geriatric populations have shown promise (Pitkala et al., 2008; Flaherty et al., 2010).

The American Psychiatric Association (APA, 1999) practice guidelines recommended the use of antipsychotics as the first-line pharmacological option in the treatment of symptoms of delirium. A 2004 Cochrane review (Jackson and Lipman, 2004) on drug therapy for delirium in the terminally ill concluded that haloperidol was the most suitable medication for the treatment of patients with delirium near the end of life, with chlorpromazine being an acceptable alternative. A 2007 Cochrane review (Lonergan et al., 2007) comparing the efficacy and the incidence of adverse effects between haloperidol and atypical antipsychotics concluded that, like haloperidol, selected atypical antipsychotics were effective in managing delirium. None of the antipsychotics were found to be superior when compared with others in the treatment of delirium symptoms, and there is evidence for efficacy in the improvement of the symptoms of delirium for the atypical antipsychotics including olanzapine, risperidone, aripiprazole, and quetiapine (Breitbart and Alici, 2012a).

Clinicians are sometimes concerned that the use of sedating medications may hasten death via respiratory depression, hypotension, or even starvation. However, studies have found that the use of opioids and psychotropic agents in hospice and palliative care settings is associated with longer rather than shorter survival (Lo and Rubenfeld, 2005; Connor et al., 2007; Rietjens et al., 2008). Antipsychotics or sedatives may rarely worsen a delirium by making the patient more confused or sedated. Nevertheless, clinical experience suggests that antipsychotics are both effective and appropriate in the management of agitation, paranoia, hallucinations, and altered sensorium. A wait-and-see approach may be appropriate with some patients who present with a lethargic or somnolent type of delirium or who are having comforting hallucinations. Such an approach must, however, be tempered by the knowledge that a lethargic or hypoactive delirium may very quickly and unexpectedly become an agitated or hyperactive delirium that can worsen the suffering of the patient, family, and staff (Breitbart and Alici, 2008).

DEPRESSION

Depression is prevalent, but underrecognized, underdiagnosed, and undertreated in palliative care settings. This may be caused by multiple aspects, such as expecting patients to feel depressed and regarding this as part of a "normal" reaction to cancer or terminal illness or by not engaging a patient about his or her mood in the chance of coming across a response that is uncomfortable for the physician to handle. It is important to overcome these barriers to assessment and management of depression as even terminally ill depressed patients can be helped with timely recognition and treatment of depressive symptoms. If left untreated, depressive symptoms can not only make it difficult to manage physical distress but also result in significant existential suffering (Wilson et al., 2009). Depressive symptoms are associated with prolonged hospital stays, physical distress, poorer treatment compliance, lower quality of life, increased desire for hastened death, and completed suicide in palliative care settings (Li et al., 2011).

Rates of depression are estimated as high as 40%, whereas rates of depressive spectrum disorders have been found to be as high as 58% depending on the criteria used (Massie, 2004). Wilson et al. (2007a) in their summary of the prevalence literature conclude that approximately 5% to 20% of patients with advanced cancer meet criteria for major depression even when the most stringent criteria are used. An additional 15% to 20% of palliative care patients present with depressive disorders that are less severe; however, this can still present a major source of suffering to patients (Wilson et al., 2009). Hopko et al. (2008) showed that depressive symptoms are associated with more rapidly progressing cancer symptoms, advanced disease, and pain among cancer patients. Depression typically worsens the distress experienced from physical and psychosocial symptoms, and can interfere with effective coping (Weinberger et al., 2010).

The diagnosis of depression is difficult in palliative care settings (Wilson et al., 2009) because the symptoms of cancer and the side effects of treatment overlap with the symptoms of depression. Weight loss, sleep problems, anergia, poor concentration, and thoughts of suicide may be either symptoms of depression or symptoms of advanced illness and/or its accompanying treatment side effects. Major depressive disorder is a treatable condition, which can significantly contribute to a patient's suffering, including a desire for hastened death. In addition to the complexities noted in the preceding in diagnosis of depression in cancer patients, older adults often present with more somatic complaints as opposed to affective complaints when compared with younger adults (Kim et al., 2002; Brodaty et al., 2005; Husain et al., 2005). Depressed mood and loss of pleasure or interest are important in assessment of depression in patients with advanced illness (Roth and Modi, 2003; Spoletini et al., 2008; Weinberger et al., 2009). Almost all patients with advanced illness experience a certain degree of functional decline and disengagement from areas of interest. However, a pervasive anhedonia that extends to loss of interest and pleasure in almost all activities merits considerable attention as an important indicator of depression in palliative care settings (Wilson et al., 2009).

Treatment of depression should encompass combinations of strategies, including psychopharmacology, psychotherapy, particularly addressing existential distress, which in turn improves quality of life. Cognitive behavioral interventions in the form of individual or group psychotherapy have been proved effective in treatment of depressive symptoms in palliative care settings (Spiegel et al., 1981; Wilson et al., 2009). Kissane et al. (2007a) showed that supportive expressive group therapy among advanced breast cancer patients ameliorated and prevented new depressive disorders, reduced hopelessness, and improved social functioning. Targeted and manualized psychotherapies have been developed, including Meaning-Centered Group therapy (Breitbart et al., 2010a), Dignity therapy (Chochinov et al., 2005), Mindfulness-Based Meditation therapy (Ando et al., 2009), and a brief supportive-expressive intervention referred to as Managing Cancer and Living Meaningfully (CALM) (Nissim et al., 2011). As detailed in a *Journal of Clinical Oncology* editorial by Kissane (2007b), despite lack of evidence for prolonged survival with a variety of psychosocial interventions it has been shown through well-designed randomized controlled trials that a variety of psychotherapy interventions are effective in decreasing depressive symptoms and suffering in advanced cancer patients.

Studies of the use of antidepressants in the terminally ill are few in number. Williams and Dale (2006) completed a systematic review of randomized placebo-controlled trials of pharmacological and psychotherapeutic interventions for cancer patients with depression showing mixed results for effectiveness and tolerability of fluoxetine. A study by Stockler et al. (2007) found sertraline not to be helpful in treatment of depressive symptoms among advanced cancer patients. A Cochrane Database review (Gill and Hatcher, 2000) on antidepressants in the treatment of depression in medical illness concluded that there is evidence that antidepressants reduce depressive symptoms in medical settings. The review showed that the number needed to treat depressive symptoms with antidepressants in medically ill patients was four. In other words for one medically ill patient with depression to get relief of depressive symptoms, four medically ill patients had to be treated with an antidepressant. Although there was a trend toward more effectiveness with tricyclic antidepressants in nonrandomized trials, the tolerability of selective serotonin reuptake inhibitors (SSRIs) was better in medically ill depressed patients. Another systematic review of antidepressants in cancer patients concluded that the evidence for effectiveness of antidepressants is limited and that combined approaches, a combination of antidepressants and psychotherapeutic interventions, may be most effective in this population (Rodin et al., 2007).

Psychostimulants have been considered in treatment of depression in advanced cancer patients. Despite the paucity of evidence for antidepressant efficacy, faster onset of action, and improvement in attention, concentration, energy, and mood are the main clinical considerations to initiate treatment with a psychostimulant while monitoring closely for side effects such as anxiety, overstimulation, and confusion (Wilson et al., 2009).

In summary, it is important to note that depression has been associated with significant morbidity and shortened survival in individuals in cancer (Satin et al., 2009; Pinquart and Duberstein, 2010). The psychotherapeutic or combined interventions for depression in advanced cancer patients have revealed mixed survival results; however, it has been well-proved that treatment of depressive symptoms improves quality of life and decreases suffering in palliative care settings (Kissane, 2007b; Li et al., 2012; Pirl et al., 2012)

Psychosocial and Existential Issues

Physicians working with cancer patients are likely to encounter patients and family members facing existential challenges, which fall into multiple domains that may be expressed as various forms of despair or distress. In other words, existential concerns are intrinsic to the human experience of facing mortality in palliative care settings. Recognizing components of existential and psychological distress are important in palliative care settings as treatment targets and areas for intervention. Although we have tools and medications to assess and manage pain, depression, or anxiety, we have not, until recently, begun to have a similar mastery of the assessment and management of psychosocial and existential distress in palliative care settings. More and more clinicians and researchers from different disciplines are beginning to grapple with the issues of despair, demoralization, "desired for hastened death", loss of dignity, and loss of meaning. Interventions are being developed, and tested in controlled randomized trials, and demonstrated to be effective in relieving aspects of despair and distress among terminally ill patients beyond symptom control. Although addressing existential and spiritual issues in terminally ill patients, it is of utmost ethical importance to respect patient's autonomy and be aware of the sensitivity of existential and spiritual values and conflicts for patients. In this next section we explore hopelessness, desire for hastened death, physician-assisted suicide, demoralization, loss of meaning and dignity, all which become clinically relevant manifestations of suffering as a patient moves closer toward death.

HOPELESSNESS

Hope can be defined as a future-oriented outlook and can serve as a defense mechanism that allows a person facing terminal illness or physical illness to cope. If despair is the border between hope and hopelessness, where in this continuum the patient lies can have a significant impact on the physical and emotional well-being of the individual (Kylma et al., 2001).

Hopelessness can arise from physical and existential distress, such as pain, loss of meaning, loss of dignity, and depression. Levine (2007) characterized hopelessness as an embittered, dark state that can lead to feelings of emptiness and despair. Sullivan (2003) conceptualized hopelessness as a form of anticipatory grief that can arise in response to one's own inevitable death. Hopelessness has emerged as one of the strongest predictors of end-of-life decision making regarding issues such as physician-assisted suicide and desire for hastened death, advance directives, and use or requests for life-sustaining interventions (Rosenfeld et al., 2011).

Everson et al. (1996) conducted a longitudinal study of 2,428 middle-aged Finnish men, and demonstrated that individuals with high levels of hopelessness were slower to recover from medical interventions. Anda et al. (1993) found after studying 2,832 American adults that individuals with moderate to severe hopelessness had a 1.6-fold increase in the risk of fatal ischemic heart disease. Watson et al. (2005) in a 10-year follow-up population-based cohort study showed that hopelessness/helplessness within a few weeks of a breast cancer diagnosis had a continuing effect on disease-free survival after 10 years. Depression was not found to have an effect on the 10-year disease-free survival in the same study, highlighting the centrality of assessment and management of hopelessness in cancer patients. Measuring hopelessness in a clinical setting is challenging. Psychiatric patient population scales such as the Beck Hopelessness Scale cannot account for the symptoms that individuals with terminal illness encounter such as imagining an extended future in the context of a poor prognosis.

Rosenfeld et al. (2011), focused on the development and validation of a scale of hopelessness that applies to individuals with terminal illness. The development of the "Hopelessness Assessment in Illness Questionnaire" has considerable potential for helping assess important outcomes, such as the effectiveness of interventions designed to improve psychological adjustment or the impact of psychological states on end-of-life decisions.

Treatment of hopelessness includes psychotherapy modalities such as meaning centered psychotherapy, mindfulness, dignity-conserving therapy, cognitive-existential therapy, supportive-expressive therapy, acceptance and commitment therapy, nurse-facilitated preparation and life completion interventions, and dialectic behavior therapy (Spiegel et al., 1981; Kissane et al., 2004, 2007a; Breitbart et al., 2010a; Chochinov, 2011; Breitbart et al., 2012b; Keall et al., 2012; Sachs et al., 2013). Both individual meaning-centered psychotherapy and meaning-centered group psychotherapy interventions have been shown to improve hopelessness among advanced cancer patients (Breitbart et al., 2010a, 2012b).

DESIRE FOR HASTENED DEATH AND SUICIDE

Suicide and desire for hastened death remain among the most controversial topics in palliative care. Although several studies have explored suicidality and the desire for hastened death in the terminally ill, complex questions remain around the prevalence, assessment, and management of these phenomena (Olden et al., 2009). Physicians in palliative care settings commonly encounter a patient's desire for a hastened death. This desire may range from passive death wishes, contemplating suicide or requesting the physicians' aid in dying sooner. It may be due to patients' suffering having become intolerable. An accelerated end to life may be the only solution that a patient in despair may see. Breitbart et al. (2000) found that 17% of 92 terminally ill patients assessed in a hospice setting had a high desire for hastened death. In a Canadian study of patients with terminal cancer 39.8% of 379 patients stated that they would consider making a request for physician-assisted suicide (Wilson et al., 2007b). It is because of this common occurrence that caretakers should attempt to recognize the underlying issues that drive patients to request this. For people at the end of life, depression, hopelessness, and psychosocial distress are among the strongest correlates of desire for hastened death. Therefore it is important for clinicians to differentiate expressions of a desire for hastened death from suicidal ideation to address patient concerns and intervene appropriately (Olden et al., 2009). A prospective Dutch study in 138 terminally ill cancer patients examined the association between depression and requests for euthanasia. They found that of the 22% of patients who requested euthanasia, 23% were depressed at baseline and 44% of those depressed patients requested euthanasia compared to 15% of the non-depressed. The rate of request for euthanasia for patients with depression was 4.1 times greater than that of patients without depression (Van der Lee et al., 2005).

Breitbart et al. (2000) found a significant association between clinical depression and a desire for hastened death. Patients with depression were four times as likely to desire for hastened death as compared with those who were not depressed (47% vs. 12%). Hopelessness was also a risk factor for the desire for hastened death. Both were independent risk factors; however two-thirds of the patients with both clinical depression and hopelessness were likely to desire a hastened death. In a group of 372 AIDS patients, depression and hopelessness were identified as strong predictors of desire for hastened death (Rosenfeld et al., 2006). In the study by Wilson et al. (2007b), a current desire for hastened death was strongly associated with a diagnosis of major depression, lower religiosity, reduced functional status, and greater distress around physical, social, and psychological symptoms.

In summary depression, hopelessness, loss of autonomy, uncontrolled pain (and symptom burden), poor social support, cognitive impairment (in the form of delirium or other cognitive deficits), history of psychiatric illnesses, and concerns about being a burden to others have been identified as the main risk factors for desire for hastened death and suicide in terminally ill patients (Olden et al., 2009). Existential concerns such as loss of meaning, loss of purpose, loss of dignity, awareness of incomplete life tasks, anxiety around what happens after death merit careful assessment in palliative care settings. Existential concerns and related existential distress not only increase risk for desire for hastened death and suicide but have also been identified as potential areas for intervention to reduce distress in the terminally ill. Patients who present with suicidal ideation, intent, or plans should be assessed urgently as appropriate interventions may be critical.

Despite the increased risk of suicide among terminally ill patients, the prevalence of suicide attempts in patients with terminal illness has not been studied extensively. In a study from Norway examining the data from the Cancer Registry of Norway standard mortality ratios of 1.55 for males and 1.35 for females were identified, respectively (Hem et al., 2004). In a study from Sweden, of the 88 completed suicides among cancer patients, 14 had an uncertain prognosis and 45 had a poor prognosis (Bolund, 1985).

In addition to the risk factors detailed in the preceding for desire for hastened death, a personal and a family history of suicide should be included in assessment of patients presenting with suicidal ideation. Evaluation of the patient's mental state and symptom control for any distressing symptoms are essential. Clinicians should ascertain the reasons underlying suicidal ideation, and the seriousness of suicidal intent. Support systems should be mobilized as much and as soon as possible. In addition to the treatment of underlying factors depending on the suicide risk assessment, an inpatient admission might be required for close supervision and management of distressing symptoms.

It is notable that the completed assisted suicides are rare. Assisted suicides account for 0.2% of all the deaths (including people who weren't terminally ill, such as deaths resulting from accidents) in Oregon or about 1/500 Oregonians who die each year (Quill, 2012). It has been reported that one in six terminally ill Oregonians talk to their families about the possibility of an assisted death, whereas one in 50 talks to his or her physician, and only one in 1,000 terminally ill patients actually dies using the Oregon Death with Dignity Act (Tolle et al., 2004). These findings are supportive of the fact that most terminally ill patients want to talk about their options, but very few ultimately need a medically assisted death even in an environment in which it is legally permissible. Ganzini et al. (2008), in their cross-sectional survey of 58 Oregonians who had either requested aid in dying from a physician or contacted an aid in dying advocacy group, found that 15 patients met "caseness" criteria (i.e., diagnosis based on symptoms as opposed to a constellation of signs and symptoms) for depression. Three of 15 participants met criteria for depression. All three depressed participants died by legal ingestion within 2 months of the research interview. The authors concluded that although most terminally ill Oregonians who receive aid in dying do not have depressive disorders, the current practice of the Death with Dignity Act may fail to protect some patients whose choices are influenced by depression.

Data describing the practice of physician-assisted death in Oregon have been published each year since the law was activated in 1997, and are available online at <http://www.oregon.gov/DHS/ph/pas/>.

Physician-assisted suicide is also legal in the Netherlands, Belgium, and Switzerland, and in the States of Oregon, Washington, and Montana in the United States (Prokopetz and Lehmann, 2012). Physician-assisted suicide remains a much-debated and ethically challenging topic worldwide. In a 2003 study of American Medical Association members, 69% of the members objected to physician-assisted suicide (Curlin et al., 2008), which also appears to be a position officially held by various national and state medical associations. The proponents of legalization of physician assisted-suicide argue that open, legally permitted use of this practice in conjunction with the safeguards of standard palliative care, rigorous informed consent, diagnostic and prognostic clarity, and an independent second opinion by someone with expertise in palliative care would protect terminally ill patients against error, abuse, and coercion. Opponents of physician-assisted suicide argue that the role of the physician in the care of terminally ill patients is to spend the time, expense, and energy to provide excellent physical, psychological, and existential/spiritual interventions; in other words to "care for the dying" as opposed to "aid in dying" (Breitbart, 2010). With advances in pain and physical symptom control, the organization and delivery of palliative care, and the development of effective interventions to manage the emotional despair and existential suffering clinicians are increasingly able to humanely and effectively provide care for the dying that is consistent with goals of preserving life (not prolonging life or hastening death) and protecting patients from harm (Breitbart, 2010). Regardless of the legalization of physician-assisted suicide, the primary goal of the clinician should be to assess the complexity of each case individually with particular attention to underlying depression, hopelessness, and physical distress when faced with these requests.

Evaluating the underlying root cause of the desire for hastened death requires the healthcare provider to engage in the conversation with the patient regarding his or her wishes. He or she must clarify if the patient is having passive death wishes, if the patient is suicidal, or if the patient is exploring options for physician-assisted suicide or death. It is through the physician's empathic listening skills and communication, as well as a strong therapeutic relationship, that underlying reasons for a hastened death can be uncovered and addressed. It is important to be nonjudgmental, and convey to the patient that these topics are completely acceptable for discussion. The healthcare provider should support the patient by working through the process and attempt to problem solve, evaluate the patient for hopelessness, depressive symptoms, anxiety, and delirium, all of which can be addressed. Empathic listening skills from a provider can be a very therapeutic intervention with the patient and should be practiced (Quill 1993). If underlying depression has been detected as the driving force of a desire for hastened death, then it would be important to offer treatment for this psychiatric component. In a study by Breitbart et al. (2010b), patients with advanced AIDS ($N = 372$) were assessed for depression and desire for hastened death. Patients diagnosed with a major depressive syndrome were provided with antidepressant treatment and assessed weekly for depression and desire for hastened death. The study showed that desire for hastened death decreased dramatically in patients whose depression responded to antidepressant treatment. The authors concluded that successful treatment for depression appears to substantially decrease desire for hastened death in patients with advanced AIDS.

Based on a systematic literature review and the opinions of an expert consensus panel, recommendations for assessment and management of desire for hastened death have been summarized as follows (National Health and Medical Research Council Australia, 2003; Hudson et al., 2006; Olden et al., 2009):

◻ Be alert to your own responses as the clinician, be aware of "countertransference" issues and personal fears of death (seek supervision, be aware of how your responses influence communication, and monitor your own attitude).

◻ Be open to hearing concerns and be willing to have the conversation (be alert to verbal and nonverbal distress cues, encourage expression of feelings, actively listen without interrupting, be sensitive to explore the underpinnings of a wish to die, discuss desire for hastened death in patient's own words, acknowledge differences in response to illness).

◻ Assess potential contributing factors (lack of social support, feelings of burden, family conflicts, depression, anxiety, existential concerns, physical symptoms, cognitive impairment).

◻ Respond to specific issues (address modifiable contributing factors, recommend interventions, develop a plan to manage more complicated issues, acknowledge family fears and concerns).

◻ Be clear about what is and is not within one's professional mandate (offer care; eliminate the suffering, not the sufferer; obey the law).

◻ Conclude discussion (summarize and review important points, clarify patient perceptions, provide opportunity for questions, facilitate discussion with others, and provide appropriate referrals).

◻ Assure commitment to ongoing care (nonabandonment).

◻ After discussion, document discussion in medical records and communicate with members of the treatment team.

These recommendations are intended to be flexible guidelines and should take place over time within the context of a trusting relationship. Empathy, active listening, management of realistic expectations, permission to discuss psychological distress, and providing referral to other professionals when appropriate comprise the essential components of a therapeutic response to a desire for hastened death (Olden et al., 2009).

Expressions of desire for hastened death or requests for physician-assisted suicide are always complex, multidetermined, and frequently ambivalent. Physicians do not reliably possess the diagnostic and therapeutic skills needed to care for such patients, particularly those with existential despair, pain, and other physical symptoms. Unfortunately, guidelines don't reliably work to screen out depressed patients. In physician-assisted suicide, choice is not limited to patient choice only. Physicians and the society are obliged to make choices as well. Physicians have a choice in response to requests for physician-assisted suicide by affirming the possibility of meaning, and aligning with the part of the patient that might see the potential for meaning and value even in a diminished state, or agree that the patient's life has no further value and succumb to a shared sense of helplessness, fear, and anger.

DEMORALIZATION

The concept of demoralization is of central importance in the field of palliative care and caring for medically ill patients. Demoralization can be viewed as an inability to cope effectively with stressors.

Demoralization is characterized by loss of meaning and purpose, with helplessness, hopelessness, inability to cope, sense of personal failure, and social isolation (Kissane et al., 2009). The demoralized patient is described as impotent, isolated, despairing, alienated, rejected, and with low self-esteem, merely trying to survive (Frank and Frank, 1993). For medically ill patients, demoralization involves disempowerment and hopelessness. Psychological and social factors contribute to demoralization. Cancer patients often experience their illness as all-consuming and leading to a loss of control, which in turn leads to helplessness and hopelessness (Greer and Watson, 1987). Patients in palliative care settings often experience demoralization, given loss of control, inability to function independently at times, and feeling disempowered. Given this common occurrence it is relevant for physicians to attempt to identify and address underlying demoralization.

Demoralization is conceptualized as a morbid mental state when its distress is persistent, and when the phenomenology involves meaninglessness, helplessness, and hopelessness, with the potential to give up on life and desire death (Kissane et al., 2001). Descriptors used to conceptualize demoralization often blur lines with depressive symptoms; however, there are distinct differences between demoralization and depression. Clarke and Kissane (2002) put forth that anhedonia is not a part of the demoralization phenomenology, whereas it is one of the integral symptoms of depression. Suicidal thinking in demoralized patients is driven by hopelessness and meaninglessness, not by anhedonia.

Younger age, severe physical illness, bodily disfigurement, serious mental illness, social isolation or alienation, poor family cohesiveness, and avoidant coping styles have been associated with the development of demoralization (Kissane, 2001). In palliative care settings, poor self-esteem, cumulative losses, reduced social support, poor symptom management, prominent side effects of cancer treatments, and deteriorating physical health might predispose patients to demoralization (Kissane, 2001).

Once demoralization is recognized in a patient, multiple approaches may improve the patient's state, including continuity of care, symptom management, teasing out the relevant existential issues, inquiring about hope and meaning in a patient's life, cognitive restructuring, addressing spiritual/religious support, including support of family and friends (Kissane et al., 2009). Meaning-centered therapy, dignity-conserving therapies, interpersonal psychotherapy, cognitive behavioral therapy, and life narrative can all be used effectively in treatment of demoralization in palliative care settings (Kissane et al., 2009).

If patients are demoralized because of physical symptoms such as pain or fatigue, then treating these symptoms should be a priority to relieve suffering.

If a patient's symptoms such as depression, agitation, and anxiety persist, then treatment of these components are also helpful and instill hope. The physician's role is primarily a relationship to the patient enveloped in empathy. The ability to serve as a vector of human connection alone can protect a patient from feeling abandoned, even in the setting of incurable disease, in conjunction with symptom relief. It is important to discuss meaning and value in a person's life to help the patient find his or her own version of hope. This can be attained by assessing the existential needs of a patient when building the physician-patient relationship or speaking about goals of care. Psychotropic medications can be considered for co-morbid anxiety or depressive symptoms. Kissane et al. (2009) highlight the importance of restoring hope in patients with demoralization through valuing and affirming the story of their lives, the roles of the patient, their accomplishments, and sources of fulfillment.

LOSS OF MEANING

Meaning or having a sense that one's life has meaning involves the conviction that one is fulfilling a unique role and purpose in a life that is a gift (Breitbart and Appelbaum, 2011). Viktor Frankl, a Holocaust survivor and psychiatrist (Frankl, 1959), defined "meaning" as the manifestation of values that occur through three main paths, including creativity (e.g., work, deeds, dedication to causes), experience (e.g., art, nature, humor, love, relationships, roles), and attitude (one's attitude toward suffering and existential problems). In his seminal book, *Man's Search for Meaning*, Frankl described that "the will to meaning" is an inherent drive to connect with something greater than one's own needs, and through this one finds meaning and self-transcendence, particularly at times of intense psychological and physical suffering (Frankl, 1959). Frankl emphasized that individuals have the right to choose the meaning in their unique existence, referred to as "freedom of will," including their attitude toward suffering (Table 10.1).

A lack of meaning has been closely associated with demoralization, hopelessness, and a desire for hastened death (Breitbart et al., 2000; Kissane et al., 2001). It has been demonstrated that terminally ill patients are able to consider their lives as worth being lived as long as they are able to sustain meaning in their lives; therefore, meaning and search for meaning have become central elements of psychotherapeutic interventions in palliative care settings.

TABLE 10.1

The Sources of Meaning: Achieving Transcendence

Creativity—work, deeds, causes
Experience—nature, art, relationships
Attitude—the attitude one takes toward suffering and existential problems
Legacy—individual, family, community history

Adapted from Breitbart and Appelbaum, 2011.

Meaning-centered therapy, developed by William Breitbart and colleagues (Breitbart and Appelbaum, 2011), has applied the concepts put forth by Viktor Frankl to advanced cancer patients in the group setting and individually. Meaning-centered therapy is designed to help patients with advanced cancer sustain or enhance a sense of meaning, peace, and purpose in their lives as they confront death. Breitbart et al. (2010a) found that meaning-centered group psychotherapy (MCGP) demonstrated significant benefits compared with supportive group psychotherapy (SGP), particularly in the areas of spiritual well-being and enhancing a sense of meaning. Treatment effects were notable for 2 months after treatment ended, and reduced psychological distress. Improvements were noted in hopelessness, desire for hastened death and anxiety, and these treatment effects increased over the 2-month follow-up period. Breitbart et al. (2012) published their findings from a pilot randomized controlled trial of Individual Meaning-Centered Psychotherapy (IMCP) in patients with advanced cancer. Patients with stage III or IV cancer ($N = 120$) were randomly assigned to seven sessions of either IMCP or therapeutic massage (TM). Of the 120 participants randomly assigned, 78 (65%) completed the posttreatment assessment, and 67 (56%) completed the 2-month follow-up. At the posttreatment assessment, IMCP participants demonstrated significantly greater improvement than the control condition for the primary outcomes of spiritual well-being (including both components of spiritual well-being, namely, a sense of meaning and faith), and quality of life. Significantly greater improvements for IMCP patients were also observed for the secondary outcomes of symptom burden and symptom-related distress, but not for anxiety, depression, or hopelessness. At the 2-month follow-up assessment, the improvements observed for the IMCP group were no longer significantly greater than those observed for the TM group.

The authors concluded that IMCP has clear short-term benefits for spiritual suffering and quality of life in patients with advanced cancer; therefore, clinicians working with advanced cancer patients should consider IMCP as an approach to enhance quality of life and spiritual well-being.

Meaning-Centered Psychotherapy: Session Topics and Themes

Session #1: Concepts & Sources of Meaning
* *Introductions to Intervention and Meaning*
Session #2: Cancer & Meaning
* *Identity—Before and After Cancer Diagnosis*
Session #3: Historical Sources of Meaning
* *Life as a Living Legacy (past)*
Session #4: Historical Sources of Meaning
* *Life as a Living Legacy (present-future)*
Session #5: Attitudinal Sources of Meaning
* *Encountering Life's Limitations*

Session #6: Creative Sources of Meaning
  * *Actively Engaging in Life (via: creativity and responsibility)*
Session #7: Experiential Sources of Meaning
  * *Connecting with Life (via: love, beauty, and humor)*
Session #8: Transitions
  * *Reflections and Hopes for Future*

LOSS OF DIGNITY

Patients often experience loss of control, loss of sense of self, feeling demoralized, marginalized, and devalued by the experience of chronic illness and their failing health. Patients often draw upon what they have lost through their suffering and feel a fragmented sense of being. Terminally ill patients struggle with many existential concerns from which significant distress can arise, such as loss of meaning, value, or dignity, which can diminish hope. Dignity is defined as the quality or state of being worthy, honored, or esteemed. In palliative care settings it is essential for patients to feel that they are respected or worthy of respect despite the physical and psychological distress brought about by the illness. Maintaining feelings of physical comfort, autonomy, meaning, spiritual comfort, social connectedness, and courage are also essential components of maintaining dignity in palliative care patients (Chochinov et al., 2002, 2004). A fractured sense of dignity has been found to be associated with increased risk of hopelessness, depression, loss of will to live, and desire for hastened death (Chochinov, 2002).

Chochinov (2002) has designed a novel intervention termed "dignity therapy" to address existential and psychosocial distress among terminally ill patients. This therapy type allows the patient to discuss issues that matter most or that they would most want remembered. Sessions are transcribed and edited, with a returned final version that they can bequeath to a friend or family member. Chochinov et al. (2005) reported that of 100 patients who completed the study, 91% reported feeling satisfied or highly satisfied with the intervention (dignity therapy); with 86% reporting that the intervention was helpful or very helpful. Seventy-six percent indicated that it heightened their sense of dignity and 68% indicated that dignity therapy increased their sense of purpose, and 67% indicated that it heightened their sense of meaning. Forty-seven percent of participants indicated that dignity therapy increased their will to live. Chochinov et al. (2011) reported their findings of the effect of dignity therapy on distress and end-of-life experience in terminally ill patients from a randomized controlled trial. Patients (aged ≥18 years) with a terminal prognosis (life expectancy ≤6 months) who were receiving palliative care in a hospital or community setting (hospice or home) in Canada, the United states, and Australia were randomly assigned to dignity therapy, client-centered care, or standard palliative care. No significant differences were noted in the distress levels before and after completion of the study in the three groups. For the secondary outcomes, patients reported that dignity therapy was significantly more likely than the other two interventions to have been helpful, improve quality of life, increase sense of dignity, change how their family saw and appreciated them, and be helpful to their family. Dignity therapy was significantly better than client-centered care in improving spiritual well-being, and was significantly better than standard palliative care in terms of lessening sadness or depression; significantly more patients who had received dignity therapy reported that the study group had been satisfactory, compared with those who received standard palliative care. Although the ability of dignity therapy to mitigate outright distress, such as depression, desire for death or suicidality, has yet to be proved, its benefits in terms of self-reported end-of-life experiences support its clinical application for patients nearing death.

LOSS OF SPIRITUAL WELL-BEING

Spirituality has been defined as the aspect of humanity that refers to the way individuals seek and express meaning and purpose and the way they experience their connectedness to the moment, to self, to others, to nature, and to the significant or sacred (Puchalski et al., 2009). Spirituality plays an important part in the lives of patients with serious illness. The importance of spiritual well-being and sense of meaning and purpose in life are increasingly recognized by clinicians who care for patients at the end of life. An Institute of Medicine (IOM) report identified spiritual well-being as one of the most important influences on quality of life at the end of life (Field and Cassell, 1997). Despite the paucity of data in this field, there are convincing data that support the essential role of spirituality in people's lives, especially in the context of terminal illness. Implementation of spiritual assessment has been considered to be an ethical mandate in the care of dying patients. Assessment of patient's spiritual beliefs, assessing the importance of spirituality in his or her life, exploring whether he or she belongs to a spiritual community, and offering chaplaincy referral or connection with the patient's religious or spiritual leaders comprise essential components of a spiritual assessment. Terminally patients may experience a number of spiritual issues, including but not limited to lack of meaning, guilt, shame, hopelessness, loss of dignity, loneliness, anger toward God, abandonment by God, feeling out of control, grief, and spiritual suffering. Although management of spiritual issues is more complex than the approach to physical or psychiatric symptoms, the general management principles include a compassionate presence, reflective listening, inquiry about spiritual values and beliefs, life review, and continued presence in addition to referral to chaplaincy (Breitbart, 2009).

SUMMARY

Existential suffering and despair can arise in the palliative care setting from a variety of psychiatric and psychological diagnostic disorders, but clearly meta-diagnostic existential concerns, such as loss of meaning, hopelessness, loss of dignity, demoralization, and even existential guilt experienced by lack of completion of life tasks are sources of despair and suffering that are in the domain of the mental health professional. Mental health palliative care providers, as well as the multidisciplinary palliative care team, now have interventions available to them to effectively intervene with not only the common neuropsychiatric complications of advanced disease, but also the existential sources of despair and suffering that affect us all because we are, after all, all too human. This chapter has attempted to provide an introduction into these areas on psychiatric and psychosocial sources of suffering. Certainly the topic is very broad, complex, and would constitute a text of its own. Ultimately the palliative care clinician must be capable of assessing and treating common psychiatric syndromes in the palliative care setting that, if not managed appropriately, cause suffering. Additionally, a new set of novel existentially oriented interventions are starting to become available to be applied to the palliative care setting. Each is somewhat unique. Perhaps one common principle among all of these novel interventions is the following: The role of the palliative care practitioner is to provide "care." The affirmation that the possibility of experiencing, rediscovering, or creating meaning exists with a cancer illness, even in the last days of life is at the heart of psychiatric, psychosocial, and existential palliative care.

References

American Psychiatric Association. (1999). Practice guideline for the treatment of patients with delirium: American Psychiatric Association. Am J Psychiatry. 156:1–20.

American Psychiatric Association. (2000). Diagnostic and Statistical Manual of Mental Disorders, 4th ed., Text Rev. Washington, DC: American Psychiatric Association.

Anda R, Williamson D, Jones D, Macera C, Eaker E, Glassman A, Marks J. (1993). Depressed affect, hopelessness, and the risk of ischemic heart disease in a cohort of U.S. adults. Epidemiology. 4:285–94.

Ando MT, Morita T, Akechi T, et al. (2009). The efficacy of mindfulness-based meditation therapy on anxiety, depression, and spirituality in Japanese patients with cancer. J Palliat Med. 12:1091–4.

Breitbart W. (2009). The spiritual domain of palliative care: who should be "spiritual care professionals"? Palliat Support Care. 7(2):139–41.

Breitbart W. (2010). Physician-assisted suicide ruling in Montana: struggling with care of the dying, responsibility, and freedom in Big Sky Country. Palliat Support Care. 8(1):1–6.

Breitbart W, Alici Y. (2008). Agitation and delirium at the end of life: "We couldn't manage him." JAMA. 300(24):2898–910.

Breitbart W, Alici Y. (2012a). Evidence-based treatment of delirium in patients with cancer. J Clin Oncol. 30(11):1206–14.

Breitbart W, Appelbaum A. (2011). in eds Watson M, Kissane D. Handbook of Psychotherapy in Cancer Care, Meaning-Centered Group Psychotherapy, 1st ed. New York: Wiley-Blackwell, pp 137–48.

Breitbart W, Gibson C, Poppito S, Berg A. (2004). Psychotherapeutic interventions at the end of life: a focus on meaning and spirituality. Can J Psychiatry. 49:366–72.

Breitbart W, Gibson C, Tremblay A. (2002). The delirium experience: delirium recall and delirium related distress in hospitalized patients with cancer, their spouses/caregivers, and their nurses. Psychosomatics. 43(3):183–94.

Breitbart W, Poppito S, Rosenfeld B, Vickers AJ, Li Y, Abbey J, Olden M, Pessin H, Lichtenthal W, Sjoberg D, Cassileth BR. (2012b). Pilot randomized controlled trial of individual meaning-centered psychotherapy for patients with advanced cancer J Clin Oncol. 30(12):1304–9.

Breitbart W, Rosenfeld B, Gibson C, Pessin H, Poppito S, Nelson C, Tomarken A, Timm A, Berg A, Jacobsen C, Sorger B, Abbey J, Olden M. (2010a). Meaning-centered group psychotherapy for patients with advanced cancer: a pilot randomized controlled trial. Psycho-oncology. Jan 19 (1):21–8.

Breitbart W, Rosenfeld B, Gibson C, Kramer M, Li Y, Tomarken A, Nelson C, Pessin H, Esch J, Galietta M, Garcia N, Brechtl J, Schuster M. (2010b). Impact of treatment for depression on desire for hastened death in patients with advanced AIDS. Psychosomatics. 51(2):98–105. doi:10.11.

Breitbart W, Rosenfeld B, Pessin H, et al. (2000). Depression, hopelessness, and desire for hastened death in terminally ill patients with cancer. JAMA. 284:2907–11.

Breitbart W, Rosenfeld B, Roth A, Smith MJ, Cohen K, Passik S. (1997). The Memorial Delirium Assessment Scale. J Pain Symptom Manage. 13(3):128–37.

Brodaty H, Cullen B, Thompson C, et al. (2005). Age and gender in the phenomenology of depression. Am J Geriatr Psychiatry 13(7): 589–96.

Buss MK, Vanderwerker LC, Inouye SK, Zhang B, Block SD, Prigerson HG. (2007). Associations between caregiver-perceived delirium in patients with cancer and generalized anxiety in their caregivers. J Palliat Med. 10(5):1083–92.

Cassel EJ. (1982). The nature of suffering and the goals of medicine. N Engl J Med. 306(11):639–45.

Chochinov HM. (2002). Dignity-conserving care—a new model for palliative care: helping the patient feel valued. JAMA. 287(17):2253–60.

Chochinov HM, Hack T, Hassard T, Kristjanson LJ, McClement S, Harlos M. (2004). Dignity and psychotherapeutic considerations in end-of-life care. J Palliat Care. 20(3):134–42.

Chochinov HM, Hack T, McClement S, Kristjanson L, Harlos M. (2002). Dignity in the terminally ill: a developing empirical model. Soc Sci Med. 54(3):433–43.

Chochinov HM, Hack T, Hassard T, et al. (2005). Dignity therapy: a novel psychotherapeutic intervention for patients near the end of life. J Clin Oncol. 23:5520–5.

Chochinov HM, Kristjanson LJ, Breitbart W, McClement S, Hack TF, Hassard T, Harlos M. (2011). Effect of dignity therapy on distress and end-of-life experience in terminally ill patients: a randomised controlled trial. Lancet Oncol. 12(8):753–62.

Clarke DM, Kissane DW. (2002). Demoralization: its phenomenology and importance. Aust NZ J Psychiatry. 36:733–42.

Connor SR, Pyenson B, Fitch K, Spence C, Iwasaki K. (2007). Comparing hospice and nonhospice patient survival among patients who die within a three-year window. J Pain Symptom Manage. 33(3):238–46.

Curlin FA, Nwodim C, Vance JL, Chin MH, Lantos JD. (2008). To die, to sleep: US physicians' religious and other objections to physician assisted suicide, terminal sedation, and withdrawal of life support. Am J Hosp Palliat Care. 25:112–20.

De Haes J, van Knippedberg F, Neijut J. (1990). Measuring psychological and physical distress in cancer patients: structure and application of the Rotterdam Symptom Checklist. Br J Cancer. 62:1034–8.

Derogatis L, Melisaratos N. (1983b). The brief symptom inventory: an introductory report. Psychol Med. 13:595–605.

Derogatis L, Morrow GR, Fetting J, et al. (1983a). The prevalence of psychiatric disorders among cancer patients. JAMA. 249:751–75.

DiMartini A, Dew MA, Kormos R, McCurry K, Fontes P. (2007). Posttraumatic stress disorder caused by hallucinations and delusions experienced in delirium. Psychosomatics. 48(5):436–9.

Everson SA, Goldberg DE, Kaplan GA, Cohen RD, Tuomilehto J, Salonen JT. (1996). Hopelessness and risk of mortality and incidence of myocardial infarction and cancer. Psychosom. Med. 58:113–21.

Field MJ, Cassell CK (eds) (1997). Approaching death: improving care at the end of life. (Institute of Medicine report). Washington, DC: National Academy Press.

Flaherty JH, Steele DK, Chibnall JT, et al. (2010). An ACE unit with a delirium room may improve function and equalize length of stay among older delirious medical inpatients. J Gerontol A Biol Sci Med Sci. 65:1387–92.

Frankl VF. (1959/1992). Man's search for meaning, 4th ed. Boston: Beacon Press.

Frank JD, Frank JB. (1993). Persuasion and healing: a comparative study of psychotherapy, 3rd ed. Baltimore: Johns Hopkins University Press.

Gagnon P, Allard P, Gagnon B, et al. (2012). Delirium prevention in terminal cancer: assessment of a multicomponent intervention. Psychooncology. 21:187–94.

Ganzini L, Goy ER, Dobscha SK. (2008). Prevalence of depression and anxiety in patients requesting physicians' aid in dying: cross sectional survey. BMJ. 337.

Gill D, Hatcher S. (2000). Antidepressants for depression in medical illness. Cochrane Database Syst Rev. (4):CD001312. Review. Update in: Cochrane Database Syst Rev. (4):CD001312.

Greer S, Watson M. (1987). Mental adjustment to cancer: its measurement and prognostic importance. Cancer Surv. 6:439–58.

Hem E, Loge JH, Haldorsen T, Ekeberg Ø. (2004). Suicide risk in cancer patients from 1960 to 1999. J Clin Oncol. 22(20):4209–16.

Holland JC, Morrow GR, Schmale A, Derogatis L, Stefanek M, Berenson S, Carpenter PJ, Breitbart W, Feldstein M. (1991). A randomized clinical trial of alprazolam versus progressive muscle relaxation in cancer patients with anxiety and depressive symptoms. J Clin Oncol. 9(6):1004–11.

Hopko DR, Bell JL, Armento ME, et al. (2008). The phenomenology and screening of clinical depression in cancer patients. J Psychosoc Oncol 26(1):31–51.

Hudson PL, Schofield P, Kelly B, Hudson R, O'Connor M, Kristjanson LJ, Ashby M, Aranda S. (2006). Responding to desire to die statements from patients with advanced disease: recommendations for health professionals. Palliat Med. 20(7):703–10.

Husain MM, Rush AJ, Sackeim HA, et al. (2005). Age-related characteristics of depression: a preliminary STAR*D report. Am J Geriatr Psychiatry. 13(10):852–60.

Inouye SK, Vandyck C, Alessi C, Balkin S, Siegal AP, Horwitz RI. (1990). Clarifying confusion: the confusion assessment method, a new method for the detection of delirium. Ann Intern Med. 113(12):941–8.

Jackson KC, Lipman AG. (2004). Drug therapy for delirium in terminally ill patients. Cochrane Database Syst Rev. 2:CD004770.

Jaspers K. (1955). Reason and existenz. trans William Earle. New York: Noonday Press.

Keall RM, Butow PN, Steinhauser KE, Clayton JM. (2012). Nurse-facilitated preparation and life completion interventions are acceptable and feasible in the Australian palliative care setting: results from a phase 2 trial. Cancer Nurs. [Epub ahead of print].

Kiely DK, Jones RN, Bergmann MA, Marcantonio ER. (2007). Association between psychomotor activity delirium subtypes and mortality among newly admitted postacute facility patients. J Gerontol A Biol Sci Med Sci. 62(2):174–9.

Kierkegard S, Hong H, Hong E. (1983). Fear and trembling/repetition. Princeton, NJ: Princeton University Press.

Kim Y, Pilkonis PA, Frank E, Thase ME, Reynolds CF. (2002). Differential functioning of the Beck depression inventory in late-life patients: use of item response theory. Psychol Aging. 17(3):379–91.

Kissane D, Clarke D, Street A. (2001). Demoralization syndrome: relevant psychiatric diagnosis for palliative care. J Palliat Care 17:12e21.

Kissane DW, Grabsch B, Clarke DM, Smith GC, Love AW, Bloch S, Snyder RD, Li Y. (2007a). Supportive-expressive group therapy for women with metastatic breast cancer: survival and psychosocial outcome from a randomized controlled trial. Psychooncology. 16(4):277–86.

Kissane DW, Love A, Hatton A, Bloch S, Smith G, Clarke DM, Miach P, Ikin J, Ranieri N, Snyder RD. (2004). Effect of cognitive-existential group therapy on survival in early-stage breast cancer. J Clin Oncol. 22(21):4255–60. Epub 2004 Sep 27.

Kissane DW. (2007b). Letting go of the hope that psychotherapy prolongs cancer survival. JCO 5689–90.

Kissane DW, et al. (2009). in eds Chochinov H, Breitbart W. Handbook of psychiatry in palliative medicine, dignity, meaning, and demoralization: emerging paradigms in end-of-life care, 2nd ed. New York: Oxford University Press, pp 101–12.

Kolva E, Rosenfeld B, Pessin H, Breitbart W, Brescia R. (2011). Anxiety in terminally ill cancer patients. J Pain Symptom Manage. 42(5):691–701.

Kylma J, Vehvilainen-Julkunen K., Lahdevirta J. (2001). Hope, despair, and hopelessness in living with HIV/AIDS: a grounded theory study. J Adv Nurs. 33:764–75. doi:10.1046/j.1365- 2648.2001.01712.x.

Levin T, Alici Y. (2010). in eds. Holland et al. Psycho-oncology, anxiety disorders. New York: Oxford University Press.

Levine R. (2007). Treating idealized hope and hopelessness. Intl J Group Psychother. 57:297–317. doi:10.1521/ijgp.2007.57.3.297.

Li FR. (2012). Evidence-based treatment of depression in patients with cancer. JCO 1187–96.

Li M, Boquiren V, Lo C, et al. (2011). in eds Davis M, Feyer P, Ortner P, et al. Supportive oncology, depression and anxiety in supportive oncology, 1st ed. Philadelphia: Elsevier, pp 528–40.

Lo B, Rubenfeld G. (2005). Palliative sedation in dying patients: "we turn to it when everything else hasn't worked." JAMA. 294(14):1810–6.

Lonergan E, Britton AM, Luxenberg J, et al. (2007). Antipsychotics for delirium. Cochrane Database Syst Rev 2:CD005594.

Massie MJ. (2004). Prevalence of depression in patients with cancer. J Natl Cancer Inst Monogr. (32):57–71.

Meagher DJ, Moran M, Raju B, et al. (2007). Phenomenology of delirium: assessment of 100 adult cases using standardised measures. Br J Psychiatry. 190:135–41.

Moorey S, Greer S, Bliss J, Law M. (1998). A comparison of adjuvant psychological therapy and supportive counselling in patients with cancer. Psychooncology. 7(3):218–28.

Morita T, Hirai K, Sakaguchi Y, Tsuneto S, Shima Y. (2004). Family-perceived distress from delirium-related symptoms of terminally ill cancer patients. Psychosomatics. 45(2):107–13.

National Health and Medical Research Council Australia. (2003). Clinical Practice Guidelines for the Psychosocial Care of Adults with Cancer.

Nissim R, Freeman E, Lo C, et al. (2011). Managing Cancer and Living Meaningfully (CALM): a qualitative study of a brief individual psychotherapy for individuals with advanced cancer. Palliat Med [epub ahead of print].

Olden et al. (2009). in eds Chochinov H, Breitbart W. Handbook of psychiatry in palliative medicine, suicide and desire for hastened death in the terminally ill, 1st ed. New York: Oxford University Press, pp 101–12.

Pinquart M, Duberstein PR. (2010). Depression and cancer mortality: a meta-analysis. Psychol Med. 40:1797–810.

Pirl, Greer, Traeger, et al. (2012). Depression and survival in metastatic non–small-cell lung cancer: effects of early palliative care. JCO 1310–5.

Pitkala KH, Laurila JV, Strandberg TE, et al. (2008). Multicomponent geriatric intervention for elderly inpatients with delirium: Effects on costs and health related quality of life. J Gerontol A Biol Sci Med Sci. 63:56–61.

Prokopetz JJ, Lehmann LS. (2012). Redefining physicians' role in assisted dying. N Engl J Med. *367*(2):97–9.

Quill TE. (1993). Doctor, I want to die. Will you help me? JAMA. 270:870–3.

Quill TE. (2012). Physicians should "assist in suicide" when it is appropriate. J Law Med Ethics. 40(1):57–65.

Rietjens JA, van Zuylen L, van Veluw H, van der Wijk L, van der Heide A, van der Rijt CC. (2008). Palliative sedation in a specialized unit for acute palliative care in a cancer hospital: comparing patients dying with and without palliative sedation. J Pain Symptom Manage. 36(3):228–34.

Rodin G, Katz M, Lloyd N, Green E, Mackay JA, Wong RK. (2007). Treatment of depression in cancer patients. Curr Oncol. 14(5):180–8.

Rosenfeld B, Breitbart W, Gibson C, Kramer M, Tomarken A, Nelson C, Pessin H, Esch J, Galietta M, Garcia N, Brechtl J, Schuster M. (2006). Desire for hastened death among patients with advanced AIDS. Psychosomatics. 47(6):504–1276/appi. psy.51.2.98.

Rosenfeld B, Pessin H, Lewis C, Abbey J, Olden M, Sachs E, Amakawa L, Kolva E, Brescia R, Wein S, Breitbart W. (2011). Assessing hopelessness in terminally ill cancer patients: development of the Hopelessness Assessment in Illness Questionnaire. Psychol Assess. 23:325–36.

Roth AJ, Kornblith AB, Batel-Copel L, Peabody E, Scher HI, Holland JC. (1998). Rapid screening for psychologic distress in men with prostate carcinoma: a pilot study. Cancer. 82(10):1904–8.

Roth A, Massie MJ. (2009) in eds Chochinov H, Breitbart W. Handbook of psychiatry in palliative medicine, anxiety in palliative care, 2nd ed. New York: Oxford University Press, pp 69–80.

Satin JR, Linden W, Phillips MJ. (2009). Depression as a predictor of disease progression and mortality in cancer patients: a meta-analysis. Cancer 115:5349–61.

Spiegel D, Bloom JR, Yalom I. (1981). Group support for patients with metastatic cancer: a randomized outcome study. Arch Gen Psychiatry. 38:527–33.

Spiller JA, Keen JC. (2006). Hypoactive delirium: assessing the extent of the problem for inpatient specialist palliative care. Palliat Med. 20(1):17–23.

Spoletini I, Gianni W, Repetto L, Bria P, Caltagirone C, Bossù P, Spalletta G. (2008). Depression and cancer: an unexplored and unresolved emergent issue in elderly patients. Crit Rev Oncol Hematol. 65(2):143–55.

Stagno D, Gibson C, Breitbart W. (2004). The delirium subtypes: a review of prevalence, phenomenology, pathophysiology, and treatment response. Palliat Support Care. 2(2):171–9.

Stockler MR, O'Connell R, Nowak AK, Goldstein D, Turner J, Wilcken NR, Wyld D, Abdi EA, Glasgow A, Beale PJ, Jefford M, Dhillon H, Heritier S, Carter C, Hickie IB, Simes RJ. (2007). Zoloft's effects on symptoms and survival time trial group. Effect of sertraline on symptoms and survival in patients with advanced cancer, but without major depression: a placebo-controlled double-blind randomised trial. Lancet Oncol. 8(7):603–12.

Sullivan MD. (2003). Hope and hopelessness at the end of life. Am J Geriatr Psychiatry. 11:393–405.

Tolle SW, et al. (2004). Characteristics and proportion of dying Oregonians who personally consider physician-assisted suicide. J Clin Ethics. 15:111–18.

Trzepacz PT. (1999). The Delirium Rating Scale: its use in consultation-liaison research. Psychosomatics. 40(3):193–204.

van der Lee ML, van der Bom JG, Swarte NB, Heintz AP, de Graeff A, van den Bout J. (2005). Euthanasia and depression: a prospective cohort study among terminally ill cancer patients. J Clin Oncol. 23(27):6607–12. Epub 2005 Aug 22.

Watson M, Homewood J, Haviland J, Bliss JM. (2005). Influence of psychological response on breast cancer survival: 10-year follow-up of a population-based cohort. Eur J Cancer. 41(12):1710–4.

Weinberger MI, Roth AJ, Nelson CJ. (2009). Untangling the complexities of depression diagnosis in older cancer patients. Oncologist 14(1):60–66.

Weinberger MI, Whitbourne SK. (2010). Depressive symptoms, self-reported physical functioning, and identity in community-dwelling older adults. Ageing Int. 35(4):276–85.

William S, Dale J. (2006). The effectiveness of treatment for antidepressant/depressive symptoms in adults with cancer: a systematic review. Br J Cancer 94(3):372–90.

Wilson KG, Chochinov HM, McPherson CJ, Skirko MG, Allard P, Chary S, Gagnon PR, Macmillan K, De Luca M, O'Shea F, Kuhl D, Fainsinger RL, Karam AM, Clinch JJ. (2007b). Desire for euthanasia or physician-assisted suicide in palliative cancer care. Health Psychol. 26(3):314–23.

Wilson KG, Chochinov HM, Skirko MG, Allard P, Chary S, Gagnon PR, Macmillan K, De Luca M, O'Shea F, Kuhl D, Fainsinger RL, Clinch JJ. (2007a). Depression and anxiety disorders in palliative cancer care. J Pain Symptom Manage. 33(2):118–29.

Wilson KG, et al. (2009). in eds Chochinov H, Breitbart W. Handbook of psychiatry in palliative medicine, diagnosis and management of depression in palliative care, 2nd ed. New York: Oxford University Press, pp 39–68.

Yalom ID. (1980). *Existential psychotherapy.* New York: Basic Books.

Zigmond A, Snaith R. (1983). The hospital anxiety and depression scale. Acta Psychiatr Scaninavia. (67):361–70.

11

Capacity and Shared Decision Making in Serious Illness

Ronald M. Epstein and Vikki A. Entwistle

> ... *a large acquaintance with particulars often makes us wiser*
> *than the possession of abstract formulas, no matter how deep*
> (James, 1902)

Clinicians who are committed to whole-person care generally wish to find ways to promote effective interventions (those that research has shown are likely to secure benefit and avoid harm) and also to respect individual patients' needs, values, and preferences to the greatest degree possible. These desires reflect the ethical principles of beneficence ("What's best for this patient?"), nonmaleficence ("How can I avoid harming this patient"), and respect for autonomy ("How can I help this patient live life on his or her own terms?"). Yet, in the context of advanced and life-limiting illness, there are important challenges to achieving these goals, particularly when patients have limited capacity to reason and participate actively in discussions about their care.

In situations of serious illness for which palliative care is—or is likely to become—appropriate, diagnostic and prognostic information is often complex, clinical options and their risks and benefits are often uncertain, and the patient's values and goals of care sometimes only come into focus as the situation evolves. The patient's cognitive capacity may wax and wane, depending on fatigue, emotional overload, his or her clinical conditions, and medications. Family members are often involved in decision making, yet it can be difficult for clinicians to tell to what degree other people are enabling or undermining the patient's autonomy. Patients' and family members' desire for choice and autonomy may also vary.

In this chapter we explore these challenges and consider a range of approaches to promote collaborative decision making with seriously ill patients. The first section considers the characteristics of decisions in palliative care. The second section examines factors that influence patient involvement in decisions. The third section considers social aspects of decision making—how clinicians, family members, friends, and online communities can enhance or limit patients' autonomy. The fourth section focuses on decisions involving patients with severely limited capacity to participate in decisions regarding their care, considering the principles underlying different forms of surrogacy. The fifth section addresses ways in which effective communication can help resolve ethical problems in palliative care. The chapter concludes with some recommendations for clinical practice.

The Characteristics of Decisions in Palliative Care: Ethical Dilemmas and Ethical Problems

All difficult situations faced by patients with serious illness and their families potentially have ethical ramifications. These are more likely to be recognized as "ethical issues" when someone perceives some kind of conflict or tension. Conflict or tension can arise when the various parties involved in the patient's care assign different levels of importance to competing values (e.g., comfort and longevity; alertness and symptom control) or particular healthcare options. These parties might include patients, families/friends, members of the healthcare team, regulatory bodies and/ or payers. In addition, these parties might themselves feel torn among competing views and perspectives.

Ethical issues can be viewed as dilemmas or problems (Gracia, 2001). Taking a "dilemmatic" view, situations are seen as involving a choice between two or more incompatible options, and the task is to pick the "best" answer. For example, clinicians might wonder, should they follow a patient's previously stated wishes to avoid prolonged life support or follow the wishes of the patient's appointed healthcare proxy, who insists that this exceptional circumstance warrants mechanical ventilation? A dilemmatic view assumes that all options are known, discrete, mutually exclusive, and unlikely to change over time (at least before a new situation emerges for which a separate decision will be needed). Taking this view, the clinician can engage in a decision analysis that combines the clinical evidence and the patient's preferences for the options and their likely outcomes. Ultimately the task is seen as that of identifying which of the available options is "best."

Many discussions of shared decision making reflect a dilemmatic view of decision situations. But palliative care situations often do not comport with a dilemmatic approach. These might be better conceptualized as "problems" (Gracia, 2001). Choices need to be made (some action needs to be taken), but the options are not all immediately and clearly known, discrete, or mutually exclusive. This can be illustrated with the case of Ruth.

CASE PRESENTATION

Ruth, a retired nurse, is hospitalized with advanced emphysema and worsening shortness of breath, so much so that she has some difficulty talking. Because of the effort of breathing, Ruth is extremely fatigued. She wakens when spoken to, but drifts off to sleep a minute or two later. During a similar previous episode of shortness of breath, she spent 2 weeks in the intensive care unit intubated with ventilator support.

Recognizing that intensive interventions may impose burdens incommensurate with her values and goals, one clinician presents Ruth with a dichotomous choice between "ventilator" and "no ventilator," interpreted by her nurse as "doing everything" and "making you comfortable." Some patients might be able to choose between these options, but Ruth is not. As Ruth develops greater awareness of her situation, she indicates that she fears prolonged life support, does not want to suffer and yet does not want to "give up" quite now. Ruth wants to see a particular grandchild who cannot arrive for 2 days. She expresses discomfort both with "doing everything" and with "comfort care." Different members of her care team then offer additional options: one proposes a "trial of intubation" that would be reconsidered after an agreed time (Quill & Holloway, 2011), and another proposes BiPAP (mechanical ventilation that is less invasive but also has lower potential for life prolongation). It is clarified that with any of these options, she could be given a small amount of morphine with the hope of achieving an acceptable level of comfort while maintaining alertness. Ruth elects a trial of BiPAP and morphine. She also makes clear that if her heart were to stop, she would not want to be resuscitated.

After her grandson's visit, Ruth becomes more withdrawn. She says she is "tired" of BiPAP but cannot focus sufficiently to answer other questions about her care. She appears uncomfortable, and accepts higher doses of morphine to control her shortness of breath. Her family suggests stopping the BiPAP when it appears that she is deriving no further benefit in terms of quality of life and it is merely prolonging her death.

DISCUSSION

In this case, the clinicians initially constructed dilemmatic-type choices for Ruth. But it became clear that they need not have done so. The options they presented first were unduly limited (Wirtz, Cribb, & Barber, 2006). Ruth was constrained to either "doing everything" or "providing comfort care only." Other relevant options and goals could have been mentioned.

Because the options are not all always known at the outset, clinicians may need to "muddle through" these situations (Lindblom, 1959). They will base their decisions on intermediate outcomes, recognizing that these are provisional and iterative; goals might only come into focus as clinicians, patients, and families interpret the evolving situation and intermediate outcomes, and identify the next sets of possible courses of action. To share decision making with patients and family members (to the extent that this is possible and desired), clinicians need to help them to interpret how the situation might be changing, and allow new goals to come into focus (e.g., in Ruth's case, to relieve suffering even when it involves sedation).

Experienced clinicians need a capacity to improvise and construct new options when the situation does not fit readily within dilemmatic and decision analytic ways of thinking. Aristotle recognized this capacity as an aspect of *phronesis,* or practical wisdom (Aristotle, 2009). Clinicians who practice with phronesis can navigate the best possible course of action in a particular situation in a particular context at a particular time—all the while recognizing that in other contexts and at other times, a similar clinical presentation might require different actions. When we think about palliative care situations as problem situations and recognize the value of practical wisdom, we can acknowledge that although ethical principles might provide general guidance, the territory is at least partially unknown and there might be more than one ethically reasonable path through it.

Ruth's situation also illustrates that options need not be presented as inseparable "packages" such as "doing everything" or "comfort care." For example, choosing mechanical ventilation does not oblige either acceptance or refusal of cardiac resuscitation. To individualize care, the possibilities for unpacking options should be examined to support the identification of courses of action most concordant with each patient's goals, context, and situation.

In serious illness, potentially salient information can be vast, complex, and uncertain and (in part) distressingly absent. Questions about how to present information and options to patients arise even when clinicians consider only those options that will clearly be available. It is sometimes assumed that providing patients with "full" information about each option is a prerequisite for shared decision making and an ethical mandate for clinicians. But there is no guarantee that when a clinician provides "full" information a patient will become "fully informed." And the goal of a "fully informed" patient is particularly elusive—and perhaps inappropriate—in serious illness (Epstein, Korones, & Quill, 2010). The case of Gloria can illustrate this.

CASE PRESENTATION

Gloria is a 47-year-old engineer with advanced heart failure. She reported a worsening cough to her primary care physician, and an x-ray and subsequent CT scan revealed massive enlargement of the lymph nodes adjacent to her lungs. The diagnostic possibilities included sarcoidosis, lymphoma, and carcinoma. Sarcoidosis is a benign condition that generally carries a good prognosis when managed with steroid medications. Lymphoma is more serious; there are dozens of types of lymphoma, each with different prognoses. Many chemotherapy options might be incompatible with Gloria's heart failure regimen. Carcinoma with nodal involvement carries a poor prognosis.

During the consultation in which the CT scan results were presented, Gloria and her partner had numerous questions about the treatment options for each of the three diagnostic possibilities and their subsets. Her primary care physician wondered how much information to provide and when about these options.

DISCUSSION

In Gloria's and similar cases, it may be ethically correct and desirable to adopt an incremental approach recognizing that providing too much information might lead to confusion and distraction from more pressing issues. To engage in decision making, the clinician should first help the patient understand whether there is a pressing need to establish a firm diagnosis, provide some basic information about each of the diagnostic possibilities, and promise more information and discussion once the situation is clearer and the next stage in the course of action can be considered.

Finally, clinicians do have to be cognizant of the ways in which a patient's options can be constrained by nonclinical issues, such as insurance regulations, finances, and distance from medical centers (Meier & Morrison, 2002). Questions about whether and how these constraints should be discussed with patients or family members are complex and challenging (Entwistle, Sheldon, Sowden, & Watt, 1998). Honesty might generally be a good policy. Patients who are told about locally unavailable or expensive options can sometimes mobilize resources to access them. However, an attempt to inform may backfire by engendering false hope and unnecessary distress. This represents another problem situation that requires practical wisdom to help steer a reasonable course.

Psychological Aspects of Preferences and Decision Making

Having briefly reviewed the characteristics of decision situations in palliative care, we now turn to the psychological aspects of these situations, focusing particularly on issues relating to patients' preferences and the ways that patients' family, friends, and clinicians influence courses of action. Bob's case illustrates some of the issues that can arise.

CASE PRESENTATION

Bob was a 52-year-old craftsman and a practicing Buddhist. He was recovering well from extensive surgery to remove a highly aggressive but localized malignant melanoma, and had completed an advance directive stating that he did not want "extraordinary measures" if his disease were to progress and he were to become incapacitated.

Two months later, after a 2-week subtle cognitive decline, Bob had a severe headache and was diagnosed with a solitary brain metastasis. A neurosurgeon told Bob and his wife that a prognosis of a few weeks could be potentially extended to a few months with surgery. Bob agreed to have surgery, although he was somewhat passive in the decision-making process. It was not clear whether his passivity was caused by emotional terror, tumor-related cognitive compromise, and/or power differentials between himself and the neurosurgeon. He improved after surgery and his thinking cleared.

A few weeks later, Bob became more fatigued and a brain scan revealed a second metastatic lesion. Bob opted for further treatment, this time with stereotactic radiosurgery. After the procedure, he enrolled in a home hospice program; saying that he had "come to terms," and that he wanted a peaceful "death with dignity."

A few weeks later still, Bob felt "fuzzy" and returned to the neurosurgeon for follow-up. The surgeon offered a high-risk procedure on the first metastasis that had re-grown. At the prompting of his wife, Bob agreed to surgery. He dis-enrolled from hospice, and tolerated the procedure well with improved cognition.

Within a few weeks, Bob became aloof and passive, and his wife increasingly made decisions on his behalf. He never asked for prognostic information and when information was offered, he quickly changed the topic. After two more procedures with minimal improvement he was told that the best course at this point was to "wait and see." He re-enrolled in hospice, and died at home 3 weeks later.

DISCUSSION

In this scenario, Bob's (and his wife's) treatment preferences and ideas about the goals of his care changed several times. As with many patients with advanced cancer, his trajectory of decision making was "erratic" and nonlinear (de Kort, Pols, Richel, Koedoot, & Willems, 2010). For example, he opted for more and less aggressive care at different points in his disease trajectory. This is partially because the salience of each option also changed; surgery and radiosurgery were used first to increase longevity and then to improve mental clarity.

Bob's changing cognitive and affective states played a role in his desire for information, understanding of risk and uncertainty, clarification of goals of treatment and the ways decisions were made. Bob, like many others, faced with serious illness, experienced cognitive difficulties owing to disease factors (e.g., cerebral metastases), emotional reactions (e.g., terror, helplessness), and the care environment (Cassell, 1982; Greenberg, Pyszczynski, & Solomon, 1986; Cassell, Leon, & Kaufman, 2001). In the presence of these factors, provision of large amounts of disease and treatment-related information may paradoxically overwhelm him and undermine his ability to participate in decision making (Hoffman, 2005; Peters & Dieckmann, 2007). And, unlike Gloria, who was seeking information, Bob was not; he may feel assaulted by information, potentially further undermining his self-trust and ability to participate in decision making and his trust that his clinicians can respect and work with him (McCleod, 2002). Yet, shared understanding is critical.

The majority of patients with advanced cancer receiving palliative chemotherapy falsely believe that it is likely to substantially extend life and many believe that the treatment is potentially curative (Weeks et al., 2012). These misconceptions limit the degree to which patients can exercise their autonomy. Clinicians often struggle about what to say to patients when the prognosis is poor regardless of treatment. In this case, Bob was offered a "wait-and-see" approach. Saying "wait and see" rather than acknowledging a very limited prognosis is ethically tenuous. Such an approach requires that the clinician balance respecting a patient's desire not to know his prognosis, avoiding deception and ensuring that the patient make decisions based on sufficient understanding. Although Bob chose hospice at this point, other patients might not if they had an inaccurate understanding of the situation.

Cognitive and emotional overload can impair information processing and decision making in a variety of ways. People experiencing such overload may have greater difficulty understanding risks and benefits of different options. They are more susceptible to framing and ordering effects and tend to simplify complex issues, become less flexible, and make hasty decisions.

People experiencing cognitive overload may also have greater difficulty managing the uncertainties that are intrinsic to serious illness (Epstein et al., 2007; Epstein & Street, 2007a,b). Uncertain situations are those in which all options are not known and probabilities cannot be expressed with precision (Volz & Gigerenzer, 2012). Cognitive neuroscience provides some clues about why managing uncertainty is so difficult. There is growing evidence that decision making relies on two parallel systems or processes. The first system or process involves emotions, gut feelings, intuitions, and rules of thumb. It operates relatively quickly and is often called the heuristic system. This system is a double-edged sword. People who cannot engage these affective aspects of decision making often make poor decisions (Damasio, 1994; Gigerenzer, 2007; Evans, 2008). Yet, unexamined affect can also lead peoples' reasoning astray.

The second system involves the kind of deliberative reasoning that is associated with standards of logic. It is often called the "analytic" system, and is invoked, for example, when clinicians or patients are encouraged to adopt formal decision analytic steps such as assigning numerical probabilities and values to the possible outcomes of several different options. These kinds of steps can often help decision making, but quickly become unmanageable when many of the probabilities and values are missing or unclear.

Conditions involving uncertainty and cognitive overload can affect both systems. They tend to impair peoples' ability to regulate their emotional reactions that otherwise might be informative. They limit the extent to which people appreciate how their emotions are affecting their decisions (Meier & Morrison, 2002). They also impair reasoning ability (de Neys, 2006).

Furthermore, cognitive overload impairs people's ability to imagine the future and to underestimate their ability adapt to unforeseen circumstances. Consequently, patients may "mis-imagine the unimaginable" (Ubel, Loewenstein, Schwarz, & Smith, 2005), for example, their ability to enjoy quality of life after a colostomy for cancer. Clinicians can offer correctives to patients' unchallenged beliefs about their adaptability and resilience, and through introducing curiosity and uncertainty, help decision making to be more completely informed (Epstein, 2012; Epstein & Gramling, 2012). For this reason, patients' provisional decisions should not necessarily be taken at face value until it is clear that they are sufficiently informed. To promote autonomy in these circumstances, clinicians should provide cognitive and emotional support to help patients and families avoid premature closure, and effectively engage in effective deliberation and explore their feelings.

Given the dynamic nature of clinical situations, options, emotions, and social influences in palliative care settings, it is not surprising that patients' preferences for interventions, including care at the end of life, frequently change. For example, more than one-third of patients change their end-of-life preferences even when their clinical condition is stable, and more do so when additional information is provided about their condition (Fagerlin & Schneider, 2004; Fried, O'Leary, Van, & Fraenkel, 2007). Importantly, physicians, family members, and patients themselves cannot reliably identify who will have stable preferences and who will not. One explanation of this "preference instability" has to do with the distinction between global values and situation-specific values (Fischhoff, 1991; Schneiderman, Pearlman, Kaplan, Anderson, & Rosenberg, 1992). Consider Julia's situation.

CASE PRESENTATION

During her entire adult life, Julia, a successful businesswoman, would say to family members when seeing incapacitated people obviously suffering from neurocognitive disorders, "I'd never want to live like that," and "If I get that way, shoot me." Her healthcare proxy and living will reflect these wishes. Now at age 80, Julia has slowly progressive Parkinson's disease; she requires a wheelchair for distances greater than 30 feet, occasionally drools, and has mild dementia which is noticeable only to close friends and family. Yet, she maintains an independent existence, still works part time, and maintains an active social life. She now has pneumonia, potentially reversible with intubation and antibiotics. She clearly opts for hospitalization, and would want to be resuscitated if she could have a good chance of returning to her current baseline.

DISCUSSION

In Julia's case, her global values—not wanting to live in a severely impaired state—tended to remain stable, but they lacked the specificity to inform decisions in previously unimagined situations. Until she was actually in the situation, she could not imagine being quite impaired yet still enjoying a good quality of life.

Finally, in some situations, patients' preferences may appear to be at odds with their stated values (Fischer & Arnold, 1994), sometimes referred to as "mis-wanting." First, consider a patient with advanced cancer who is offered fourth-line "palliative" chemotherapy. The patient is told that treatment may improve quality of life in 10% of patients, may involve some side effects in up to 30%, and is not intended to prolong life. The patient's stated goal is a "death with dignity," yet he requests the treatment. Second, consider a patient with chronic pain. She states a goal of pain relief and acknowledges that her pain is uncontrolled, yet is reluctant to increase her pain medications (Falzer et al., 2012). In both situations, accepting the patient's stated preference at face value—to proceed with fourth-line chemotherapy or not to increase pain medications—might seem to be "respecting the patient's autonomy." However, deeper exploration might reveal factors contributing to the patient's acceptance or refusal of treatment. Patients often have unchallenged beliefs about prognosis or the benefits of treatment (Weeks et al., 2012). They may not have considered palliative options or may be acquiescing to social pressure. Patients commonly refuse pain medications because of stoicism, or fear—of stigmatization, addiction, or acknowledging that the disease is progressing. Deliberation might help them seek more detailed information about the benefits and risks of particular treatments and reconsider their goals of care. Reflective questions (Table 11.1) can challenge patients to explore their beliefs and values (Schei, 2006), enhance patients' self-awareness (Meyers, 1989), their ability to access and interpret gut feelings (Gigerenzer, 2007), and improve their ability to forecast how they might feel about a decision (Halpern & Arnold, 2008; Wilson & Gilbert, 2010). Exploring patients' reasoning in a collaborative and respectful way can also help make explicit the conditions under which preferences might change, and ultimately promote their *phronesis* and autonomy (Emanuel & Emanuel, 1992).

Ethical Reflections on the Roles of Clinicians, Family, and Friends in Decision Making

Social influences become more important as illness advances; patients become more reliant upon and may be more easily influenced by the input of others (Emanuel et al., 1999). In Bob's case, his wife took greater responsibility for decisions when Bob was more cognitively compromised. At times she helped him to organize his thinking, facilitating deliberations among the patient, physician, and family; at other times, when he was more disengaged and passive, she assumed a role of surrogate decision maker and it was not always clear whether her decisions reflected his values or her own.

This case raises a strong and widely shared concern that decisions should be shaped primarily by what matters to individual patients themselves. This concern is associated with the concept of personal autonomy, and the biomedical-ethical principle of respect for autonomy. In this section, we explain the difference between individualistic and relational views of autonomy, and consider how relational views can help clinicians assess the appropriateness of their own and family members' roles in decisions about patients' care.

TABLE 11.1

Clarifying and Reflective Questions

Enhancing patients' self-awareness

"Right now, what's most important to you?"
"Who knows you the best? What would they say about the current situation? Do you agree with that?"
"Putting it all together, how do you think you'll feel about this decision in a month or two?"
"Do you usually make decisions by yourself, or do you talk things over with someone else? Who would that be?"

Exploring conditions under which preferences might change

"What if I could find a medication that did not make you sleepy or constipated?"
"Do you feel that taking these medications is a sign of weakness?"
"Are you considering this medication because you believe it is the best approach?"

The concept of personal autonomy refers to a widely held value that each person should be able to be his or her own person and live life on his or her own terms rather than under the control of others. When considered in this broad sense, personal autonomy is relatively easy to "get" as a concept, and readily recognized as "a good thing." But the questions of what people need to "achieve" personal autonomy, how we can tell whether someone is autonomous, and how we can respect and promote other people's autonomy present notoriously difficult philosophical and practical challenges. However, equating personal autonomy with highly independent individual choice (particularly strong in North American culture) and action can be problematic (Mackenzie & Stoljar, 2000). Our personal values, ideas, and ways of reasoning about how we would like to live our lives are often strongly influenced by our past and present social situations, cultures, and relationships, even if we can't clearly recognize those influences. We therefore need to question whether and how it is meaningful to think that any of our values, choices, or actions can be considered our "own."

An important set of alternative "relational" ways of thinking about personal autonomy can be very helpful for clinicians who are concerned to respect or support patients' autonomy (Mackenzie, 2008; Entwistle, Carter, Cribb, & McCaffery, 2010). Relational accounts of autonomy vary, but all emphasize the significance of interactions with other people (interdependence) and de-emphasize individual independence. Clinicians taking a relational view would consider how social influences—past and present—might support or undermine a person's capability to have a voice in the clinical decisions that affect their lives. The question of which values, choices, or actions are genuinely a person's own remains difficult, but relational accounts stress that an individual's capability for autonomy is socially shaped and guide us to distinguish autonomy-supporting from autonomy-undermining social influences.

Taking a relational view, friends, family, and clinicians can be autonomy-supportive when they help the patient to recognize and articulate their needs and values, and when they offer their perspectives in ways that allow the patient to remain in the driver's seat while being enabled to craft and articulate their preferences (Entwistle, Cribb, & Watt, 2012). This kind of support can be particularly important when patients are weakened, frightened, or overwhelmed by illness. To varying degrees, research suggests that supportive others actually can help patients think through complex situations, identify possibilities and intermediate goals, recall important information, break down the complexity into digestible chunks, sound out and refine their views, and feel more confident about making or contributing to decisions (Meegan & Berg, 2002a).

The term "collaborative cognition" is used to express the notion that an individual's decision making results from interdependent thinking processes; thinking is shared in such a way that the solution to a problem is not uniquely his or her own (Meegan & Berg, 2002b; Rapley, 2008). Collaborative cognition can involve patients, family members, clinicians, and others. Relational understandings of autonomy allow us to recognize that if those others are appropriately supportive, patients' autonomy need not be "lost" during collaborative cognition or reasoning processes. The concept of "shared mind"—in which ideas and perspectives have emerged from the interactions among two or more individuals (Zlatev, Racine, Sinha, & Itkonen, 2008)—goes one step further by including affective resonance as well as cognition. In fact, "shared mind" can strengthen autonomy and help extend range of ways in which people weakened by illness can be enabled to have a voice (Epstein & Street, Jr., 2011).

Relational understandings of autonomy can refresh thinking about the biomedical-ethical principle of respect for autonomy and its application in palliative care contexts. The principle is conventionally considered with a focus on autonomous choices (Beauchamp & Childress, 2001)—choices that are given some thought (rather than made habitually and without reflection) and made with sufficient information or understanding and with sufficient freedom from controlling influence. This definition is often taken in combination with the kind of dilemmatic view of decision situations considered in the first section of the chapter. As a result, clinicians who want to share decisions tend to inform patients about their (limited number of) options and then let them choose, or elicit their preferences and ensure these shape the decision. However, we have noted that reliance on patients' expressed preferences can be difficult and problematic. Thus, we consider it an ethical obligation of clinicians to provide patients not only with information, but also with adequate support through the decision situations they face. The (especially North American) cultural idealizations of self-sufficient responsible individuals are often unrealistic for patients with serious illness. If they are simply informed about their treatment options and then expected to choose among them without recommendations or support, such patients are particularly likely to feel "abandoned to their rights to choose" (Davies & Elwyn, 2008). Even when people understand the information they are given about options, they may lack confidence in expressing their views, struggle with conflicting priorities, be fearful of disappointing their physician, or worry about blaming themselves for making the wrong choice if things do not go well (Adams, Elwyn, Legare, & Frosch, 2012; Frosch, May, Rendle, Tietbohl, & Elwyn, 2012).

These observations call upon clinicians to re-conceptualize their roles and the roles of family members and friends with regard to patient decision making. Clinicians may, for example, need to offer information, opinions, and recommendations about options while empowering and enabling patients to engage in deliberation that might generate novel and creative solutions to complex problems. Given the importance to most people of family relationships, clinicians might also need to facilitate the achievement of at least some degree of shared mind. Communication to promote shared mind might include discussing and agreeing on what issues are of greatest importance; involving helpful others; sharing relevant information without overloading everyone with unnecessary details; seeking to appreciate the patient's perspectives or affective state; and confirming with the patient (if possible) or others, that any agreed course of action reflects the patient's values to the best of everyone's knowledge.

Surrogacy, Including Advance Directives

In the previous sections, we acknowledged that seriously ill patients' capacity to participate in their own care varies. Here, we consider surrogacy—situations when others make decisions on the patient's behalf while attempting to respect the wishes and autonomy of patients whose capacity is severely impaired and who are quite unable to participate directly in decisions regarding their care.

Patients can lack capacity in varying ways and to different degrees, and their lack can be temporary or permanent. Young children, people with moderate dementia or cognitive disabilities, those with mental illness, and those who are unable to talk can often understand aspects of their illnesses and express wishes that should be respected, even if they lack the fuller capacity to make decisions that depend on a deeper understanding of the situation. Importantly, physicians should not underestimate what capacities patients do have, and should be aware of their own reasons for considering that a patient might lack full decision-making capacity. Stereotypical judgments and difficulties with communication sometimes may lead them to invoke surrogacy inappropriately for patients whose culture or health beliefs differ from their own. Particular care is needed that physicians do not invoke lack of capacity to avoid difficult discussions with the patient and turn to (possibly easier) discussions with a family member.

Ethical issues can arise when subjective factors influence how and when surrogacy is invoked. Clinicians may have a strong sense of "normal practice." That is, they might assume that all patients would "naturally" want a particular option or assume that they understand patients' values; thus, information from family members and others might not be sought. Often surrogacy is only enacted when no realistic life-extending options exist, or only when there is a conflict between the physician's treatment recommendations and the stated desires of a patient with questionable capacity.

Beauchamp and Childress describe three standards for surrogate decision making: substituted judgment; "pure autonomy"; and best interest approaches (Beauchamp & Childress, 2001). We outline each and discuss their ethical ramifications in the following.

SUBSTITUTED JUDGMENT

A principle of substituted judgment is invoked when a trusted relative or friend is appointed to make decisions on the patient's behalf. The appointment is sometimes documented as a legally recognized health care proxy or power of attorney (Bomba, 2011). The appointed persons are tasked with choosing what patients themselves would want if they could speak for themselves—not what the surrogate decision makers would want for themselves in a similar situation and not necessarily what they would generally consider to be in the patient's best interest.

Although the general principles of substituted judgment are clear, in practice substitute judgments can be hard to make. Psychologically, surrogates may find it difficult to distinguish their own values from those of the patient. They might preferentially recall those instances when the patient expressed values concordant with their own and forget those in which their views were discordant. Yet the personal knowledge that friends and relatives can bring to a clinical situation often improves on the knowledge that a clinician might have about the patient's wishes. Furthermore, even if there is one appointed surrogate, other family members and friends are often involved in discussions about the appropriate course of action. If these discussions result in a coherent consensus about how the patient might have responded to the current situation, this potentially represents the patient's wishes and interests more adequately than the surrogate alone could do. It takes considerable skill to navigate such discussions if there is distress or discord in the family, but efforts to bring together various perspectives are ethically justified because they foster a broader understanding of the patient and their context.

"PURE AUTONOMY" APPROACHES, INCLUDING PHYSICIAN ORDERS FOR LIFE-SUSTAINING TREATMENTS AND LIVING WILLS

"Pure autonomy" approaches are so called because they attempt to enable patients to direct their own care even when they are no longer able to express their wishes directly (Beauchamp & Childress, 2001). They involve some kind of advance specification and documentation of the patient's preferences—for example in the form of Physician Orders for Life Sustaining Treatments (POLST) and living wills. These documents attempt to capture patients' clearly expressed advance wishes that can be enacted without relying on the (presumably imperfect) input of their family members, friends, and clinicians.

CASE PRESENTATION

Dwayne was a 51-year-old machinist when he had a catastrophic neurological injury caused by an automobile accident while intoxicated. On the first day, he weakly squeezed a family member's hand; thereafter, his neurological function deteriorated and he became completely unresponsive to voice or touch. On a New York State Health Proxy Form, Dwayne's son was his designated surrogate; in addition, on the form, Dwayne had checked a box indicating that he did not wish to have extraordinary measures if his situation was hopeless or with little or no chance for recovery. All of his family members described him as valuing his independence. He had recently witnessed the death of another relative, and stated that if he "ended up like this" he would not want "all those machines to keep me alive."

Dwayne's son consulted reputable websites that suggested that neurological recovery after trauma can take up to 30 days to manifest. A neurologist indicated that improvement would be very unlikely, but that there have been cases of recovery after a few weeks of unresponsiveness if there was not further deterioration during that time. Consultants differed on their definition of recovery, some focusing on re-appearance of brainstem reflexes, and others focusing on ability to interact meaningfully with others.

Even though there was no sign of improvement in neurological functioning, his surrogate and several other family members interpreted Dwayne's wishes to justify a 30-day trial of mechanical ventilation after which they would decide. The ICU team, however, interpreted Dwayne's prior statements to indicate that life support should be stopped; "recovery" would almost definitely mean a minimally conscious or severely impaired state that the patient indicated he would not want. An ethics consultation was called, and the son reiterated his wishes, which were contested by some family members and supported by others. At 30 days, with no improvement evident, the family instructed the care team to stop ventilator support and focus on comfort measures only.

DISCUSSION

Dwayne's situation illustrates ways in which the implementation of advanced care planning can be complex and contentious, even when the patient and others had thought that his prior wishes were stated clearly. Dwayne had appointed a surrogate and also indicated directives regarding specific wishes for his care should he lack capacity. Yet, the surrogate argued that this specific situation was one that the patient could not have anticipated and he deserves every reasonable chance to recover, whereas in the eyes of the clinical team and some family members, the patient's wishes were clearly stated and applicable to the current situation, and were not being heeded by the surrogate. Dwayne's situation points out some important limitations to living wills, and other means of providing enduring and clear representations of patients' wishes should they lose decision-making capacity.

Living wills have proved problematic in other ways. Even with strong encouragement from clinicians, living wills are completed rarely. Even when living wills have been completed and are available, they have had surprisingly little influence on clinical care (Haidet et al., 1998; Fagerlin & Schneider, 2004). Statements in living wills are usually general and made when the patient is healthy. These often cannot account for unanticipated unique features of each specific situation. Vague language, such as "extraordinary measures," is subject to interpretation. In some dire circumstances such as Dwayne's, a very small percentage of patients can experience some recovery, so no situation is truly hopeless. Furthermore, patients rarely update living wills, and one-third of patients change their preferences over time, leaving clinicians and family to wonder whether values expressed several years previously still apply (Fried et al., 2007). In practice, many clinicians use living wills after the fact to justify decisions that have largely been made, but do not use them to guide those choices in real time.

Recognizing these challenges, there have been attempts to create clearer, more comprehensive living will documents using a series of case scenarios to discern patients' thresholds for aggressive care (Doukas & McCullough, 1991). Although thoughtfully constructed, these scenarios can take a long time to complete, patients find them difficult, and many patients' preferences change even within a 2-month period of stable health (Schubart et al., 2012). Although some patients use living wills as a catalyst for useful discussions of their values and preferences, until they have proved to affect clinical care, the authors do not favor targeting resources to the completion of living wills, preferring instead to focus on naming surrogates and on providing more specific instructions when the patient's clinical condition warrants them.

One means for providing more explicit situation-specific instructions is a POLST document. Usually created by patients who are already seriously ill, they document specific treatments that patients have said that they do or do not want (e.g., resuscitation, intubation, hospitalization, antibiotics, and artificial hydration and nutrition) and, unlike hospital DNR orders, are valid in inpatient, outpatient, and home settings. Because they are supposed to be completed and re-evaluated during serious illness episodes, they can be relatively up to date representations of patients' wishes. Physician Orders for Life-Sustaining Treatments can also be created by healthy people (in Oregon, after age 75) or surrogates. In the latter case they would best be considered as examples of substituted judgment or best interest approaches.

"BEST INTEREST" STANDARDS

Situations frequently arise in which decisions must be made for patients who have lost capacity and have no advance directives and whose wishes and values in this domain are unknown. These situations can occur for patients who have been socially isolated, who have no living relatives, who have communication difficulties, or who have been estranged from their families. In these circumstances, decisions can only be guided by a "best interest" standard—what most people would choose who have a full understanding of the situation under the same set of circumstances. Like substituted judgment and pure autonomy standards, best interest should also consider the dignity and uniqueness of each person, the likelihood that interventions might improve the patient's health or functioning and relief of the patient's suffering. In these circumstances, clinicians should not shy away from limiting burdensome treatments for which the possible benefits in terms of survival or quality of life are marginal at best; for example, clinicians should advocate for comfort care for someone with irreversible brain injury and widely metastatic cancer. Situations in which the patient never had the capacity to reason and participate in decisions (e.g., profound intellectual disability since birth, severe autism) are subject to complex legal protections to prevent undertreatment. Discussion of these cases is beyond the scope of this chapter.

Effective Communication

Although many of the ethical issues around decision making in serious illness are nuanced and complex, in our view most of the resolution of ethical problems lies in good communication—that which addresses real issues in an ongoing way with patients and the people who matter to them. Physicians typically do a poor job of communicating prognosis, engaging in discussions about advance directives, and assessing patients' beliefs and values (Tulsky, Fischer, Rose, & Arnold, 1998). Understanding the illness and the context, recognizing disagreements, engaging in give-and-take deliberations, and committing to achieving consensus in an evolving situation often generate greater wisdom than the application of abstract principles and rules. Particularly important is not assuming that mutual understanding has occurred. False consensus can be avoided by asking the patient and relevant others to state their understanding and at that point to reconcile differences and bring ethical problems and ethical dilemmas into sharper relief.

Clinicians, patients, and families have many opportunities to address many of these issues prospectively. Patients with serious illnesses are frequently accompanied to visits by family members. Ethical practice also includes emotional preparation for unpredictable, harsh and unanticipated crises, and promising individualized care, presence, and compassion. Clinicians can pre-empt some of the inevitable angst raised by these situations by preparing patients and their families for difficult moments and difficult dialogues by indicating that "there will come a point when we will have to consider..." a particular option or conundrum (Perkins, 2007). Such discussions can engage family members explicitly by preparing them for a potential decision-making role in the patient's care. It is important to balance hope ("We're hoping for the best...") and predictability ("...and some of the hurdles we have are predictable...") with the realistic possibility of an uncertain future ("...but sometimes unexpected things can happen and we'd have to make a decision quickly...") and the need for surrogate decision making ("...and it's important that I have some guidance about what to do.") (Back, Arnold, & Quill, 2003). At critical points in evolving clinical situations, better-prepared patients may be more able to express their wishes about their desired level of input into and responsibility for decisions. Such discussions may also avoid patients feeling bludgeoned with information and decision-making burdens that they do not want (Davies & Elwyn, 2008). This is not to say that such discussions are easy or pleasant. In fact, patients may seem more satisfied when clinicians collude in avoiding unpleasant truths (Weeks et al., 2012); but the consequences of deception or avoidance can result in poor decisions and distrust (Fallowfield, Jenkins, & Beveridge, 2002).

Physician self-awareness of their own distress is important; avoidance of emotional topics is common (Morse, Edwardsen, & Gordon, 2008; Pollak et al., 2010), and linked to physician discomfort, feelings of inadequacy and "empathic distress" (Halpern, 2001; Larson & Yao, 2005). Becoming more mindful can help physicians "turn towards dissonance" (Makowski & Epstein, 2012), develop resilience, and yet remain psychologically present in the face of suffering (Cassell, 1982; Epstein, 1999).

Discussions of prognosis and advance directives in the context of palliative care consultations have shown some promise in averting inappropriately aggressive care, and improving both quality and quantity of life (Temel et al., 2007). Strong patient-physician relationships can provide the scaffolding for such discussions, but do not substitute for them—physicians are not particularly accurate in their predictions of patients' advance care wishes, and family members are often inaccurate as well. Although such discussions are essential, clinicians should recognize that values and preferences may change when people are confronted with serious illness.

Evidence favors a two-step approach (Bomba, Kemp, & Black, 2012). First, people should designate a surrogate or proxy while healthy so that the authority for decision making is clear. This designation should be accompanied by a discussion of general values and preferences that might guide the surrogate's decision. The second step occurs when the person is diagnosed with a serious illness. This step should include a discussion among the patient, relevant family members, and friends, and the patient's clinical care team to understand the patient's wishes and complete a POLST document. Research on the use of POLSTs produced like this suggests that they are generally enacted appropriately in both hospital and nonhospital settings (Bomba et al., 2012).

Some seriously ill patients do not wish to discuss prognosis, diagnosis, and/or treatment options at all, and in some cultures, such discussions are considered inappropriate (Blackhall, Murphy, Frank, Michel, & Azen, 1995; Carrese & Rhodes, 2000; Kagawa-Singer & Blackhall, 2001; Frank et al., 2002), because of beliefs that patients would be harmed in some way. These views should be explored and respected if they are clearly held by the patient, whether or not the patient belongs to a culture that supports those beliefs; patients have rights not to know and to defer decisions to family members. "Consensual surrogacy"—the patient permitting and even directing that others make decisions on her behalf—is ethically acceptable under these circumstances. We take the view that all clinical encounters are cross-cultural. Yet, it is a mistake to assume that all members of a culture share a particular set of values; individuals often have differing views. To probe these issues, a clinician might ask, "People have different feelings about how to talk about their illness. What would be your preference—talk with you alone, with you and your family, or just with your family?" Discretion, cultural brokerage, and practical wisdom should guide the content and timing of such inquiries.

Conversely, surrogacy sometimes is enacted tacitly or explicitly when patients still do have capacity and desire to participate in decisions regarding their care. In these situations family members "speak for" or "speak as" the patient (Mazer, Cameron, DeLuca, Mohile, & Epstein, 2012) and thus may derail the patient's involvement in care, so-called "pseudo-surrogacy." We have observed several examples of pseudo-surrogacy in conversations relating to prognosis and treatment choices in seriously ill patients. In one such example, a physician addressed a patient about hospice. Before the patient could answer, a family member interrupted "speaking for" the patient saying, "we're not ready for that…"; the clinician never clarified if the patient actually agreed with the family member's statement (Mazer et al., 2012). Although we actively support family members' involvement in care, and often such involvement is helpful, clinicians have an obligation to ascertain with the patient, if possible, that family members and friends are supporting and not undermining their autonomy. This may involve speaking to the patient separately from the family; sometimes passive patients are reluctant to contradict what their family members have suggested, even if they disagree.

Conclusion

In this chapter, we have attempted to provide a broader and more nuanced description of the nature of ethical concerns in decisions faced by patients and families confronting serious illness. We have also characterized the exercise of autonomy as an interactional process that often depends on the input of and facilitation by others. Respect for autonomy relates to more than decision making; it is about enabling patients to engage meaningfully in care. Similarly, although a two-step approach is a practical protocol to anticipate possible scenarios in which a patient could not express and enact his or her wishes, enacting surrogate decision making requires flexibility and imagination, not just following rules. Ethical mandates thus go beyond simply supplying information about options and asking patients and their families to choose. Clinicians can help to enable patients and their families to achieve the skills, opportunities, self-confidence, and trusting relationships within which their voices can be heard.

Acknowledgments

We wish to thank Bill Ventres, MD, PhD, who offered very helpful critique of a draft of this manuscript, and Carol Moulthroup for her assistance with editing and formatting.

References

Adams, J. R., Elwyn, G., Legare, F., & Frosch, D. L. (2012). Communicating with physicians about medical decisions: a reluctance to disagree. *Arch. Intern. Med.*, *172*(15), 1184-6. doi:10.1001/archinternmed.2012.2360.

Aristotle (2009). *The Nicomachean Ethics/Aristotle,* translated by David Ross, revised *with an introduction and notes* by Leslie Brown. New York: Oxford University Press.

Back, A. L., Arnold, R. M., & Quill, T. E. (2003). Hope for the best, and prepare for the worst. *Ann. Intern. Med., 138*, 439–43.

Beauchamp, T. & Childress, J. (2001). *Principles of Biomedical Ethics*, 5th ed. New York: Oxford University Press.

Blackhall, L. J., Murphy, S. T., Frank, G., Michel, V., & Azen, S. (1995). Ethnicity and attitudes toward patient autonomy. *Jama, 274*, 820–5.

Bomba, P. (2011). Landmark legislation in New York affirms benefits of a two-step approach to advance care planning including MOLST: a model of shared, informed medical decision-making and honoring patient preferences for care at the end of life. *Widener Law Rev., 17*, 475.

Bomba, P. A., Kemp, M., & Black, J. S. (2012). POLST: an improvement over traditional advance directives. *Cleveland Clin. J. Med., 79*, 457–64.

Carrese, J. A. & Rhodes, L. A. (2000). Bridging cultural differences in medical practice. The case of discussing negative information with Navajo patients. *J. Gen. Intern. Med., 15*, 92–6.

Cassell, E. J. (1982). The nature of suffering and the goals of medicine. *N. Engl. J. Med., 306*, 639–45.

Cassell, E. J., Leon, A. C., & Kaufman, S. G. (2001). Preliminary evidence of impaired thinking in sick patients. *Ann. Intern. Med., 134*, 1120–3.

Damasio, A. R. (1994). *Descartes' Error: Emotion, Reason, and the Human Brain*. New York: G. P. Putnam's Sons.

Davies, M. & Elwyn, G. (2008). Advocating mandatory patient "autonomy" in health-care: adverse reactions and side effects. *Health Care Anal., 16*, 315–28.

de Kort, S. J., Pols, J., Richel, D. J., Koedoot, N., & Willems, D. L. (2010). Understanding palliative cancer chemotherapy: about shared decisions and shared trajectories. *Health Care Anal., 18*, 164–74.

de Neys, W. (2006). Dual processing in reasoning: two systems but one reasoner. *Psychol. Sci., 17*, 428–33.

Doukas, D. J. & McCullough, L. B. (1991). The values history. The evaluation of the patient's values and advance directives. *J. Fam. Pract., 32*, 145–53.

Emanuel, E. J. & Emanuel, L. L. (1992). Four models of the physician-patient relationship. *Jama, 267*, 2221–6.

Emanuel, E. J., Fairclough, D. L., Slutsman, J., Alpert, H., Baldwin, D., & Emanuel, L. L. (1999). Assistance from family members, friends, paid care givers, and volunteers in the care of terminally ill patients. *N. Engl. J. Med., 341*, 956–63.

Entwistle, V. A., Carter, S. M., Cribb, A., & McCaffery, K. (2010). Supporting patient autonomy: the importance of clinician-patient relationships. *J. Gen. Intern. Med., 25*, 741–5.

Entwistle, V. A., Cribb, A., & Watt, I. S. (2012). Shared decision-making: enhancing the clinical relevance. *J. R. Soc. Med, 105*, 416–21.

Entwistle, V. A., Sheldon, T. A., Sowden, A., & Watt, I. S. (1998). Evidence-informed patient choice. Practical issues of involving patients in decisions about health care technologies. *Int. J. Technol. Assess. Health Care, 14*, 212–25.

Epstein, R. M. (1999). Mindful practice. *Jama, 282*, 833–9.

Epstein, R. M. (2013). Whole mind and shared mind in clinical decision-making. *Patient Educ. Couns., 90*(2), 200–6.

Epstein, R. M. & Gramling, R. E. (2012). What is shared in shared decision making? Complex decisions when the evidence is unclear. *Med. Care Res. Rev., 70*(1), 94–112.

Epstein, R. M., Hadee, T., Carroll, J., Meldrum, S. C., Lardner, J., & Shields, C. G. (2007). "Could this be something serious?" Reassurance, uncertainty, and empathy in response to patients' expressions of worry. *J. Gen. Intern. Med., 22*, 1731–9.

Epstein, R. M., Korones, D. N., & Quill, T. E. (2010). Withholding information from patients—when less is more. *N. Engl. J. Med., 362*, 380–1.

Epstein, R. M. & Street, R. L. (2007a). A framework for patient-centered communication in cancer care. In *Patient-Centered Communication in Cancer Care* (pp. 17–38). Bethesda, MD: National Cancer Institute, NIH.

Epstein, R. M. & Street, R. L. (2007b). Decision-making in cancer care. In *Patient-Centered Communication in Cancer Care* (pp. 161–72). Bethesda, MD: National Cancer Institute, NIH.

Epstein, R. M. & Street, R. L., Jr. (2011). Shared mind: communication, decision making, and autonomy in serious illness. *Ann. Fam. Med., 9*, 454–61.

Evans, J. S. (2008). Dual-processing accounts of reasoning, judgment, and social cognition. *Annu. Rev. Psychol., 59*, 255–78.

Fagerlin, A. & Schneider, C. E. (2004). Enough. The failure of the living will. *Hastings Cent. Rep., 34*, 30–42.

Fallowfield, L. J., Jenkins, V. A., & Beveridge, H. A. (2002). Truth may hurt but deceit hurts more: communication in palliative care. *Palliat. Med., 16*, 297–303.

Falzer, P. R., Leventhal, H. L., Peters, E., Fried, T. R., Kerns, R., Michalski, M., et al. (2012). The practitioner proposes a treatment change and the patient declines: what to do next? *Pain Pract.*

Fischer, G. S. & Arnold, R. M. (1994). Measuring the effectiveness of ethics education. *J. Gen. Intern. Med., 9*, 655–6.

Fischhoff, B. (1991). Value elicitation: is there anything in there? *Am. Psychol., 46*, 835–47.

Frank, G., Blackhall, L. J., Murphy, S. T., Michel, V., Azen, S. P., Preloran, H. M. et al. (2002). Ambiguity and hope: disclosure preferences of less acculturated elderly Mexican Americans concerning terminal cancer—a case story. *Cambridge Quart. Healthcare Ethics, 11*(2):117–26.

Fried, T. R., O'Leary, J., Van, N. P., & Fraenkel, L. (2007). Inconsistency over time in the preferences of older persons with advanced illness for life-sustaining treatment. *J. Am. Ger. Soc., 55*, 1007–14.

Frosch, D. L., May, S. G., Rendle, K. A., Tietbohl, C., & Elwyn, G. (2012). Authoritarian physicians and patients' fear of being labeled "difficult" among key obstacles to shared decision making. *Health Aff. (Millwood), 31*, 1030–8.

Gigerenzer, G. (2007). *Gut Feelings: The Intelligence of the Unconscious.* New York: Penguin.

Gracia, D. (2001). Moral deliberation: the role of methodologies in clinical ethics. *Med. Health Care Philos., 4*, 223–32.

Greenberg, J. M., Pyszczynski, T., & Solomon, S. (1986). The causes and consequences of the need for self-esteem: a terror management theory. In R. F. Baumeister (Ed.), *Public Self and Private Self* (pp. 189–212). New York: Springer-Verlag.

Haidet, P., Hamel, M. B., Davis, R. B., Wenger, N., Reding, D., Kussin, P. S., et al. (1998). Outcomes, preferences for resuscitation, and physician-patient communication among patients with metastatic colorectal cancer. SUPPORT Investigators. Study to Understand Prognoses and Preferences for Outcomes and Risks of Treatments. *Am. J. Med., 105*, 222–9.

Halpern, J. (2001). *From Detached Concern to Empathy: Humanizing Medical Practice*. New York: Oxford University Press.

Halpern, J. & Arnold, R. M. (2008). Affective forecasting: an unrecognized challenge in making serious health decisions. [Review] [83 refs]. *J. Gen. Int. Med., 23*, 1708–12.

Hoffman, J. (2005, August 14). Awash in information, patients face a lonely, uncertain road. *New York Times*. http://www.nytimes.com/2005/08/14/health/14patient.html?pagewanted=all&_r=0 (Last accessed today. Oct 15 2013).

James, W. (1902). *The Varieties of Religious Experience: A Study in Human Nature*, reprint edition 1961. New York: Norton.

Kagawa-Singer, M. & Blackhall, L. J. (2001). Negotiating cross-cultural issues at the end of life: "You got to go where he lives." *Jama, 286*, 2993–3001.

Larson, E. B. & Yao, X. (2005). Clinical empathy as emotional labor in the patient-physician relationship. *Jama, 293*, 1100–6.

Lindblom, C. E. (1959). The science of "muddling through." *Pub. Admin. Rev., 19*, 79–88.

Mackenzie, C. (2008). Relational autonomy, normative authority and perfectionism. *J. Soc. Philos., 39*, 512–33.

Mackenzie, C. & Stoljar, N. (2000). *Relational Autonomy: Feminist Perspectives on Autonomy, Agency and the Social Self*. New York: Oxford University Press.

Makowski, S. K. & Epstein, R. M. (2012). Turning toward dissonance: lessons from art, music, and literature. *J. Pain Symptom. Manage., 43*, 293–8.

Mazer, B. L., Cameron, R. A., DeLuca, J. M., Mohile, S. G., & Epstein, R. M. (2012). Speaking for and speaking as: pseudo-surrogacy in physician-patient-companion medical encounters in advanced cancer. unpublished work

McCleod, C. (2002). *Self-Trust and Reproductive Autonomy*. Cambridge, MA: MIT Press.

Meegan, S. P. & Berg, C. A. (2002a). Contexts, functions, forms, and processes of collaborative everyday problem solving in older adulthood. *Int. J. Behav. Dev., 26*, 6–15.

Meegan, S. P. & Berg, C. A. (2002b). Contexts, functions, forms, and processes of collaborative everyday problem solving in older adulthood. *Int. J. Behav. Dev., 26*, 6–15.

Meier, D. E. & Morrison, R. S. (2002). Autonomy reconsidered. *N. Engl. J. Med., 346*, 1087–9.

Meyers, D. (1989). *Self, Society and Personal Choice*. New York: Columbia University Press.

Morse, D. S., Edwardsen, E. A., & Gordon, H. S. (2008). Missed opportunities for interval empathy in lung cancer communication. *Arch. Intern. Med., 168*, 1853–8.

Perkins, H. S. (2007). Controlling death: the false promise of advance directives. *Ann. Intern. Med., 147*, 51–7.

Peters, E. & Dieckmann, N. (2007). Less is more in presenting quality information to consumers. *Med. Care Res. Rev., 64*, 169–90.

Pollak, K. I., Arnold, R., Alexander, S. C., Jeffreys, A. S., Olsen, M. K., Abernethy, A. P., et al. (2010). Do patient attributes predict oncologist empathic responses and patient perceptions of empathy? *Support. Care Cancer, 18*, 1405–11.

Quill, T. E. & Holloway, R. (2011). Time-limited trials near the end of life. *Jama, 306*, 1483–4.

Rapley, T. (2008). Distributed decision making: the anatomy of decisions-in-action. *Sociol. Health Illness, 30*, 429–44.

Schei, E. (2006). Doctoring as leadership: the power to heal. *Perspect. Biol. Med., 49*, 393–406.

Schneiderman, L. J., Pearlman, R. A., Kaplan, R. M., Anderson, J. P., & Rosenberg, E. M. (1992). Relationship of general advance directive instructions to specific life-sustaining treatment preferences in patients with serious illness. *Arch. Intern. Med., 152,* 2114–22.

Schubart, J., Green, M. J., Whitehead, M., Farace, E., Lehmann, E., & Levi, B. H. (2012). Reliability of a computer based decision aid for advance care planning. *J. Palliat. Med., 15,* 637–42.

Temel, J. S., Jackson, V. A., Billings, J. A., Dahlin, C., Block, S. D., Buss, M. K. et al. (2007). Phase II study: integrated palliative care in newly diagnosed advanced non-small-cell lung cancer patients. *J. Clin. Oncol., 25,* 2377.

Tulsky, J. A., Fischer, G. S., Rose, M. R., & Arnold, R. M. (1998). Opening the black box: how do physicians communicate about advance directives? *Ann. Intern. Med., 129,* 441–9.

Ubel, P. A., Loewenstein, G., Schwarz, N., & Smith, D. (2005). Misimagining the unimaginable: the disability paradox and health care decision making. *Health Psychol., 24,* S57–62.

Volz, K. G. & Gigerenzer, G. (2012). Cognitive processes in decisions under risk are not the same as in decisions under uncertainty. *Frontiers Decision Neurosci., 6,* 1–6.

Weeks, J. C., Catalano, P. J., Cronin, A., Finkelman, M. D., Mack, J. W., Keating, N. L., et al. (2012). Patients' expectations about effects of chemotherapy for advanced cancer. *N. Engl. J. Med., 367,* 1616–25.

Wilson, T. D. & Gilbert, D. T. (2010). Affective forecasting: knowing what to want. *Psychol. Sci., 14,* 131–4.

Wirtz, V., Cribb, A., & Barber, N. (2006). Patient-doctor decision-making about treatment within the consultation—a critical analysis of models. *Soc. Sci. Med., 62,* 116–24.

Zlatev, J., Racine, T. P., Sinha, C., & Itkonen, E. (2008). *The Shared Mind: Perspectives on Intersubjectivity*. Philadelphia: John Benjamins.

SECTION IV

Difficult Decisions Near the Very End of Life

12

Withholding and Withdrawing Life-Sustaining Treatments

Robert D. Truog

Many of the most difficult and challenging aspects of palliative care revolve around decisions to withhold or withdraw life-sustaining treatments. In this chapter I will examine whether there are ethical, psychological, or practical differences between decisions to withhold or withdraw a treatment. I will also explore whether there are relevant distinctions among different types of therapies that may be withheld or withdrawn, focusing especially upon cardiac pacemakers and feeding. Finally, I will examine a few principles for managing symptoms in end-of-life care, with particular attention to strategies for withdrawal of mechanical ventilation and some pearls and pitfalls associated with the use of sedatives and analgesics at the end of life.

Many of my perspectives on these topics have been shaped by more than 25 years of experience working as a physician in a large pediatric intensive care unit (ICU). This focus on children and the ICU setting has clearly influenced my approach to these issues, but I have studied, observed, and consulted widely in the field of palliative care across the entire spectrum of age and clinical context, and I have tried to ensure that my treatment of these topics is sufficiently inclusive to be relevant to palliative care practitioners in all settings. All of the cases that I have included are real; I have altered them only for brevity and to protect confidentiality.

The Distinction between Withholding and Withdrawing Life-Sustaining Treatments

Clinicians frequently report that they prefer to withhold treatments, rather than to withdraw them. A few years ago I was involved in a case that highlighted several aspects of this distinction.

CASE PRESENTATION

Eve was a 2-year-old girl with holoprosencephaly, a congenital malformation of brain development that had, in her case, resulted in arrested cognitive development at the **187** *level of a newborn, with no hope of improvement. Her parents had a close relationship with their neurologist, had agreed to limit her treatment to comfort measures only (including no attempts at resuscitation), and had even signed consent for an autopsy to be performed after she died.*

One evening they brought her to the emergency room for upper respiratory infection symptoms. As part of their evaluation, the resident in charge of her care obtained a blood gas. Because Eve appeared to be in only mild respiratory distress, her parents were shocked when the resident returned a short time later and told them that the blood gas showed Eve to be in impending respiratory failure. The resident told the parents that although the clinical team was willing to abide by their decision to offer comfort care only, she wanted the parents to know that without intubation and ventilation Eve would likely die in the next hour or so. Despite their considered decisions about not wanting her to be resuscitated, faced with her imminent death they reversed their decision and requested resuscitation.

Three days later, in the ICU, she had been diagnosed with respiratory syncytial virus (RSV) bronchiolitis, a common respiratory illness in children. She was improving, and it appeared she would be ready to extubate within the next several days. Her parents, however, now deeply regretted their decision to have her intubated, and requested that she be extubated immediately, recognizing that this would almost certainly lead to her death. The ICU staff was nearly universally opposed, insisting that her favorable trajectory and likely recovery made withdrawal of ventilation at this point unethical.

DISCUSSION

There is much to learn from this case, but I will focus on the question, "If the clinicians were willing to abide by the parent's decision to withhold intubation at the time of Eve's admission, why were they unwilling to consider withdrawal of ventilation 3 days later?"

Philosopher Dan Brock has written about why it is illogical to make this kind of distinction between withholding and withdrawing life-sustaining treatments.[1] To paraphrase one of his thought experiments, imagine an elderly man with a properly executed do-not-attempt-resuscitation (DNAR) order who lives at home with his wife. He develops respiratory distress, and an ambulance takes him to a nearby emergency room. In the first version of the story, his wife arrives at the hospital shortly after the ambulance, shows the physician the DNAR order, and her husband is admitted to the ward for palliative care. In the second version of the story, his wife is delayed in traffic, and arrives at the emergency room only after the physician has already intubated her husband and placed him on a ventilator. The physician, who was willing to withhold ventilation in the first version of the story, is refusing to remove the endotracheal tube and the ventilator, now that they are in place. As Brock explains, do not the very same circumstances that justified not placing the patient on the ventilator now justify taking him off of it? How can the mere fact that his wife was delayed in traffic be sufficient reason to justify keeping him intubated, contrary to his expressed wishes? Thought experiments like these are taken to show that the bare difference between withholding and withdrawing cannot be a sufficient reason for treating otherwise similar cases differently.

In addition to these philosophical considerations, there are also practical reasons for not differentiating between withholding and withdrawing. Consider decisions such as whether to initiate resuscitation for premature babies born at the threshold of viability. If we hold the view that treatments must be continued once they have been started, we will be very cautious about initiating resuscitation for babies we think might not survive, because this might commit them to a long but ultimately futile course of intensive medical care. On the other hand, if we are willing to withdraw treatment once we have begun it, we might be more willing to initiate resuscitation in the delivery room as a trial of therapy, knowing that the baby could be removed from mechanical ventilation and transitioned to palliative care if the clinical trajectory turned out not to be favorable.

In many cases involving life-sustaining treatments, there may also be ambiguity about what counts as a "withholding" versus a "withdrawing." For example, when a patient makes a decision to stop undergoing hemodialysis, should this be framed as a decision to *withdraw* from a dialysis program (generally three times a week), or a decision to *withhold* the next and all subsequent dialysis treatments? Pushing the point further, when a patient chooses to no longer receive mechanical ventilation, is this a decision to *withdraw* the ventilator, or a decision to *withhold* the next and all subsequent breaths? Although we may have intuitions about how to frame the decision in each case, either view is logically plausible. These differences are important in some cultural and religious traditions. For example, one view in orthodox Judaism is that life-sustaining treatments may be withheld but not withdrawn. In order to respect this view while still permitting patients to receive trials of mechanical ventilation, Halakhic scholars have proposed that ventilators be equipped with timers that would allow them to function for a set period of time (such as a week). If a decision is made to not continue ventilation after that point, then the timer causes the ventilator to shut down, and treatment can be considered to have been withheld, not withdrawn.[2]

Despite these arguments, the fact remains that many clinicians are much more uncomfortable withdrawing therapy than they are withholding it. In everyday life we feel much greater responsibility for our acts than for our omissions; for example, an act of homicide is deemed far worse than withholding contributions to Oxfam, even though either may result in the loss of a life. Hence we are psychologically predisposed to feel greater moral responsibility for acts of withdrawing as opposed to omissions of withholding.

Thus far I have been examining the case of Eve through the philosophical lens of whether the clinicians can justify their reluctance to withdraw mechanical ventilation from Eve, even though they were willing to withhold it at the time of admission. Another way of looking at this dilemma, however, is to see it as a conflict between competing narratives.

In the context of end-of-life care, patients and their families may have a commitment to telling a certain kind of story, and their story may be very different from the one that the clinicians would like to construct. In Eve's case, her parents wanted to tell a story that reflected their core values. They wanted their story to show how they had lovingly cared for her as long as possible, that they were able to protect her from harm, and made sure that she was able to die in peace. They anticipated that her death was likely to occur in the context of a respiratory infection, and were angry with themselves that in a moment of crisis they were unable to follow through on their convictions (and perhaps also angry that the medical staff did not do more to help them live up to their convictions). They did not understand what the medical staff meant when they insisted that Eve was getting "better," because the treatments being provided were incapable of doing anything to improve Eve's profound neurological disability. Their decision to institute mechanical ventilation and ICU care was therefore profoundly at odds with the narrative they were trying to create, and hence they were adamant that the plan of care be immediately corrected.

Eve's clinicians, however, had an interest in constructing a different story: one to be told on morning rounds, in case conferences, and informally among colleagues. They wanted to tell a story that showed they were doing "good medicine." In their story, a child with only mild evidence of respiratory distress was correctly discovered to have impending respiratory failure. A differential diagnosis was considered, the correct laboratory studies were sent, and the illness was quickly diagnosed as RSV bronchiolitis. The patient was promptly intubated, the ventilator was managed skillfully, and now the patient was expected to make a complete recovery. The only problem with their being able to tell this triumphant narrative is that her parents were inexplicably demanding that their treatments be terminated prematurely! It is not hard to imagine why, in the context of this narrative, the clinicians might conclude that the parents were not behaving rationally and would resist their demands.

As it turned out, the clinical team came to see that there were many reasons to support the parents' request to extubate Eve and to redirect the goals of her care. Despite success with the management of her viral respiratory infection, she was not getting "better" in any sense that was relevant to either Eve or her parents. Mechanical ventilation was therefore withdrawn later that day, and Eve had a peaceful death, surrounded by friends and family, with the need for only a minor footnote to the loving narrative that her parents had sought to create.

Ethical Distinctions Among Different Types of Therapies That May Be Withheld or Withdrawn

Although the withdrawal of many types of treatment has become well accepted, some persist in provoking controversy. Decisions to disable cardiac pacemakers and to discontinue feedings are among those that continue to stir debate. Unlike situations where a treatment is being withdrawn because its use has become futile (as in the withdrawal of mechanical ventilation in the face of intractable respiratory failure), in these cases the treatment that is being withdrawn is continuing to function very effectively (i.e., pacing the heart and providing nutrition). In other words, the rationale for withdrawing the treatment is not that the treatment itself is no longer working, but that other considerations (most commonly, neurological disability) justify the decision to withdraw. In this sense, withdrawal of the pacemaker or tube feedings may seem a matter of convenience, because if the patient were not dependent upon the pacemaker or the tube feedings, death could not be effected by their withdrawal. Whether this distinction is ethically relevant is debatable, but it does seem to make a difference in the way caregivers perceive withdrawal of these therapies.

IMPLANTED PACEMAKERS

One class of life-sustaining treatments that has provoked a great deal of debate has been the use of implantable pacemakers.

Case Presentation

A 19-year-old man had undergone repair of complex congenital heart disease as an infant at a children's hospital. He had severe conduction disturbances, and was pacemaker dependent. He had moderate mental retardation, and his parents functioned as his medical decision makers. He had begun to have recurrent strokes, and was becoming increasingly obtunded. His parents asked that all life-sustaining therapy be discontinued, and that he be allowed to die. They asked that his pacemaker be removed, or at least disabled. They understood that this would result in his immediate death.

Discussion

This case forces us to think about how cardiac pacemakers compare to other forms of "life-sustaining therapy."[3] Are cardiac pacemakers analogous to ventilators, such that each pulse of the pacemaker is like each breath of the ventilator? If so, then is turning off a pacemaker no different from turning off a ventilator? Or, once it is surgically implanted, do pacemakers become just another part of the body, like the kidneys or the liver? Or should we consider them to be foreign, but nonetheless nonremovable, like an aortic graft or a transplanted kidney? Are there ethically relevant distinctions between surgically removing the pacemaker, re-programming it so that it stops functioning, or choosing to allow the batteries to run out without replacing them?

Guidelines from the American College of Cardiology and the American Heart Association state that although physicians should not be obligated to deactivate a pacemaker, honoring this request "should not be regarded as either physician-assisted suicide or euthanasia."[4] Other commentators disagree with this position, arguing that a pacemaker is "an integrated part of the person," and that "to stop pacing in such a patient is a deliberate act that is intended to hasten death." They go on to say that "for those who are not opposed to physician-assisted suicide, this distinction may not be morally relevant, but for those opposed to this practice, the distinction is glaring."[5]

Although acknowledging that deactivation of pacemakers may make many clinicians uncomfortable with the feeling that they have crossed the line from "allowing to die" to "causing death," I believe it is difficult to build an argument for why cardiac pacing is fundamentally different from other forms of life-sustaining treatment (such as mechanical ventilation or dialysis), and I agree with those who hold that patients or surrogates should have the right to request that these devices be disabled when they perceive that the burdens of continuing their use outweigh the benefits.

WITHDRAWING TUBE FEEDINGS

Following the Supreme Court decision in Cruzan in 1990, withdrawal of tube feedings has become much more common and less controversial, especially in the care of adults with advanced forms of dementia and other neurological disability. Endorsement of this practice has been much slower in pediatrics, however, and many children's hospitals continue to refuse requests to withdraw tube feedings in situations that would be commonplace in adult hospitals. C. Everett Koop, a pediatric surgeon and former US Surgeon General, was frequently quoted for characterizing withdrawal of tube feedings in children as "starving a child to death."[6]

The reasons for this difference in the care of adults versus children are multifactorial, but certainly relate, in part, to the fact that small children universally require assistance in eating. Choosing to provide this assistance to healthy children, but to withhold it from disabled children, may feel discriminatory. Unlike in adults, feeding is a reciprocal, dyadic, social activity between the caregiver and the child, and is a gratifying source of satisfaction to both the feeder and the child. Furthermore, successfully feeding and supporting the growth and development of a child is indicative of good parenting, whereas failure to do these things may imply that the parenting is negligent. Although none of these considerations raise fundamental differences between decisions to withdraw tube feedings in children versus adults, they may help ethicists and palliative care clinicians better understand the frequent reluctance of parents and pediatricians to consider this as an option for end-of-life care.[7]

WITHHOLDING ORAL FEEDINGS

Case Presentation

The well-known case of Terry Schiavo involved a young woman who lapsed into a persistent vegetative state at the age of 27, living in this condition for the last 15 years of her life. Both her personal and court-appointed physicians expressed the opinion that there was no hope for improvement or rehabilitation, an assessment that was ultimately confirmed by her autopsy. Her husband, Michael Schiavo, contended that it was his wife's wish that she not be kept alive through unnatural, mechanical means. He therefore requested that her tube feedings be withdrawn, a decision that was ultimately supported by the courts over the objections of her parents. She died on March 31, 2005, 13 days after her feeding tube was removed.

Less well-known is the fact that Schiavo's parents repeatedly pointed out that her ability to swallow was never tested, contending that it was possible for her to be safely hand-fed. They also unsuccessfully petitioned the courts to be permitted to attempt hand-feeding if and when her gastrostomy feeds were discontinued.[8]

Discussion

A central finding of the Cruzan case in 1990 was that patients have the right to refuse any unwanted medical treatment, even if life sustaining. The Supreme Court also accepted the view that tube feedings are a "medical treatment." Hence, patients have the right to refuse tube feedings, following the same logic supporting the rights of patients to refuse mechanical ventilation.[9]

As Schiavo's parents recognized, patients in a persistent vegetative state often retain rudimentary swallowing reflexes and many of them can be successfully hand-fed.[10] The process is typically very laborious and time consuming, and few nursing facilities would be able to support the many hours that would be required each day to provide this intensity of care. Yet to my knowledge no one has ever argued that oral feedings can be considered a "medical treatment." So in those cases in which patients are being nourished through a feeding tube as a matter of *convenience* rather than a matter of *necessity*, the current consensus about the rights of patients to refuse unwanted medical treatments cannot be used to justify the withholding of oral feedings.

Thos Cochrane and I have argued that the current consensus about rights to refuse medical treatments may be based upon an unsupported distinction between natural and artificial interventions.[11] One interpretation of the holding in Cruzan is that patients may refuse unwanted medical treatments because they are "artificial." If this is the case, then we may conclude that patients do not have a right to refuse "natural" interventions, like hand-feeding. If so, then Schiavo's parents were correct in their view that Terry should have been tested for her ability to be hand-fed and offered this as an option, if she were capable.

Alternatively, one could argue that patients have a right to refuse any unwanted interventions, whether medical or not, and whether artificial or natural. As discussed elsewhere in this volume, many patients have voluntarily chosen to stop eating and drinking.[12] Although one might worry that this would lead to thirst and starvation, the actual experience appears to be quite the opposite, with slow dehydration leading to the production of sedating metabolites, followed by a comfortable and peaceful death.

Of course, individuals who choose to voluntarily stop eating and drinking differ from those like Terry Schiavo, in that these individuals have made this decision for themselves, whereas for patients like Schiavo someone else has made the decision on their behalf. Although this is an important distinction, and points out the need for careful procedures to protect these vulnerable patients, both law and ethical practice in the United States support the view that patients do not lose their right to make medical decisions when they become incapacitated. Instead, they retain this right, but their decisions must be effected through the authority of their surrogate decision maker. Just as withdrawal of tube feedings were vigorously debated in the 1990s, I believe that debates about withdrawal of oral feedings may become more prominent in the future.

Principles for Managing Symptoms in End-of-Life Care

About one-third of deaths in the United States occur in hospitals, many of these involving the withdrawal of mechanical ventilation and use of medications for sedation and comfort. End-of-life care, like any other medical procedure, needs to be done meticulously and with attention to detail.[13,14] Just as checklists and protocols have been shown to improve care around medical procedures like the placement of central catheters and endotracheal tubes, so have these techniques been found useful in improving care at the end of life.[15,16] Two areas that often generate controversy concern approaches taken toward ventilator withdrawal, and certain practices surrounding the administration of medications during end-of-life care.

VENTILATOR MANAGEMENT: TERMINAL EXTUBATION
VERSUS TERMINAL WEAN[13,14]

In 1983 Ake Grenvik described an approach for withdrawal of mechanical ventilation that he labeled a "terminal wean."[17] As the technique has evolved, today terminal weaning can be defined as a process of slowly decreasing the patient's ventilator settings while leaving the endotracheal tube in place. Over a period of 5 to 10 minutes, the ventilator rate is reduced to zero and the oxygen concentration is decreased to 21% (room air). The patient is carefully observed for any signs of air hunger or other distress, and sedation is titrated as necessary to keep the patient comfortable.

This approach is typically contrasted with terminal extubation. Using this approach, the endotracheal is removed after premedicating the patient to block any acute air hunger or distress that might accompany the sudden withdrawal of mechanical support. The amount of sedation that should be given for this premedication is determined by clinical judgment, but for patients who have been receiving sedation on a regular basis, should be at least equivalent to what the patient has received over the previous hour. Once the tube is removed, additional medication is titrated as necessary.

Each approach has advantages and drawbacks. By leaving the endotracheal tube in place, terminal weaning avoids any problems with airway obstruction from the soft tissues of the pharynx, gurgling or choking on secretions, or the development of gasping respirations. By gradually reducing the ventilator settings, air hunger is more easily controlled and prevented. Many clinicians prefer this approach because it feels less active, reducing the sense of moral burden for both the clinician and the family.

On the other hand, terminal extubation has a different set of advantages and drawbacks. By quickly removing the endotracheal tube, the dying process is not prolonged; the patient is free of unwanted interventions, allowing for a more natural interaction between the patient and family. This is particularly true for children, where parents may be able to hold their child without any tubes or awkward connections to the ventilator.

The preferred approach is heavily influenced by the physician's specialty, with surgeons and anesthesiologists preferring terminal weaning, whereas internists and pediatricians prefer terminal extubation.[18] This is potentially problematic, because it suggests that the preferences and comfort of the physician may supersede the actual needs and desires of the patient and family.

Another way of looking at the process is to see these two approaches as a false dichotomy. Instead, consider that ventilated patients are receiving three distinct modalities of support: an artificial airway to keep the airway patent, supplemental oxygen to support blood oxygen levels, and a ventilatory rate to maintain normal carbon dioxide levels. Rather than being locked into one of the two prototype approaches described in the preceding, clinicians should learn how to "mix and match" withdrawal of these three modalities of support to meet the unique needs of each individual patient.

For example, a patient who is deeply comatose or brain-dead could have all three modalities removed at once, because there is no risk of the patient experiencing air hunger or distress. On the other hand, a conscious patient might be best managed by first decreasing the supplemental oxygen level, titrating additional sedation as necessary, slowly reducing the ventilator rate to zero, and finally removing the endotracheal tube when the patient is no longer conscious.

Sedation and Analgesia in End-of-Life Care[13,14]

Many of the principles for providing patients with sedation and analgesia during end-of-life care involve application of the doctrine of double effect, which is described and examined elsewhere in this volume. In this section, I will describe two cases from my experience that illustrate some of the pearls and pitfalls of medicating patients at the end of life.

Opioids (like morphine or fentanyl) and benzodiazepines (like lorazepam or midazolam) are the most commonly used medications to treat patients during end-of-life care in the hospital. Although standard doses of these medications are generally sufficient to make patients comfortable, clinicians need to be prepared for what to do when this typical approach does not work. The greatest concern arises with the small number of patients who have an acute crescendo of pain, air hunger, or other distress during the withdrawal of life support. In the midst of this emotional event, the clinicians may panic. This may prompt them to make unwise choices, such as giving the patient a paralytic agent or a lethal drug like potassium chloride, choices that would likely be regarded as illegal and outside the parameters of double effect.

Instead, clinicians should remember two approaches that are fully compatible with double effect and with US law. First, we can and should provide the patient with whatever dose is necessary to achieve comfort—there are no maximal doses! Especially when patients have been receiving opioids and benzodiazepines as a part of their clinical management, they may require unexpectedly large doses to gain control of their symptoms. As long as the dose is necessary to make the patient comfortable, it is within the parameters of law and ethics.

Second, neither law nor ethics limit the choice of sedatives and analgesics to just opioids and benzodiazepines. Again, patients who have been receiving these agents as part of their clinical care may be highly tolerant to their effects. Even worse, they may not respond to what would seem like a much larger dose of what they have already been receiving, perhaps because they have reached a "ceiling effect" from the medication related to saturation of the pharmacological receptors. In these cases it can be very helpful to switch to another class of drug. For example, I have found propofol to be a very effective agent, particularly in patients who have been receiving large amounts of opioids and benzodiazepines. The medication acts rapidly and predictably (perhaps because of actions on different receptors), allowing for effective titration and rapid control of distressing symptoms.

CASE PRESENTATION

An internist was providing end-of-life care for an elderly woman in the hospital across the street from his office. During the day he went back and forth from his office to her hospital bed, titrating incremental doses of sedation to keep her comfortable. By late that evening, she had been unconscious and unresponsive for several hours, but continued to breathe at a low rate of four to six times per minute. Her family was exhausted and fully prepared for her death. The hospital did not have any house staff, and the physician worried that if he went home, the nursing staff would not be able to follow through on the excellent palliative care that he had been providing during the day.

He decided to administer a dose of vecuronium, a neuromuscular blocking agent that rapidly causes paralysis. Within moments the patient appeared to relax, and then stopped breathing. Although the family did not understand the implications of her having received the vecuronium, they were grateful for her care, and after some minutes of grieving together, the physician and the family both left the hospital.

The next morning, the physician received a call from the hospital president. The nurse who had been caring for the patient had reported the use of the vecuronium. The hospital president was sympathetic to the physician's motivations, but felt compelled to suspend his hospital privileges and report the event to both the district attorney and the state medical board.

Six months later, after a grand jury investigation and a review by the medical board, no charges were filed, and his medical license was conditionally reinstated. The hospital, however, did not renew his hospital privileges. The physician ultimately decided not to return to clinical practice.

DISCUSSION

This case, a true story, contains an important lesson. It is not enough to rely on instinct and good intentions in providing end-of-life care. Although the physician appeared to be acting out of compassion for the patient and the family, and although it is unlikely that the vecuronium unduly hastened the patient's death or caused her any distress or suffering, the physician should have known that the principles of end-of-life care require the proportionate use of sedatives and analgesics, titrated to the patient's degree of discomfort. Vecuronium and other neuromuscular blocking agents do not have any analgesic effects; hence, the intention of the physician cannot be to make the patient comfortable, but expressly to cause death. All clinicians who do palliative care should know that neuromuscular blocking agents should never be included on the pharmacological menu in end-of-life care.

In this chapter I have tried to highlight what I see as some of the most interesting and controversial issues surrounding the withholding and withdrawing of life-sustaining treatments in palliative care. I hope this discussion will help to ensure that the care we provide to the dying and those with life-threatening conditions is delivered with same high level of expertise and compassion as the care we provide in all other medical settings.

References

1. Brock DW. Death and dying. In: Veatch R, ed. *Medical Ethics.* 2nd ed. Sudbury MA: Jones and Bartlett Publishers; 1997:363–94.
2. Ravitsky V. Timers on ventilators. Br Med J 2005;*330*:415–7.
3. Mueller PS, Hook CC, Hayes DL. Ethical analysis of withdrawal of pacemaker or implantable cardioverter-defibrillator support at the end of life. Mayo Clinic proceedings Mayo Clinic 2003;78:959–63.
4. Epstein AE, DiMarco JP, Ellenbogen KA, et al. ACC/AHA/HRS 2008 Guidelines for Device-Based Therapy of Cardiac Rhythm Abnormalities: a report of the American College of Cardiology/American Heart Association Task Force on Practice Guidelines. Circulation 2008;117:e350–408.

5. Zellner RA, Aulisio MP, Lewis WR. Should implantable cardioverter-defibrillators and permanent pacemakers in patients with terminal illness be deactivated? Circ Arrhythm Electrophysiol 2009;2:340–4.

6. Koop CE, Schaeffer FA. Whatever happened to the human race? Wheaton IL: Crossway Books; 1979.

7. Diekema DS, Botkin JR. Clinical report—Forgoing medically provided nutrition and hydration in children. Pediatrics 2009;124:813–22.

8. Quill TE. Terri Schiavo—a tragedy compounded. N Engl J Med 2005.

9. Annas GJ. "Culture of life" politics at the bedside—the case of Terri Schiavo. N Engl J Med 2005;352:1710–5.

10. Mitchell SL, Buchanan JL, Littlehale S, Hamel MB. Tube-feeding versus hand-feeding nursing home residents with advanced dementia: a cost comparison. J Am Med Dir Assoc 2003;4:27–33.

11. Truog RD, Cochrane TI. Refusal of hydration and nutrition: irrelevance of the "artificial" versus "natural" distinction. Arch Intern Med 2005;165:2574–6.

12. Bernat JL, Gert B, Mogielnicki RP. Patient refusal of hydration and nutrition: an alternative to physician-assisted suicide or voluntary active euthanasia. Arch Intern Med 1993;153:2723–7.

13. Truog RD, Cist AF, Brackett SE, et al. Recommendations for end-of-life care in the intensive care unit: the Ethics Committee of the Society of Critical Care Medicine. Crit Care Med 2001;29:2332–48.

14. Truog RD, Campbell ML, Curtis JR, et al. Recommendations for end-of-life care in the intensive care unit: a consensus statement by the American Academy of Critical Care Medicine. Crit Care Med 2008;36:953–63.

15. Rubenfeld GD. Principles and practice of withdrawing life-sustaining treatments. Crit Care Clin 2004;20:435–51.

16. Treece PD, Engelberg RA, Crowley L, et al. Evaluation of a standardized order form for the withdrawal of life support in the intensive care unit. Crit Care Med 2004;32:1141–8.

17. Grenvik A. "Terminal weaning": discontinuance of life-support therapy in the terminally ill patient. Crit Care Med 1983;11:394–5.

18. Faber-Langendoen K. The clinical management of dying patients receiving mechanical ventilation: a survey of physician practice. Chest 1994;106:880–8.

13

Medical Futility: Content in the Context of Care

Peggy L. Determeyer and Howard Brody

An 88-year-old patient, Mr. Norbert Johnson, has been in the Intensive Care Unit for 1 week. He was admitted with respiratory distress resulting from multiple years of COPD and a deteriorating ejection fraction. On previous admissions for these symptoms, he has always recovered within a few days to return to his normal activities, which include living alone with some assistance from friends and family. However, during this admission, the antibiotics are ineffective, and his kidney and liver functions are declining, which have resulted in encephalopathy and loss of decision-making capacity. Family members have been kept up to date with the patient's condition, and continue to insist that full treatment continue, because he has always recovered from prior acute events. Mr. Johnson's attending physician suggests that a "Do Not Resuscitate" (DNR) order be implemented, but the family is resistant. They are concerned that the staff will not work as diligently to help their loved one to recover. As days pass and the patient is not improving, the medical care team is becoming more frustrated with the family, believing that the care for the patient is becoming medically inappropriate. Some of his physicians raise the specter of futility in conversations with each other.

Medical futility is not a new concept. The physician's obligation to place limits on treatment extends as far back as the ancient Greeks, who required that the physician restrict treatment in those with incurable diseases.[1] In modern medicine, it is sometimes more difficult to recognize the limits of treatment for practitioners and patients, their family members, or surrogates. This chapter will examine the definition of "futility," identify core ethical values, and discuss procedural approaches. Our overall goal is to identify an ethical understanding of futility that leads in practice to optimal communication and trust.

What is Futility?

Futility is derived from the Latin *futillis*, referring to a vessel that is wide at the top and narrow at the bottom so that it is "leaky" and "easily pours out." Though unreliable as a container, when placed in the context of its use as a religious object, the vessel did meet its purpose. Similarly, medical treatment must also be placed in the context of the goals of care. Thus, the term medical futility requires further exploration. For Mr. Johnson, mechanical ventilation, antibiotics, and other medical treatments are supporting life by maintaining circulation and respiration. As such, the treatments themselves are not futile. If, however—as discussions with the family suggest—the goal of care that they accept is not the mere maintenance of circulation, but Mr. Johnson's recovery to his previous baseline functional status, then these treatments may indeed be futile. Consequently, the statement, "Treatment X is futile" is always an incomplete sentence; it requires the addition of the phrase, "... for purposes of achieving goal Y."

Schneiderman and Jecker have proposed a quantitative definition of futility as "any effort to provide a benefit to the patient that is highly likely to fail and whose rare exceptions cannot be systematically produced."[2] They suggest that if in the last 100 cases, no one has recovered, the treatment might be considered to be futile for that condition.[3] The challenge in using such a metric is that few medical cases are exactly alike, and thus the predictive factors become murky. No physician can predict with certainty that a patient will not recover. In the conversation with Mr. Johnson's family, the family's data point that he has always "bounced back" previously becomes difficult for physicians to contest. A California study of three tertiary hospitals noted that nearly two-thirds of patient surrogates doubted the physicians' futility predictions.[4] Another study found that nearly 80% of respondents believed that miracles still occur.[5] Thus, the attempt to establish quantitative measures as the sole reference for establishing futility may lead to further uncertainty and disagreement, rather than the desired clarity.

In addition to considering the statistical likelihood that a treatment will work, Schneiderman and Jecker also support the qualitative definition of medical futility provided by the University of California San Diego Medical Center as "any treatment without a realistic chance of providing an effect that the patient would ever have the capacity to appreciate as a benefit, such as merely preserving physiologic functions of the permanently unconscious patient" or any treatment that "has no realistic chance of achieving the medical goal of returning the patient to a level of health that permits survival outside the acute care setting at UCSD Medical Center."[6] These definitions, however, create problems by specifying the goals of care as part of the definition of futility. We agree, as noted, that the concept of futility is ultimately incomplete until the goal is specified. But it seems a clearer approach first to state what futility means, and then later address which goals might or might not be acceptable.

We prefer to define futility in qualitative terms as an intervention that has no reasonable likelihood of achieving the agreed-upon goals. This definition captures the basic concept for futility, and avoids taking a stand on controversial issues that are better addressed separately and not by definitional fiat. People may disagree on what counts as reasonable evidence that a treatment will not work in a given case. They may also disagree on what goals of treatment are acceptable, and to whom. It is better to address these disagreements head-on rather than to try to finesse them by taking a stand on those points within the definition itself.

As a minor point, because of this definition, we object to the terms "futile *care*" and even "futile *treatment*." The terms "care" and "treatment" imply something that has a reasonable chance of working and so cannot be consistent with futility. Though "futile intervention" is more awkward, we believe it to be more correct.

Gillon objects to the term "futility" because he considers it ambiguous, and notes that it can become pejorative when applied to medical treatment.[7] We would reply that the notion, "it won't work" is not ambiguous at all, however difficult it may be to apply in any given circumstance. Moreover, to say that something has no reasonable chance of working is indeed a pejorative comment, but if true, is merited. Finally, Gillon's objections appear to suggest that we could dispense with the term "futility" and be none the worse. But a little reflection will show that "futility" is an unavoidable concept within medical practice. One striking example is the decision to cease CPR. There has been a great deal of debate about when and if the medical staff can unilaterally decide not to begin CPR on the basis of futility, but there has been virtually no debate that the staff is fully entitled to decide when to stop CPR on the basis of futility. After some period of time has passed, and considering the patient's status and medical history, the team makes a determination that continuing CPR has no reasonable chance of working. To date, we are aware of no one who has suggested that this latter decision should require the consent of the family. If that stance is appropriate, and we believe that it is the only sensible approach to take, then medical staff both need to and are entitled to make futility judgments.

What Are the Core Ethical Values?

Judgments of medical futility are relevant to three core ethical values: patient autonomy, professional integrity, and respectful treatment of patients and families.

Patient autonomy has appropriately become a core value in modern medicine, and extends to the right of the patient's surrogate to act on the patient's behalf. We must then ask whether the exercise of autonomy in treatment decisions has any limits; and brief reflection will show that it must. We could probably readily agree that patients have no "right" to demand antibiotics for viral colds, or gall bladder surgery when they have no signs of gall bladder disease. In those areas of medicine, we can readily see that autonomy does not include a right to demand or receive interventions that predictably won't work.

The reason for this limitation is clear when we ask what patients have an autonomous right to demand and receive; and presumably the answer is *good medical care*. What counts as "good" medicine must incorporate elements of patient autonomy: When reasonable options exist, patient values and preferences should guide the decision. As we have noted, an intervention is futile only in relation to a specified goal and respect for patient autonomy implies a right of patients and surrogates to determine the appropriate goals of care. But at some point, what counts as "good" medical care becomes a matter of scientific and professional judgment and not a matter of pure patient preferences. Whenever that point is reached, patient autonomy does include a right to refuse "good" medical care, as in the case of a Jehovah's Witness refusal of a medically indicated blood transfusion. However, merely invoking "autonomy" cannot justify forcing a practitioner to provide a patient with an intervention that is not included in the scope of good medical practice.

Decisions about antibiotics for colds and gall bladder surgery are uncontroversial because they are not life-or-death decisions; on the other hand, the debate over futility versus autonomy has generally focused on end-of-life care. Clearly, the stakes are higher when a questionable treatment may be the patient's last chance of survival, although the general principle does not change simply because death may be imminent.

If patient autonomy, by itself, cannot resolve debates over medical futility, what other values are relevant? The two values that seem critical to us (professional integrity and respectful treatment of patients and families) are not generally listed in standard works on principles of bioethics. Yet we believe that without appeal to those values, we cannot really make sense of the decisions health providers are called upon to make.

Professional integrity provides the medical practitioner with the authority and responsibility unilaterally to refuse to provide interventions that fall outside the realm of good medical practice. One category of interventions that violate integrity is those that (based on the best available evidence) predictably won't work. To require that professionals administer such interventions is basically asking them to be fraudulent—to perform a charade of treatment.[8] Futility is, however, only one example of interventions that transgress professional integrity. Integrity accords to professionals a prerogative to declare some goals of treatment to be outside the legitimate boundaries of professional practice. Providing narcotics for known addicts, and anabolic steroids for body-builders, are not futile in any sense but may still legitimately be regarded as unprofessional. Our focus in this chapter, however, will be on interventions that violate professional integrity specifically because they are futile.

If, however, we set up the futility debate as a struggle between patient autonomy and professional integrity, we create an adversarial posture that violates a third value of good practice—respectful treatment of patients and their surrogates. Research on futility determinations suggests that a common response of patients and families that tends to make the issue less tractable is their sense of the health team's lack of respect for their wishes and values. This can occur in any case but is exacerbated when the treatment team and the patient and family come from different cultural or religious backgrounds, especially when one community (such as minority groups in the United States) has long-standing reasons to distrust a white medical establishment. Although professional integrity is an important value, it is not the sole value in professional practice. Rather than demand an unchallenged prerogative to defend their integrity even at the cost of appearing to disrespect the patient and family, caregivers would be on firmer ethical ground to try to find ways that appropriately balance both values. This in turn leads to the importance of respectful and trust-building communication, which is the main practical solution to problems of futility.

Legal Procedural Approaches

Some states have established a legal process for dealing with medical futility, with the most well-publicized being the Texas Advance Directives Act (TADA), enacted in 1999 and amended in 2003. This legislation establishes procedures for reviewing cases that are deemed to involve futile interventions.[9]

- ¤ The family must be given written information about hospital policy on the ethics consultation process, with 48 hours' notice for the meeting and be invited to participate.
- ¤ The ethics consultation committee must provide a written report detailing its findings to the family. If the ethics consultation process fails to resolve the dispute, the hospital, working with the family, must try to arrange transfer of the patient to another physician or institution willing to give the treatment requested by the family.
- ¤ If no such provider can be found after 10 days, the hospital and physician may unilaterally withhold or withdraw therapy that has been determined to be futile.
- ¤ The patient or surrogate may ask a state court judge to grant an extension of time before treatment is withdrawn. This extension is to be granted only if the judge determines that there is a reasonable likelihood of finding a willing provider of the disputed treatment if more time is granted.
- ¤ If the family does not seek an extension or the judge fails to grant one, futile treatment may be unilaterally withdrawn by the treatment team with immunity from civil and criminal prosecution.

The TADA represents a major legislative accomplishment in that at least briefly, right-to-life interests and healthcare organizations agreed upon a common strategy and backed the legislation. It provides a clear procedure backed by law, and appears not to have been misused, in that no patient whose therapy was labeled "futile" in such proceedings has ever recovered. On the other hand, a criticism of the TADA is that the decision-making is placed in the hands of hospital ethics/ review committees, which may not be adequately independent of the interests of the hospital and staff. Texas providers reportedly find the process time-consuming and complex, to the extent that many physicians do not want to undertake the futility process. The most serious criticism, however, is that the procedure seems at the beginning to establish an adversarial relationship between caregivers and family, and could thereby undermine rather than encourage respectful communication.

The Children's Hospital of Boston has taken a similar approach to TADA, but has included an appeals avenue to the courts, including offers to assist the family in obtaining independent legal advice—a process they regard as fairer.[10]

Ohio has taken a different approach. If the patient has a valid advance directive and is deemed to be terminally ill or has been in a persistent vegetative state for more than 12 months, two physicians can agree to withdraw or withhold treatment. In the absence of an advance directive, physicians may refuse to provide futile interventions, but are obligated to transfer the patient to another physician. If this is not feasible, petitions are made to the Ohio Probate Court for withholding or withdrawing treatment.[11]

Either the Texas or Ohio procedures provide a means for contesting Mr. Johnson's family's refusal to consider less aggressive treatment. The question is whether these approaches predictably maximize the core ethical values that we have identified. Our view is that legalistically oriented procedures are needed as a last resort when good-faith efforts at communication break down. But, applied too early in the unfolding of a case like Mr. Johnson's, there is little guarantee that the procedures will advance either professional integrity or the respectful treatment of patients and families. For that outcome, we suggest a strategy that focuses more centrally on communication and building trust.

What Procedures Best Balance Key Values?

A general approach to futility disagreements that we believe is more likely to lead to a resolution that respects all of the core ethical values is based on a report from the American Medical Association's Council on Ethical and Judicial Affairs:[12]

- Communicate clearly and compassionately to the patient and/or family the staff's views on prognosis and treatment options.
- If the family requests treatments that the staff believes to be futile, explore their reasons.
- If the request is based on disagreement over medical facts (the prognosis or the effectiveness of treatment), seek a second medical opinion.
- If the request is based on a different view of the goals of care, clarify the different goals and discuss which are most appropriate for the patient and which are within the bounds of professional integrity.
- If the above process has not led to agreement, seek input from the institutional ethics committee.
- If the ethics committee agrees that the requested intervention is futile, and the family continues to request it, seek transfer of care within the institution to another physician willing to provide that treatment.
- If an internal transfer cannot be arranged, seek transfer to another institution willing to provide that treatment.

◻ If all transfers prove impossible, the treating staff may at this point unilaterally withdraw or withhold the futile intervention. At any time in the process, the family may choose to involve the court system.

We believe that if this approach is implemented, several beneficial outcomes are likely:

◻ At each step of the way, helpful, open communication between the treating staff and the patient or family is encouraged.

◻ The ultimate right of the staff to decline to provide futile interventions is recognized and reinforced.

◻ Only in rare instances will it become necessary for the staff to make a unilateral decision to withhold or withdraw the requested intervention, as most cases will be resolved before that point is reached.

Staff sometimes forget that time is on their side if a judgment of medical futility is well-grounded. As time passes, the family is more likely to see clear evidence of no improvement and therefore come to accept the information the staff is providing them. A protracted process may initially appear disrespectful of professional integrity, but maximizes the likelihood that the dispute will be resolved with the family feeling well respected. We think it more important that the patient and family receive respectful treatment in a setting in which the ultimate prerogative of professionals to maintain their integrity is recognized, rather than withdrawing interventions by some arbitrary deadline.

The difficulties in having these protracted conversations are twofold: Medical providers do not like to have these discussions, and many families do not like to do so either. In the worst combination of cases, this presents caregivers who are not comfortable in providing bad news with family members who are not equipped to make difficult decisions. A number of studies have confirmed the former, including one in which physicians acknowledge that they are uncomfortable with having discussions regarding a patient's DNR status and oncology fellows acknowledge that they have not received adequate training in delivering bad news, even though they are frequently called upon to do so.[13] It is the responsibility of the members of the medical team to provide thoughtful, careful, empathic information to the patient or surrogate so that decisions can be made that are congruent with the patient's condition, and better training of all staff toward this end seems indicated. Staff trained and experienced in the techniques of palliative care are often much better able to conduct these challenging conversations and can offer assistance to other providers.

Mr. Johnson's case suggests two ways in which staff may fail to provide optimal communication and build trust. First, although it seems that regular communication has occurred, it is not clear from the case description that the providers focused adequately on the family's key concerns. This family was quite helpful in indicating their thought process—because Mr. Johnson had previously looked just as bad on admission but recovered to go home, they see no reason why the same happy outcome should not occur again. Focusing on this issue, staff could have begun early on the process of laying out two scenarios—one in which Mr. Johnson repeated this previous pattern, and one in which this hospitalization sadly proved to be his terminal event. Each day, the providers could have shared with the family the clues they were looking for to see which scenario was unfolding. When, some days into the admission, the caregivers announced their concerns that this would be the hospitalization that Mr. Johnson would not survive, the family would not be surprised at this determination and would be fully apprised of the reasoning behind it.

A second bit of helpful advice for Mr. Johnson's care team comes from one of the most important papers written about ethics and futility.[14] Patients and families feel respected and build trust in the caregivers when told first what *is* going to be done for them, and when the discussion does not lead off with what is *not* going to be done. For a variety of reasons, it has become common practice in American hospitals for the DNR order to serve as a stand-in or substitute for a shift in the overall plan of care from a curative to a palliative strategy, rather than communicating the expectation that doing CPR probably will not work. However, when Mr. Johnson's family is confronted with this proposal to shift care plans with the DNR order as the *first* request made by the staff, it is very hard for them not to interpret this as a sign of abandonment.

A much better way to facilitate communication and trust is to address the new plan of care directly as a positive set of treatments to be applied to the care of the patient. Again, this is where lessons from palliative care practice can be especially beneficial, and illustrates why patients and families do so much better when assigned to receive early palliative care consultation.[15] A conversation that begins, "Mr. Johnson is unfortunately not responding to the treatment plan that we started with, and so we wonder if it's now time to switch to a better plan that will attend to his needs and assure that his suffering is not unnecessarily prolonged" may work much better than, "We recommend writing a DNR order." If the family sees the value of and accepts a plan of care that will avoid treatments that won't work and potentially segue to a plan of palliation, it is much easier to explain why CPR does not play a role in that care plan.

Even well-trained and compassionate caregivers encounter the occasional patient or family that insists upon clearly futile interventions despite prolonged efforts at reasoned communication. Not unusually, this resistance takes one of two forms—"do everything" and "we are hoping for a miracle." Fortunately, recent studies have suggested specific strategies for responding respectfully to families who take these stands with regard to medical futility.[16]

Conclusions

Even as we debate criteria and policies for determining futility, the basic concept is clear—the continuation of the treatment will not work. Fundamentally, it is not possible to eliminate the concept. However, futility can never be placed on a stand-alone basis—it is always in the context of the goals of therapy for a definition to be applied. When the goals are misunderstood, it is more likely that communications will break down. The preferred mode is always to establish those targets at the onset with careful and respectful communications. When that occurs, futility moves into the background; instead, patients, surrogates, and care teams can move as a cohesive unit towards providing optimal patient care.

Notes

1. D. W. Amundsen, "The Physician's Obligation to Prolong Life: A Medical Duty without Classical Roots," *Hastings Center Report* 8, no. 4 (1978).
2. Lawrence J. and Nancy S. Jecker Schneiderman, *Wrong Medicine: Doctors, Patients, and Futile Treatment*, Second ed. (Baltimore: The Johns Hopkins University Press, 2011), p. 11.
3. Ibid., p. 15.
4. Zier et al., "Surrogate Decision Makers' Responses to Physicians' Predictions of Medical Futility," *Chest* 136, no. 1 (2009).
5. Eric W. Widera et al., "Approaching Patients and Family Members Who Hope for a Miracle," *Journal of Pain & Symptom Management* 42, no. 1 (2011).
6. L. J. Schneiderman and N. S. Jecker, *Wrong Medicine: Doctors, Patients, and Futile Treatment*, p. 18.
7. R. Gillon, " 'Futility'—Too Ambiguous and Pejorative a Term?," *Journal of Medical Ethics* 23, no. 6 (1997).
8. Brody, Howard. "Medical Futility: A Useful Concept?" In: *Medical Futility and the Evaluation of Life-sustaining Interventions*, ed. Marjorie B. Zucker and Howard D. Zucker. New York: Cambridge University Press, 1997, pp. 1-14.
9. Texas, "Texas Advanced Directives Act," in *Procedure if not Effectuating a Directive or Treatment Decision* (1999, Amended 2003). http://www.statutes.legis.state.tx.us/Docs/HS/htm/HS.166.htm
10. Robert D. Truog, "Counterpoint: The Texas Advance Directives Act Is Ethically Flawed: Medical Futility Disputes Must Be Resolved by a Fair Process," *Chest* 136, no. 4 (2009). It should be noted that several Texas cases have been appealed to the courts, and in one publicized case, Texas Children's Hospital also provided the plaintiff, the patient's mother, with independent legal advice.
11. Ohio, "Consenting to Withholding or Withdrawing Life-Sustaining Treatment from Patient," in *2133.08* (1991, Amended 2012). http://codes.ohio.gov/orc/2133.08
12. "Medical Futility in End-of-Life Care: Report of the Council on Ethical and Judicial Affairs," *JAMA* 281, no. 10 (1999).
13. See D. P. Sulmasy, J. R. Sood, and W. A. Ury, "Physicians' Confidence in Discussing Do Not Resuscitate Orders with Patients and Surrogates," *Journal of Medical Ethics* 34, no. 2 (2008) and Mary K. Buss et al., "Hematology/Oncology Fellows' Training in Palliative Care: Results of a National Survey," *Cancer* 117, no. 18 (2011).
14. Lawrence J. Schneiderman, Kathy Faber-Langendoen, and Nancy Jecker, "Beyond Futility to an Ethic of Care." *American Journal of Medicine* 96:110–114, 1994.

15. Jennifer S. Temel, Joseph A. Greer, Alona Muzikansky, et al., "Early Palliative Care for Patients with Metastatic Non–small-cell Lung Cancer." *New England Journal of Medicine* 363:733–42, 2010.

16. Widera et al., "Approaching Patients and Family Members who Hope for a Miracle"; Timothy E. Quill, Robert M. Arnold, and Anthony L. Back, "Discussing Treatment Preferences with Patients who Want 'Everything,'" *Annals of Internal Medicine* 151:345–49, 2009.

14

Palliative Sedation

J. Andrew Billings

Palliative sedation (PS) is a recent concept in clinical medicine with a checkered history and multiple meanings.[1] Diverse procedures may be subsumed under this term, and inconsistent definitions have led to misunderstandings and confusion, including mistaking PS for physician aid-in-dying or voluntary euthanasia.[2] Different meanings may also lead to different ethical implications. This chapter parses the multiple definitions of the term, but is primarily about what has come to be known as palliative sedation to unconsciousness (PSU) or continuous deep sedation.

Palliative sedation is founded on a fundamental premise in palliative care: Patients near the end of life should receive meticulous comfort measures aimed at preventing and alleviating physical, psychosocial, and existential/spiritual distress. This premise is based on an ethical and professional duty to prevent and relieve suffering. The goals of patient comfort and of respecting patient wishes in end-of-life decision making are nearly universally imperative for expert palliative care clinicians and they rank these goals very much higher than concerns about possible effects of treatment on length of survival.[3] In the rare situation in which a dying patient faces intractable suffering despite all reasonable approaches to providing comfort, and when the patient finds his or her quality of life unacceptable such that unconsciousness and death would be preferable, clinicians may consider offering palliative sedation to unconsciousness as a "treatment of last resort,"[4] especially if withholding or withdrawing life-sustaining measures will not accomplish the desired "good death."

Case Presentation

Eric was a 51-year-old, previously healthy, single attorney who presented to the emergency room with complaints of headache and fatigue. An MRI revealed a right frontal lobe mass with extensive surrounding edema. He was begun on steroids and phenytoin. On stereotactic brain biopsy, the mass proved to be a glioblastoma multiforme. Surgical resection was not possible, given the extent of his disease. His hospital course was complicated by aspiration pneumonia, likely from leptomeningeal disease causing cranial nerve dysfunction. He refused a tracheostomy, which was considered essential if he were to tolerate radiation therapy.

The patient was referred to the Palliative Care Service while continuing chemotherapy with his neurooncologist. He appeared to have an accurate picture of his illness and was coping reasonably well. On his second visit, Eric asked his palliative care physician if she could assist him by hastening dying.

History

Palliative sedation was first recognized as a distinct clinical entity in the late 1980's[5] and early 1990s.[6,7] It was initially referred to simply as a "continuous opioid infusion,"[5] "sedation in the management of refractory symptoms,"[8] or "severe sedation"[9] and later as "total sedation," "double-effect euthanasia,"[10] or "terminal sedation,"[11] the latter term currently being the most used label in the literature. The ethical similarity of PSU to physician-assisted dying and euthanasia was captured in the term, "slow euthanasia."[12] In the following years, a more descriptive term, "sedation for intractable distress in the dying patient" was proposed but never caught on.[13]

Recently, avoiding the pejorative implications of "terminal"—including the grim association of "terminal" with "terminating" as well as the suggestion that this practice is "terminal" in the sense of occurring only in the very last days of life—"palliative sedation" has become the preferred label. The term allows consideration of sedation that does not necessarily end in death or that occurs only in the last few days of life. "Palliative sedation" has the disadvantage that it does not clearly convey the clinical indication for which the procedure is primarily used—imminently terminal illness with severe, irremediable suffering.

Definitions

Palliative sedation is generally defined as "the use of sedative medications to relieve [or prevent] intolerable and refractory distress by the reduction in patient consciousness."[1]

A few important clarifications about an ethical approach to PSU are necessary.

IMMINENT DEATH

First, the procedure, as reviewed here and widely understood, is only applied to patients near the end of life.

Separate ethical arguments may be required to justify the inclusion of this "imminence condition." The underlying ethical argument for including imminence boils down to the feeling that the patient is going to die soon anyway, so alleviating intractable suffering is more important than concerns about hastening death a little. Conversely (and independent of concerns about intractable, intolerable suffering discussed below), the more that days of living are lost, the more the sanctity of life is violated. In this familiar framework, death of a child is more tragic than death of an elderly person.

The stipulation of imminent death is necessarily vague, since no bright line exists for the beginning of the end of life. Such vagueness invites criticisms about a "slippery slope" that would allow PSU for healthier patients or persons who simply want to end their lives.

Indeed, some of the ethical justifications for PSU could be valid for patients who are not imminently dying. Ethical formulations about PSU regularly fail to delineate clear reasons why sedation for impending death differs substantially from PSU for patients who are not imminently dying[14] or are not even considered terminal. Arguments for and against restricting PSU to the terminally ill have been reviewed elsewhere,[15] and Cellarius[16] has described "early" palliative sedation, a term that attempts to distinguish continuous deep sedation when death is not imminent from its use very near anticipated death. As palliative care moves "upstream," serving patients earlier in the course of their illnesses, the vagueness of the "imminence condition" may become more problematic.

Similarly, a common ethical objection to PSU stresses the uncertainty of prognostication and the risk of applying the procedure to someone who would otherwise have had a long survival. Critics also suggest that opening the door to continuous deep sedation in dying patients will eventuate in the poor, disabled, elderly, or minorities being pressured to use PSU in order to end their lives prematurely.

INFORMED CONSENT

Second, normal procedures for informed consent should be carried out. For a decisionally incapacitated patient, substituted judgment is sought from a health care surrogate and, in general, from the close family. Such consent may be foregone in extraordinary circumstances,[17] such as catastrophic terminal events associated with highly distressing symptoms refractory to conventional measures. But failure to follow a strict protocol for informed consent, as has been reported in the Netherlands,[18] constitutes an objection to allowing PSU. Are patients and their families subtly persuaded or actually coerced into choosing this option? Can PSU be carried out without the consent of the patient, even a decisionally competent patient? These concerns about informed consent for PSU are similar to those about voluntary euthanasia, and contrast with physician aid-in-dying for which hastening of death necessarily involves at least voluntary participation of the patient.

INTRACTABLE, INTOLERABLE SUFFERING

Third, the procedure is reserved for patients with intractable, intolerable suffering. This implies that every other reasonable attempt at alleviating suffering has been attempted, ideally reflecting consultation with palliative care specialists and experts in the type of suffering experienced by the patient.[19] Commentators on PSU often cite the need for a second opinion about the appropriateness of the procedure, and may also stress the importance of psychiatric consultation. Perhaps PSU should not be offered to patients until they have tried or at least considered all imaginable alternatives for managing intractable suffering. This might include, for instance, a full course of electroconvulsive therapy for refractory depression or interventional pain procedures that are invasive, risky, experimental, or even unlikely to benefit the patient.

Critics object that some patients with remediable suffering will be improperly given PSU, simply because the quality of their care is suboptimal. Distress is often difficult to judge in obtunded patients, leading to considerable subjectivity about the need for additional sedation. Rather than focusing on the very few patients who will want PSU (or other controversial means of humanely hastening death), critics argue that resources should be directed to promoting excellent palliative care and further research on alleviating suffering.

When the reason for considering PSU is psychosocial or existential/spiritual suffering, new ethical and clinical questions may arise. These forms of suffering, like pain and dyspnea, are subjective but are less palpable to an outside observer. Is this kind of suffering as "real" as pain? How much is intolerable? Indeed, even with physical pain, how much suffering is unbearable? Would patients report that they are in terrible emotional distress because they know that such claims would entitle them to PSU? Is it the health profession's duty to try to alleviate all kinds of distress, rather than seeing some suffering in this world as inevitable, unfortunate?

A "LAST RESORT"

Finally, palliative sedation to unconsciousness is, along with voluntarily stopping eating and drinking, physician aid-in-dying, and voluntary euthanasia, a "treatment of last resort."[20-22] This implies that no other reasonable clinical option is available to manage intractable, intolerable suffering, especially other professionally accepted means of clouding consciousness or hastening death, such as withholding or withdrawing of life-sustaining measures.

But patients may choose a plan of care that leads to suffering, such as when they refuse interventions that could alleviate discomfort (e.g., a nasogastric tube that might alleviate vomiting from an obstructive gastrointestinal lesion) or lead to a gentle death (e.g., stopping dialysis). The notion of a "last resort" might be a reflection not only of the capabilities or limitations of clinical medicine—the notion of intractability described above—but also of individual patient decisions about their care. Ethical concerns may arise if the patient refuses what the healthcare team considers reasonable options for managing suffering near the end of life, including such widely accepted practices as withholding or withdrawing life supports. And what if the patient is unwilling to consider treatments (e.g., amputation for a gangrenous limb) or assume the risks and side effects of interventions (e.g., neurosurgical procedures that risk paralysis or cognitive impairment)?

Similarly, as in the case of patients who choose to voluntarily stop eating and drinking, should the subsequent symptoms—distress from hunger and thirst that patients seems to have brought upon themselves—be palliated with continuous deep sedation?

Types of Palliative Sedation

At least three categories of sedation in dying patients have been described,[4] and four additional subcategories also need to be delineated.

ORDINARY SEDATION

Ordinary sedation is commonly applied in a wide range of patients in varying stages of diseases, typically to lessen anxiety or promote sleep.

PROPORTIONATE PALLIATIVE SEDATION

Proportionate palliative sedation (PPS) uses the minimum amount of sedation necessary to relieve refractory symptoms at the end of life. Unconsciousness is not a goal, though increases in sedation may lead to mental clouding. Indeed, reports in the literature suggest that a significant number of sedated patients near the end of life are receiving doses of sedatives that exceed usual practices.[23]

Ethical controversy about PPS is minimal unless sedation leads to unconsciousness or, in the absence of artificial hydration and nutrition, leads to the inability to eat, drink, or otherwise maintain one's life. In these situations, especially as the level of sedation increases, PPS melds with PSU, and the relevant ethical issues are discussed under that category.

PALLIATIVE SEDATION TO UNCONSCIOUSNESS

Palliative sedation to unconsciousness is a more controversial practice that may be considered for occasional cases of intractable suffering near the end of life, typically after all other measures to control symptoms have been exhausted and when withdrawal or withholding of life-sustaining measures will not lead to a peaceful death. The goal is unconsciousness because, as far as is known, only such deep sedation is certain to prevent and treat the patient's physical and psychological suffering. Palliative sedation to unconsciousness could also be considered "proportionate," because deep sedation is believed to be the level of consciousness necessary to achieve adequate relief of refractory symptoms.

Familiar instances of "turning up the morphine drip" without evidence of patient distress and with the often-unacknowledged purpose of hastening death should not be considered ethically equivalent to PSU.

The drugs used to produce unconsciousness here are typically sedatives or anesthetics and, depending on clinical circumstances, analgesics, usually added on to whatever sedatives or opioids were already being used.[25] The term is almost universally used to describe a level of sedation that may depress respiration (and increase the risk of aspiration) but does not include assisted breathing by invasive or noninvasive techniques to sustain adequate ventilation. Indeed, these latter options are not discussed in the clinical literature and would not seem appropriate for an imminently terminal patient.

SUBCATEGORIES FOR PSU

Temporary versus Continuous Sedation

Is the patient to be continued on palliative sedation until death or is the plan to attempt to reduce sedation and awaken the patient at a later time? Is death going to be accepted as a natural part of the illness if it occurs during PS or is death going to be "fought off" by providing artificial hydration and nutrition or even ventilator support during the process?

Conceivably, temporary sedation would allow for symptoms to resolve or for some treatment that alleviates symptoms to take effect, and then PSU would no longer be necessary. Providing PSU while providing fluids and nutrition and with the intent to reawaken the patient is a medical procedure that can be justified by the usual weighing of the benefits and burdens of the therapy; no special ethical examination is required. Such a procedure is used, for instance, in severely burned patients who may even require intubation and mechanical ventilation due to respiratory depression from analgesics and sedatives. (Temporary sedation in palliative care is similar to the recently discredited use of deep sedation or anesthesia for immediate withdrawal from addictive drugs.[24])

Because temporary PSU has been mentioned in the palliative care literature but not reported beyond a few cases studies, it will not be discussed further; in the following comments, PSU will be assumed to be applied continuously without a plan for reversal or recovery. Critics may consider such protracted sedation a violation of the patient's dignity and an unfair burden on the family as they wait for the patient to die. Is it fair to the family to draw out the process when the certain outcome is death?

Provision versus Withholding/Withdrawing of Fluid and Nutritional Support

The provision of fluids and nutrition for a patient receiving continuous PSU makes little sense from some ethical perspectives because it merely prolongs survival in an irreversibly meaningless state. An expert panel of the Royal Society of Canada suggests using the term, "terminal sedation," only when deep sedation is associated with not providing fluids and nutrition.[25] However, insofar as concerns are raised

about hastening death with PSU, as discussed later (and despite widespread acceptance of withholding fluids and nutrition in similar situations), fluid and/or nutritional support might sometimes be instituted for the comfort of the family or staff.

Target Level of Sedation

What degree of depression of consciousness is considered adequate for alleviating
symptoms? For instance, should the patient be sedated so as not to appear to be in
distress or should the patient receive deep sedation or anesthesia to fully relieve any
possible distress?[26] How do we make sense of the studies suggesting that patients
recall the experience of being under general anesthesia and suffer distress after-
wards?[27] Yet deep sedation or anesthesia risks hypotension, respiratory depression,
and aspiration, and thus may pose an increased risk of hastening or causing death?

This issue will not be discussed further here except to express concern that severe
physical insults, such as suffocation, probably require deep sedation or anesthesia to
assure that the patient does not suffer, yet such a depression of consciousness might
contribute to an earlier death. Sedation that merely reduces the appearance of distress while not alleviating severe suffering—similar to the effect of neuromuscular
blockade[28]—would be unethical because it would leave the patient in anguish.

Preemptive Palliative Sedation to Unconsciousness

Certain end-of-life procedures, most notably terminal extubation in conscious patients, are highly likely to lead to severe distress, and clinicians routinely
increase sedation for critically ill patients undergoing withholding or withdrawal of
life-sustaining treatments.[29] For instance, an alert patient with amyotrophic lateral
sclerosis and respiratory failure will experience suffocation if removed from ventilatory support.[30] Titration of sedatives and analgesics in response to symptoms assures
that such a patient suffers while waiting for the medication to take effect, so preemptive palliative sedation is required for a humane terminal extubation. High doses of
sedatives assure that the patient does not suffer needlessly, though death is likely to
be hastened by a short period of time. The patient dies quickly, which looks and feels
like euthanasia. The levels of sedating medications are also similar to those employed
for euthanasia. Thus, the practice is humane but controversial.[26,27,30] To allow such
suffering when it could be alleviated would be unethical.[31]

Terminal extubation must be contrasted to a situation in which extubation has
a chance of leading to survival, including instances where minimal sedation may be
required. In such instances, clinicians must balance the risk of permitting suffering
against the possibility of allowing survival.

Epidemiology and Usual Practices

Despite the best efforts of palliative care teams, a small number of patients experience intolerable and refractory symptoms, such as pain or dyspnea, especially in the

last few days of life.[8,32] An American study noted requests for euthanasia in about 4% of palliative care patients,[33] evidence that such patients experience considerable suffering despite expert clinical care. Thus, without the option of PSU or other means of humanely hastening death, some patients will face intractable suffering near the end of life.

Early reports in the 1990s indicated that continuous sedation to unconsciousness was already prevalent in both Italian home care[6] and a Canadian palliative care unit.[34] Because of variations in the definition of PS, reports of its incidence range from 0% to 86%.[35] Recent data that specifically address PSU indicate that the procedure is used in as few as 2.5% of deaths in Denmark and as many as 8.5% in Italy.[36] Its prevalence is gradually increasing in the Netherlands where PSU accounted for 7.1% to 8.2% of deaths in 2005 and 12.2% in 2010[37,38] whereas PSU in Belgium was reported in 14.5% of deaths in 2007 compared with 8.2% in 2001.[39] The frequency of PS in hospice programs was 0% to 44%.[20]. No reliable data are available from the United States.

In a large, multicenter Japanese study, the authors cite the primary reasons for PSU (in order of frequency) as fatigue, dyspnea, delirium, "psycho-existential suffering," troubling bronchial secretions, and pain.[40] In a Dutch specialized palliative care unit, terminal restlessness and dyspnea were the primary indications for PSU.[41] In other studies, breathlessness, pain, and agitated delirium or restlessness represent the bulk of indications; a small percentage of PSU is prescribed for insomnia, itching, bleeding, and nausea/vomiting.[42]

Hesitation to use PS for existential suffering has been noted,[43] but in some series, "mental anguish" or "psychological distress" accounts for as many as 40% of cases; in contrast, about 3% of cases of physician-assisted suicide in this study were performed for psychiatric reasons.[44]

The prevalence of clinician reports of debilitating physical complaints in PSU contrasts strikingly with data on physician aid-in-dying. In Oregon, the major reason for requesting assisted suicide was a desire for control of the circumstances of death and to die at home, as well as worries about loss of dignity and future losses of independence.[45]

Beyond these data, little or no information is available on why the patients themselves choose PSU, its impact on family involvement and bereavement, or how the procedure is viewed by clinicians.[46] Because of the unregulated practice of PSU in most countries, facts about the procedure are clouded in uncertainty, and a case can be made that formal reporting of the procedure to hospitals, the board of health, or similar civil authorities and to researchers would provide valuable oversight of PSU.

Typical medications used for PSU include benzodiazepines, barbiturates, neuroleptics, and general anesthetics, often combined with opioids.[47,48] The success rate in controlling individual symptoms is reported to be 60% to 96%.[49,50] In the Japanese study, patients generally were deeply sedated an hour after the initiation of continuous deep sedation, whereas death occurred in 3 days or less for 77% of patients. Four percent of patients apparently experience fatal complications related to sedation, whereas 20% experienced respiratory and/or circulatory suppression.[40,49]

Case Presentation Continued

On further questioning, Eric stated that he wished to avoid undue suffering and to minimize being a burden to his family. He strongly rejected the possibility of living in a facility and expressed deep fear of "losing my mind and who I am as a person."

A thorough clinical evaluation confirmed that Eric was not suffering physically and that he was not depressed or confused. His longstanding primary care physician believed that the request for control over his death was very consistent with Eric's temperament: "A brain tumor is the worst thing that could happen to such an independent brilliant man." His siblings supported his request, noting that independence and a need for control had suited him well as a successful "self-reliant" professional. Still, they encouraged him to remain alive so they could enjoy his company and say goodbye.

Eric was referred to hospice. The palliative care physician served as primary physician. Over a 1-month period, the patient repeated his entreaty for help to quickly end his psychological suffering.

Normative Ethics and Palliative Sedation to Unconsciousness

In the clinical and ethics literature now, palliation sedation to unconsciousness is generally considered morally acceptable when the guidelines described above are followed. On both procedural and ethical grounds, PSU can usually be clearly distinguished from other modes of more directly and explicitly hastening death, such as voluntarily stopping eating and drinking, physician aid-in-dying, and voluntary euthanasia.[20] International and national consensus statements have been issued that support the practice.[25,51-55]

But exceptions are notable. Many of the ethical concerns or objections to PSU have already been outlined above in reviewing the clinical ambiguity of various definitions and corollary delineations about the procedure. A fundamental critique arises from the principle of nonmaleficence—the professional obligation to do no harm—or from foundational beliefs and associated moral arguments against killing or hastening death: "thou shalt not kill." Attendant concerns arise that PSU will be used improperly or that it is likely to evolve along the slippery slope into euthanasia. For instance, in 2003, 17% of physicians recognized the procedure as legally permitted, but objected to it on religious or moral grounds.[56] Another critic, reflecting some of the concerns noted above, claimed:

> *Terminal sedation seems consistent with traditional medical care but often is a form of euthanasia. Moreover, it is a practice that is ethically more problematic than assisted suicide or voluntary euthanasia.*[57]

The grounds for ethical acceptance of palliative sedation can be viewed in a variety of moral frameworks:

JUSTIFIABLE KILLING

To begin the discussion of formal ethics, I find the formulation of Brock[58] (and later by Miller and Truog[59]) the most convincing and broadly applicable framework for beginning to understand the morality of PSU and its relationship to other acts that hasten death near the end of life. In brief, certain forms of killing and hastening death are permissible in our society, with examples being killing in war, execution for certain crimes, withholding or withdrawing life supports, and terminating pregnancy. The distinction between these acts and impermissible acts, such as homicide or involuntary euthanasia, is one of moral values, not a strict and inviolable prohibition against killing or hastening death. (This view is nicely captured in the title of a book review, "Doctors Do Quite a Lot of Killing. Get Over It."[60]) Likewise, just as accidental homicide is distinguished from involuntary manslaughter, some fatal mistakes in medical practice (a surgeon nicking the aorta or an internist unwittingly prescribing a medication that leads to anaphylaxis) are more easily forgiven than clinical negligence. A dialogue about the permissibility of PSU (or physician aid-in-dying or voluntary euthanasia) should not be based on simple rules, such as "doctors must not kill,"[61] but rather on a fuller exploration of moral values.

THE RULE OF DOUBLE EFFECT

The rule of double effect is a very useful ethical concept that is regularly employed, mostly implicitly, in clinical practice. Indeed, practically all discussions of the ethics of PSU center on the rule of double effect,[62] such that it allows many clinicians to carry out the procedure without ethical doubts. The clinical literature is, at best, bland and monolithic in its approach to justifying the procedure: In a review of a small number of recent articles in the English literature, this rule was used exclusively in papers from the United States and included in all papers from outside the country, though, interestingly, papers from the European countries where assisted dying is legalized addressed a much broader range of ethical concepts. The almost exclusive reliance on double effect to justify PSU reflects a poverty of moral discourse.[62]

As formally defined, the rule (or doctrine or principle) of double effect requires that:

(1) The act is morally good or at least indifferent.
(2) The intent of the act is only to cause a good effect.

(3) A bad effect may be foreseen but is not intended and would have been avoided if a satisfactory alternative method to achieve the good effect could be found.

(4) The desirable effect follows from the intended effect, not from the bad effect.

(5) A proportionately grave reason exists for seeking the good effect and thus compensates for risking or permitting the bad effect.

The rule of double effect can provide a ready justification for PSU:

(1) Providing sedation to alleviate suffering is morally good.

(2) The intent of palliative sedation is only to alleviate intractable suffering.

(3) Death associated with sedation is a foreseen but not intended outcome and would have been avoided if a satisfactory alternative method to alleviate intractable suffering could be found.

(4) The alleviation of intractable suffering follows from the sedation, not from causing or hastening death.

(5) Seeking to alleviate intractable suffering is a proportionately grave reason for initiating palliative sedation, and thus compensates for the risk of causing or hastening death.

Multiple critiques of the rule of double effect as it generally applies to end-of-life decisions, particularly its reliance on assessing intentions (as opposed to behavior) and its failure to recognize ambivalence, have been put forward,[63,64] but the rule has also has been strenuously defended.[65-67] I will not reiterate these issues except to say that the rule of double effect, as turned to in most biomedical discussions of hastening death, is deeply flawed. It represents a handy justification for carrying out acts without suitable ethical deliberation, especially on the morality of hastening death. As applied, it relies on the assumption that intentionally hastening death is never permissible. Using the rule of double effect intelligently requires much deeper consideration of basic ethical judgments needed to employ it properly, including ethical decisions about acceptable modes of treatment, permissible intentions, moral means, and the weighing of the proportional benefit or harm of intended and unintended effects.[68]

Death is an inevitable consequence of PSU. Without reawakening the patient and/or without providing fluid and nutritional support, the procedure surely leads to death. Saying the intention is exclusively to alleviate symptoms requires turning a blind eye to the obvious result: PSU is also intended to lead inevitably to a peaceful death and can hasten death, especially when death is imminent but not expected in a few days or a week. As stated by Orentlicher, "death results from the physician's intentional actions."[69] To say death is foreseen but not intended when death is inevitable requires bizarre mental machination.

As commonly used, the rule specifies that causing death is an immoral act rather than, at times, a desirable outcome. Indeed, the principle of double effect is irrelevant to end-of-life situations if hastening death is considered to be an acceptable act under certain circumstances, as discussed above in the work of Brock and others.

IS PSU ETHICALLY DIFFERENT FROM VOLUNTARY EUTHANASIA?

The clinical procedure of providing PSU can be distinguished from actions that constitute voluntary euthanasia and physician aid-in-dying. But in many situations, ethical justification under the rule of double effect may simply be an excuse for seeking and providing a kind death—in other words, be a subterfuge for euthanasia, albeit slow euthanasia.

The aims of voluntary euthanasia and of PSU carried out while withholding or withdrawing life-sustaining treatments can be viewed as the same. From a utilitarian/consequentialist perspective, killing a patient slowly—by sedating him deeply and continuously and by not providing fluids or nutrition—is no different ethically than euthanasia, because the outcomes of both procedures are the same. One procedure typically kills by depressing respiration, the other by preventing eating and drinking. By performing the procedure slowly, the clinician avoids the suddenness of death and feels a diminished sense of agency, and perhaps feels better about less shortening of the patient's lifespan compared to when an intentional overdose is administered.[70] Except for the slowness of the procedure, PSU can be viewed as ethically no different than euthanasia or physician-assisted dying (hence our term, "slow euthanasia"[12]).

DO TWO RIGHTS MAKE A WRONG?

First, PSU is typically justified on the basis of the rule of double effect under which patients are entitled to sedation to unconsciousness insofar as the intent of the act is to alleviate suffering, not to cause death. But the act of providing PSU leads to the inability to eat or drink, which might be considered an unintentional but foreseen effect. Second, patients are granted the right to refuse any treatment, such as the administration of fluids and nutrition. But when patients are continuously sedated to unconscious and fluids and nutrition are also withheld, death is inevitable. In such a situation, the applicability of the rule of double effect is dubious because the "bad" effect could have been avoided by providing fluids and nutrition. And death can be viewed as ensuing from clinician-induced dehydration rather than from the underlying disease.

PATIENT RIGHTS AND CULTURAL CHANGE

The expansion of individual rights in our society constitutes a broad social movement, which, in turn, is reflected in evolving professional medical practice. The recognition of the primacy of patient choice in end-of-life care decisions grew gradually through the latter half of the 1900s. Simultaneously, end-of-life care options that were initially considered unethical became allowable in limited circumstances, and eventually became conventional practices, beginning with the acceptance of extubating ventilator-dependent patients and of foregoing CPR. As more treatments arose that could sustain life, ethical approval developed for withholding or withdrawing the provision of fluids and nutrition, stopping or foregoing dialysis, and turning off pacemakers and other cardiac assist devices. Now, hastening death under the rule of double effect has become clinically acceptable while, more recently, palliative sedation has become recognized in some circles as part of good, ethical care.[71-73]

Recognizing a right to self-determination does not necessarily mean accepting a right to receive a procedure like palliative sedation upon request. A fundamental difference exists between refusing life-sustaining treatment and requesting a life-ending treatment.[74] Thus, opponents of palliative sedation (as with physician aid-in-dying or voluntary euthanasia) may subscribe to promoting patient autonomy but not accept PSU. Or they may describe such practices as "autonomy run amok."[75]

See Figure 14.1 for a scheme that shows both a timeline of change and the degree of current acceptability of procedures that hasten death. This secular trend is likely to lead to great acceptability of PSU over time. Here, what is ethical may be defined by what is considered acceptable by society. Cultural acceptance of a

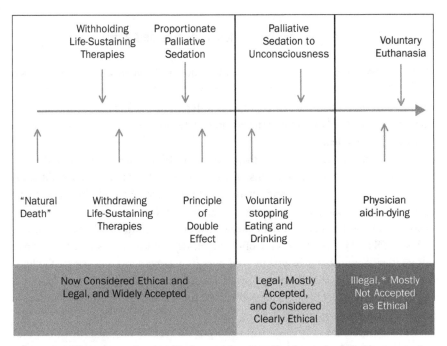

FIGURE 14.1 Changes over time in ethical approval and legality of procedures that hasten death, as well as a gradient of clinician acceptance of those procedures in the United States.

* Except in Oregon, Washington, Montana, Vermont, and a few European countries

practice is not, of course, necessarily a good ethical justification for that practice; what feels right in practice may lead subsequently to ethical rationalizations.

Legality

A series of legal cases[76,77] support the right of patients to receive relief from suffering,[78] as most clearly stated by Justice O'Connor:

> ...a patient who is suffering from a terminal illness and who is experiencing great pain has no legal barriers to obtaining medication, from qualified physicians, to alleviate that suffering, even to the point of causing unconsciousness and hastening death.[79]

In Canada, a recent report from the Royal Society of Canada Expert Panel on End-of-Life Decision-Making stresses that "terminal sedation in circumstances where it is not required to alleviate physical suffering should be considered euthanasia" but also recommended that physician-assisted suicide and voluntary euthanasia be legalized with appropriate safeguards."[25]

However, such court decisions or expert recommendations do not guarantee that the clinician performing PSU will not encounter murder accusations and legal actions.[80]

Does Palliative Sedation to Unconsciousness Hasten Death?

Although continuous PSU inevitably leads to death, the medical literature shows a curious preoccupation on whether palliative sedation hastens death.[81] A variety of studies purport to show that survival is no different for patients receiving PSU and similar patients[29,35,82] and that clinicians intend sedation to treat intolerable symptoms, not hasten death.[83]

There are four problems with these assertions. First, the bulk of the studies are retrospective but even the two arms of prospective studies are necessarily different because studies do not randomize patients into two arms. Second, the median survival is typically just a few days, making significant differences in survival unlikely; instances of longer survival are not separated out for study.[81,83] Third, the various types of PS and its indications are often not clearly defined or described so a range of practices are probably being reported. Finally, it simply makes sense that at least some patients' lives are shortened, given the known impact of deep sedation on such preterminal events as hypotension or aspiration, and the inevitable death produced by long periods of withholding fluids and nutrition.

More important, why is survival a concern? In looking at studies of withdrawal or withholding life-sustaining treatments—acts that surely can hasten death—the duration of survival is not an issue in assessing the ethics of the procedures. Would we view the procedure differently if it sometimes did hasten death?

Clinical and ethical confusion abounds on this issue. Regardless of the data, many physicians feel they are shortening life with palliative sedation, even for as long as months.[49] Dutch physicians justify PSU because they feel it does not hasten death, yet they offer it as an option to their patients early in the course of a terminal illness, whereas American physicians offer it very near the end of life and feel it might hasten death but justify the procedure by saying that they do not intend hastening.[84]

Clinical Skills: Responding to Requests for Hastened Death

Requests for palliative sedation and other means of hastening death require a detailed palliative care evaluation. First, what is leading to the request: physical, emotional, social/financial, or existential/spiritual suffering; fear of suffering, loss of control, loss of dignity, abandonment; intolerance of dependency and uncertainty, and a need for control; depression, delirium, or other major psychiatric disorders; narcissism, impulsivity, or other serious personality disorders; and so on?[19] Only with this background and assurances that every step has been taken to address the suffering and underlying meaning of the request can an ethical and clinically sensitive decision be made about the appropriateness of palliative sedation.

Case Presentation Continued

Eric's palliative care clinician requested that he speak with the team social worker and chaplain. They confirmed essentially the same story as the physician. The social worker did not identify any undue social or economic pressure that influenced the patient's choice, and the chaplain felt that Eric was spiritually and existentially at peace with his decision. The whole team carefully reviewed the case and had no further suggestions for alleviating the patient's suffering or reversing his decision.

Physician-assisted dying was illegal in Eric's state. Withdrawal of the steroids and anticonvulsants was considered but dismissed as not promising a humane dying. As a last resort, palliative sedation to unconsciousness was considered. The team was reluctant to use the procedure for emotional suffering, and noted how many patients on the service seemed to be suffering more—both physically and emotionally—than Eric. But they could not think of any reason that this sort of pain was less real and should be treated differently than overt physical suffering. They considered surreptitious assisted suicide but felt that the risk to individual providers and the Palliative Care Service was too great. They worried over the palliative care physician's attachment to and possible over-identification with Eric because the two shared a similar age and social background. After a great deal of discussion, the team agreed to offer palliative sedation to unconsciousness. One member chose not to be part of the procedure due to ethical and professional concerns.

Eric felt reassured and validated by the team's decision but hesitated to accept sedation initially, saying that he still had personal and business affairs to complete. He revised his will and made arrangements for his funeral and burial. A few weeks later, he called the palliative care physician, noting occasional choking and worsening cough with meals, as well as sudden right arm weakness. He requested immediate palliative sedation to unconsciousness at home with his family attending.

After extensive discussion with the hospice, it was agreed that the procedure would be carried out at home under supervision of the palliative care physician and nurse practitioner, assisted by the hospice staff. Eric was again offered the opportunity to change his mind, but he felt quite certain of his decision and that the time was right.

At the appointed hour, his family was present, as were the hospice chaplain and palliative care physician and nurse practitioner. An infusion of pentobarbital was initiated and slowly titrated until the patient was unresponsive to voice and chest rub. Steroids were discontinued but phenytoin was given rectally to prevent seizures that might upset his family.

Higher doses of the pentobarbital were required initially because the patient became more alert as he became dehydrated and his cerebral swelling diminished. Over the next few days, further upward titrations of the infusion were required to maintain deep sedation. The family was impatient over the prolonged course and wondered why the team could not make it go faster.

The patient died peacefully on day 4 of the procedure. The hospice nurse and chaplain consoled the family and arranged for bereavement services. The palliative care physician signed the death certificate, wrote a letter of condolence, and followed up with the family a few weeks later. Eric's death was discussed in team meeting and his name was read at a biannual palliative care memorial service, attended by his two sisters.

Safeguards

Just as the procedure for carrying out physician aid-in-dying is carefully prescribed in Oregon[85] and Washington, and safeguards for voluntary euthanasia are mandated in the Netherlands, a strong case can be made for similar protections in PSU.[86,87] Indeed, given the current ethical and legal acceptance of PSU, the procedure is utilized frequently even where other better-regulated methods for hastening death are legalized, and it has a greater potential for abuse.

Possible safeguards might include:

(1) Requirements for careful documentation of the reasons for the procedure, the completeness of the clinical evaluation, and how PSU was conducted

(2) Assurance of informed consent (or, in the case of a decisionally incapacitated patient, consent of a healthcare proxy and/or close family members)

(3) A second physician's independent opinion, ideally by a palliative care specialist, that addresses the possibility of less aggressive remedial treatments and concerns about coercion

(4) A psychiatric consultation, if feasible, in cases of depression or suspected major mental illness

(5) The ability of physicians and other potentially involved clinicians, on personal grounds, to opt out of performing the procedure while providing referral to a willing clinician

Because PSU is most often used to respond to severe and otherwise intractable suffering, a waiting period would generally not be appropriate except perhaps in cases of predominantly psychosocial and spiritual distress. Formal reporting and review by a professional or governmental body, similar to the procedure employed in Oregon for physician-aid-in dying, could potentially be intrusive and burdensome, but would not be illogical.

Conclusion

Whatever one's claims about the universality or applicability of various moral frameworks, one can usually find both objections to and support for PSU. Most ethical theories can be employed in a fashion that either justify or prohibit palliative sedation, or can identify circumstances under which the procedure is acceptable or not. In current practice, justifications for palliative sedation typically turn to the rule of double effect and the rights of the suffering patient, whereas objections cite the importance of tradition in the physician-patient relationship and the fear of the slippery slope.

Culture matters in these deliberations. Within the contemporary Western field of bioethics and academic medicine, relatively little objection to PS in general and PSU specifically is now evident. However, conservative religious groups in the West and most people outside of the wealthy, industrial democracies, including orthodox believers in the Christian, Jewish, and Muslim religions, may strongly object to any act that seems to hasten death—acts which for them may include withholding and withdrawing life support, and PSU. Objections are typically based on notions of the sanctity of life, the belief that only God should choose when someone dies, and a general respect for traditional authority—attitudes that are less prevalent in educated Western circles wherein autonomy and individual rights often hold sway in moral decisions. In another twist, Buddhists may not choose PSU because a lack of conscious awareness of suffering and death may impact on subsequent reincarnation. A pluralistic view—itself admittedly a culture-based concern—should recognize and tolerate the diversity of moral stances, both within and especially outside of Western, industrialized, wealthy democratic countries.[62]

Ethical appraisal of PSU in the United States, as with so many other moral issues, reflects our culture and history. It is a product of our era—an era in which an already existing Truth, along with other general principles or absolute or objective moral values, as traditionally pursued by philosophers, may no longer seem to be out there to be discovered by reasoning. As Richard Rorty points out,

> *Our identification with our community—our society, our political tradition, our intellectual heritage—is heightened when we see this community as ours rather than nature's, shaped rather than found, one among many which men have made. In the end, the pragmatists tell us, what matters is our loyalty to other human beings clinging together against the dark, not our hope of getting things right.*[88]

In this regard, the historical march of secularism and an associated rights-based approach that expands the role of autonomy in decisions about hastening death may, for the moment, best capture our contemporary culture's useful solution to these ethical matters. Dilemmas that trouble us now, similar to the predicaments about withholding and withdrawing life supports that unsettled us a half century ago, may become moot points.

Finally, when faced by the question, "Is it morally justifiable to leave a patient in severe distress?"[31] and lacking good alternatives to palliative sedation, our moral intuition teaches us to find reasons to justify the procedure.

References

1. Morita T, Tsuneto S, Shima Y. Definition of sedation for symptom relief: a systematic literature review and a proposal of operational criteria. J Pain Symptom Manage 2002;24:447–53.
2. Asch DA. The role of critical care nurses in euthanasia and assisted suicide. N Engl J Med 1996;334:1374–9.
3. Raijmakers NJ, Van Zuylen L, Costantini M, et al. Issues and needs in end-of-life decision making: an international modified Delphi study. Palliat Med 2012;26:947–53.
4. Quill TE, Lo B, Brock DW, Meisel A. Last-resort options for palliative sedation. Ann Intern Med 2009;151:421–4.
5. Stuart GJ, Davey EB, Wight SE. Continuous intravenous morphine infusions for terminal pain control: a retrospective review. Drug Intell Clin Pharm 1986;20:968–72.
6. Ventafridda V, Ripamonti C, De Conno F, Tamburini M, Cassileth BR. Symptom prevalence and control during cancer patients' last days of life. J Palliat Care 1990;6:7–11.
7. Truog RD, Berde CB, Mitchell C, Grier HE. Barbiturates in the care of the terminally ill. N Engl J Med 1992;327:1678–82.
8. Cherny NI, Portenoy RK. Sedation in the management of refractory symptoms: guidelines for evaluation and treatment. J Palliat Care 1994;10:31–8.
9. Bruera E, Chadwick S, Weinlick A, MacDonald N. Delirium and severe sedation in patients with terminal cancer. Cancer Treat Rep 1987;71:787–8.
10. Decisions near the end of life. Council on Ethical and Judicial Affairs, American Medical Association. JAMA 1992;267:2229–33.

11. Enck RE. Drug-induced terminal sedation for symptom control. Am J Hosp Palliat Care 1991;8:3–5.
12. Billings JA, Block SD. Slow euthanasia. J Palliat Care 1996;12:21–30.
13. Chater S, Viola R, Paterson J, Jarvis V. Sedation for intractable distress in the dying—a survey of experts. Palliat Med 1998;12:255–69.
14. Cellarius V. Terminal sedation and the "imminence condition." J Med Ethics 2008; 34:69–72.
15. Mayo DJ, Gunderson M. Vitalism revitalized: Vulnerable populations, prejudice, and physician-assisted death. Hastings Cent Rep 2002;32:14–21.
16. Cellarius V. "Early terminal sedation" is a distinct entity. Bioethics 2009;25:46-54.
17. Claessens P, Menten J, Schotsmans P, Broeckaert B. Level of consciousness in dying patients. The role of palliative sedation: a longitudinal prospective study. Am J Hosp Palliat Care 2012;29:195–200.
18. Rietjens JA, Bilsen J, Fischer S, et al. Using drugs to end life without an explicit request of the patient. Death Stud 2007;31:205–21.
19. Block SD, Billings JA. Patient requests to hasten death. Evaluation and management in terminal care. Arch Intern Med 1994;154:2039–47.
20. Quill TE, Lo B, Brock DW. Palliative options of last resort: a comparison of voluntarily stopping eating and drinking, terminal sedation, physician-assisted suicide, and voluntary active euthanasia. JAMA 1997;278:2099–104.
21. Quill TE, Lee BC, Nunn S. Palliative treatments of last resort: choosing the least harmful alternative. University of Pennsylvania Center for Bioethics Assisted Suicide Consensus Panel. Ann Intern Med 2000;132:488–93.
22. Lo B, Rubenfeld G. Palliative sedation in dying patients: "we turn to it when everything else hasn't worked." JAMA 2005;294:1810–6.
23. Sykes N, Thorns A. Sedative use in the last week of life and the implications for end-of-life decision making. Arch Intern Med 2003;163:341–4.
24. Collins ED, Kleber HD, Whittington RA, Heitler NE. Anesthesia-assisted vs buprenorphine- or clonidine-assisted heroin detoxification and naltrexone induction: a randomized trial. JAMA 2005;294:903–13.
25. Schuklenk U, van Delden JJ, Downie J, McLean SA, Upshur R, Weinstock D. End-of-life decision-making in Canada: the report by the Royal Society of Canada expert panel on end-of-life decision-making. Bioethics 2011;25 Suppl 1:1–73.
26. Billings JA. Terminal extubation of the alert patient. J Palliat Med 2011;14:800–1.
27. Billings JA. Humane terminal extubation reconsidered: the role for preemptive analgesia and sedation. Crit Care Med 2012;40:625–30.
28. Truog RD, Burns JP, Mitchell C, Johnson J, Robinson W. Pharmacologic paralysis and withdrawal of mechanical centilation at the end of life. N Engl J Med 2000;342:508–11.
29. Wilson WC, Smedira NG, Fink C, McDowell JA, Luce JM. Ordering and administration of sedatives and analgesics during the withholding and withdrawal of life support from critically ill patients. JAMA 1992;267:949–53.
30. Berger JT. Preemptive use of palliative sedation and amyotrophic lateral sclerosis. J Pain Symptom Manage 2012;43:802–5.
31. Schneiderman LJ. Is it morally justifiable not to sedate this patient before ventilator withdrawal? J Clin Ethics 1991;2:129–30.

32. Vainio A, Auvinen A. Prevalence of symptoms among patients with advanced cancer: an international collaborative study. Symptom Prevalence Group. J Pain Symptom Manage 1996;12:3–10.
33. Coyle N, Adelhardt J, Foley KM, Portenoy RK. Character of terminal illness in the advanced cancer patient: pain and other symptoms during the last four weeks of life. J Pain Symptom Manage 1990;5:83–93.
34. Fainsinger R, Miller MJ, Bruera E, Hanson J, Maceachern T. Symptom control during the last week of life on a palliative care unit. J Palliat Care 1991;7:5–11.
35. Maltoni M, Pittureri C, Scarpi E, et al. Palliative sedation therapy does not hasten death: results from a prospective multicenter study. Ann Oncol 2009;20:1163–9.
36. Miccinesi G, Fischer S, Paci E, et al. Physicians' attitudes towards end-of-life decisions: a comparison between seven countries. Soc Sci Med 2005;60:1961–74.
37. Rietjens J, van Delden J, Onwuteaka-Philipsen B, Buiting H, van der Maas P, van der Heide A. Continuous deep sedation for patients nearing death in the Netherlands: descriptive study. BMJ 2008;336:810–3.
38. Onwuteaka-Philipsen BD, Brinkman-Stoppelenburg A, Penning C, de Jong-Krul GJ, van Delden JJ, van der Heide A. Trends in end-of-life practices before and after the enactment of the euthanasia law in the Netherlands from 1990 to 2010: a repeated cross-sectional survey. Lancet 2012;380:908–15. Epub 2012 Jul 11.
39. Bilsen J, Cohen J, Chambaere K, et al. Medical end-of-life practices under the euthanasia law in Belgium. N Engl J Med 2009;361:1119–21.
40. Morita T, Chinone Y, Ikenaga M, et al. Ethical validity of palliative sedation therapy: a multicenter, prospective, observational study conducted on specialized palliative care units in Japan. J Pain Symptom Manage 2005;30:308–19.
41. Rietjens JA, van Zuylen L, van Veluw H, van der Wijk L, van der Heide A, van der Rijt CC. Palliative sedation in a specialized unit for acute palliative care in a cancer hospital: comparing patients dying with and without palliative sedation. J Pain Symptom Manage 2008;36:228–34.
42. Maltoni M, Scarpi E, Rosati M, et al. Palliative sedation in end-of-life care and survival: a systematic review. J Clin Oncol 2012;30:1378–83.
43. Dean MM, Cellarius V, Henry B, Oneschuk D, Librach L, Taskforce CSOPCP. Framework for continuous palliative sedation therapy in Canada. J Palliat Med 2012;15:870–9. Epub 2012 Jul 2.
44. Groenewoud JH, van der Maas PJ, van der Wal G, et al. Physician-assisted death in psychiatric practice in the Netherlands. N Engl J Med 1997;336:1795–801.
45. Ganzini L, Goy ER, Dobscha SK. Why Oregon patients request assisted death: family members' views. J Gen Intern Med 2008;23:154–7. Epub 2007 Dec 15.
46. Dobscha SK, Heintz RT, Press N, Ganzini L. Oregon physicians' responses to requests for assisted suicide: a qualitative study. J Palliat Med 2004;7:451–61.
47. Carter MJ, Gibbins J, Senior-Smith G, Thomas S, Guest P, Forbes K. Ketamine: does it have a role in palliative sedation? J Pain Symptom Manage 2008;36:e1–3. Epub 2008 Aug 9.
48. McWilliams K, Keeley PW, Waterhouse ET. Propofol for terminal aedation in palliative care: a systematic review. J Palliat Med 2010;13:73-6.
49. Morita T, Chinone Y, Ikenaga M, et al. Efficacy and safety of palliative sedation therapy: a multicenter, prospective, observational study conducted on specialized palliative care units in Japan. J Pain Symptom Manage 2005;30:320–8.

50. Claessens P, Menten J, Schotsmans P, Broeckaert B. Palliative sedation: a review of the research literature. J Pain Symptom Manage 2008;36:310–33.
51. Hawryluck LA, Harvey WR, Lemieux-Charles L, Singer PA. Consensus guidelines on analgesia and sedation in dying intensive care unit patients. BMC Med Ethics 2002;3:E3.
52. National Ethics Committee VHA. The ethics of palliative sedation as a therapy of last resort. Am J Hosp Palliat Care 2006;23:483–91.
53. Cherny NI, Radbruch L. European Association for Palliative Care (EAPC) recommended framework for the use of sedation in palliative care. Palliat Med 2009;23:581–93.
54. Kirk TW, Mahon MM. National Hospice and Palliative Care Organization (NHPCO) position statement and commentary on the use of palliative sedation in imminently dying terminally ill patients. J Pain Symptom Manage 2010;39:914–23.
55. Position Paper on Aid in Dying. (Accessed at http://www.amwa-doc.org/cms_files/original/Aid_in_Dying1.pdf.)
56. Curlin FA, Lawrence RE, Chin MH, Lantos JD. Religion, conscience, and controversial clinical practices. N Engl J Med 2007;356:593–600.
57. Orentlicher D. The Supreme Court and physician-assisted suicide—rejecting assisted suicide but embracing euthanasia. N Engl J Med 1997;337:1236–9.
58. Brock DW. Life And Death: Philosophical Essays in Biomedical Ethics. Cambridge: Cambridge University Press; 1993.
59. Miller FG, Truog RD, Brock DW. Moral fictions and medical ethics. Bioethics 2010;24:453–60.
60. Nelson JL. Doctors do quite a lot of killing. Get over it. Hastings Cent Rep 2012;42:46–7.
61. Kass LR. Why doctors must not kill. Commonweal 1991;118:472–6.
62. Billings JA, Churchill LR. Monolithic moral frameworks: how are the ethics of palliative sedation discussed in the clinical literature? J Palliat Med 2012;15:709–13.
63. Quill TE, Dresser R, Brock DW. The rule of double effect—a critique of its role in end-of-life decision making. N Engl J Med 1997;337:1768–71.
64. Quill TE. Principle of double effect and end-of-life pain management: additional myths and a limited role. J Palliat Med 1998;1:333–6.
65. Sulmasy DP, Pellegrino ED. The rule of double effect: clearing up the double talk. Arch Intern Med 1999;159:545–50.
66. Sulmasy DP. Commentary: double effect—intention is the solution, not the problem. J Law Med Ethics 2000;28:26–9-2.
67. Sulmasy DP, Curlin F, Brungardt GS, Cavanaugh T. Justifying different levels of palliative sedation. Ann Intern Med 2010;152:332–3; author reply 3.
68. Billings JA. Double effect: a useful rule that alone cannot justify hastening death. J Med Ethics 2011;37:437–40.
69. Orentlicher D. Terminal sedation [author reply]. N Engl J Med1998;338:1230–1.
70. Douglas C, Kerridge I, Ankeny R. Managing intentions: the end-of-life administration of analgesics and sedatives, and the possibility of slow euthanasia. Bioethics 2008;22:388–96.
71. Simon A, Kar M, Hinz J, Beck D. Attitudes towards terminal sedation: an empirical survey among experts in the field of medical ethics. BMC Palliat Care 2007;6:4.
72. Hasselaar J, Verhagen S, Reuzel R, van Leeuwen E, Vissers K. Palliative sedation is not controversial. Lancet Oncol 2009;10:747–8.

73. Billings JA, Krakauer EL. On patient autonomy and physician responsibility in end-of-life care. Arch Intern Med 2011;171:849–53.

74. Truog RD. Patients and doctors: the evolution of a relationship. N Engl J Med 2012;366:581–5.

75. Callahan D. When self-determination runs amok. Hastings Cent Rep 1992;22:52–5.

76. Washington v. Glucksberg. In: Court USS, ed. 117 SCt 2302; (1997).

77. Vacco v. Quill. In: Court USS, ed. 117 SCt 2293; (1997).

78. Burt RA. The Supreme Court speaks—not assisted suicide but a constitutional right to palliative care. N Engl J Med 1997;337:1234–6.

79. O'Connor J. Washington v. Glucksberg. 521 US 702 1997.

80. Cohen L, Ganzini L, Mitchell C, Arons S, Goy E, Cleary J. Accusations of murder and euthanasia in end-of-life care. J Palliat Med 2005;8:1096–104.

81. Thorns A, Sykes N. The use of sedatives at the end of life. Palliat Med 2001;15:347.

82. Morita T, Tsunoda J, Inoue S, Chihara S. Do hospice clinicians sedate patients intending to hasten death? J Palliat Care 1999;15:20–3.

83. Claessens P, Menten J, Schotsmans P, Broeckaert B. Palliative sedation, not slow euthanasia: a prospective, longitudinal study of sedation in Flemish palliative care units. J Pain Symptom Manage 2011;41:14–24.

84. Rietjens JA, Voorhees JR, van der Heide A, Drickamer MA. Approaches to suffering at the end of life: the use of sedation in the USA and Netherlands. J Med Ethics 2012;Sep 14 [Epub head off print].

85. The Oregon Death with Dignity Act: A Guidebook for Health Care Professionals. 2008. (Accessed at http://www.ohsu.edu/xd/education/continuing-education/center-for-ethics/ethics-outreach/upload/Oregon-Death-with-Dignity-Act-Guidebook.pdf.)

86. Braun TC, Hagen NA, Clark T. Development of a clinical practice guideline for palliative sedation. J Palliat Med 2003;6:345–50.

87. Palliative sedation protocol. Hospice & Palliative Care Federation of Massachusetts, 2004. (Accessed at http://www.hospicefed.org/hospice_pages/reports/pal_sed_protocol.pdf.)

88. Rorty R. Pragmatism, relativism and irrationalism. Proceedings and Addresses of the American Philosophical Association 1980;53:719–38.

15

Voluntarily Stopping Eating and Drinking

Emily B. Rubin and James L. Bernat

Ideally, every patient with far-advanced illness would receive optimal palliative care and comprehensive psychosocial support such that few patients ever would wish to hasten their own death. Even in areas where excellent palliative care is widely available, however, some patients with terminal illness or complex chronic medical conditions experience suffering, loss of meaning, or deterioration in quality of life to the point where they express a readiness to die and a desire to expedite the dying process.

There has been extensive discussion in both the political and bioethics arenas about the ethics of taking action to affirmatively hasten death under such circumstances and the propriety of clinicians participating in such efforts. Much of the discussion has focused on physician-assisted death (PAD) (also known as physician-assisted suicide), in which a physician provides the medical means that allow a patient to actively hasten the dying process. Less attention has been paid to the practice of voluntarily stopping eating and drinking (VSED) near the end of life. In this chapter, we discuss the practice of VSED, including the arguments in support of VSED as a legal and ethical way to hasten death when a patient with advanced illness is ready to die, the ethical distinctions between VSED and PAD, some of the benefits and disadvantages of VSED as a means of hastening death, safeguards that we believe clinicians should seek to enforce when patients consider VSED, and some of the practical challenges and potential limitations of the practice.

Definitions and Background

It is important at the outset to define what is meant by VSED. Many elderly and severely ill patients naturally lose their appetite and thirst, and sometimes the actual physical skills necessary to eat and drink, toward the end of life. This natural anorexia and loss of thirst accompanied by the cessation of eating and drinking is distinct from VSED, which is an active decision by a competent patient with advanced illness to stop eating and drinking as a mechanism of intentionally hastening his or her death. We use the medical rather than the legal concept of competence: A patient is considered "competent" to make a particular decision about his health care if she or he has the capacity to understand and appreciate the information necessary to make a rational decision.

By way of example, we first present two prototypic cases of patients who might consider VSED. The cases are abstracted from personal experience of the authors and from written personal accounts by David Eddy (1994) and Sophie Mackenzie (2012).

CASE #1 PRESENTATION

Ms. W. is a 57- year-old woman with breast cancer widely metastatic to her bones and lungs. Given the extent of her disease burden, she is not a candidate for further curative treatment and is enrolled in hospice. She has received palliative radiation, but continues to have pain that is only partially relieved by high doses of intravenous narcotics. The narcotics are causing significant nausea that is only partially relieved by antiemetics. She has difficulty controlling her bowels and bladder and is entirely dependent on others for her activities of daily living. She is dyspneic and bedbound. She has always been a very active person and physical activity has always been a source of great satisfaction for her. She finds living in a completely sedentary state, totally dependent on others, demoralizing and unsatisfying. She has come to terms with her mortality and wishes to die peacefully on her own terms without prolonging the dying process any further. She asks the hospice nurse what would happen if she were to stop eating and drinking.

CASE #2 PRESENTATION

Mrs. M. is an 84-year-old woman who was in excellent health and led a very independent and active lifestyle until a year and a half ago, when she fell and suffered a hip fracture. Her recovery was complicated by a course of severe Clostridium difficile *colitis, which required prolonged hospitalization. As she was recovering in a rehabilitation facility, she developed a significant pneumonia, which required rehospitalization. In the setting of repeated antibiotic treatment, she again developed* Clostridium difficile *infection, this time refractory to treatment. She had up to twelve diarrheal stools per day and was frequently incontinent of stool. She lost weight, became anemic, suffered from abdominal pain, weakness, and severe hip pain. She was unable to live at home by herself and was discharged from the hospital to a skilled nursing facility. She is in great discomfort and is no longer able to engage in activities that gave her life meaning and pleasure, such as daily walks and gardening. In consultation with her three grown children, she decides that she is ready to die and plans to stop eating and drinking to hasten this process.*

Depending on the individual patient circumstances, including burden of disease and baseline nutritional, hydrational, and metabolic status, death following cessation of all food and fluids, which is caused by dehydration, typically will happen in a period lasting from several days to 3 weeks (Bernat, Gert, & Mogielnicki 1993). The patient often will be awake and alert for many days following initial cessation of eating and drinking and then will become progressively less conscious in the setting of natural sedative effects from ketones or other metabolites that reduce consciousness. (Bernat et al. 1993; Quill, Lo, & Brock 1997; Truog & Cochrane 2005).

Other potential options for patients with advanced illness who wish to hasten death include PAD, which involves a physician providing the necessary medical means for a terminally ill patient to commit suicide (typically a lethal dose of an oral medication). Currently, PAD is legal in only four of the United States— Oregon, Washington, Montana, and Vermont. Palliative sedation (PS) is the practice of sedating a terminally ill patient to the point of unconsciousness in the setting of intractable suffering and stopping nutrition and hydration and any other life-sustaining treatments. Palliative sedation is widely considered to be legal based on the notion that, although it may have the secondary effect of hastening death, the primary objective of palliative sedation is to relieve intractable symptoms (Quill et al. 1997). Voluntary active euthanasia, the practice of a physician actively administering a lethal medication to a patient upon request, is not legal anywhere in the United States. These practices are discussed in detail elsewhere in this volume and we mention them only by way of comparison with VSED.

Unlike a patient who pursues PAD, a patient who elects VSED is not entirely dependent on a physician to help facilitate the process. Although a patient can stop eating and drinking without involvement of medical professionals, clinicians can nevertheless play several roles in a patient's decision to pursue VSED. Initially, the clinician can help to understand the foundation of the patient's desire to stop eating and drinking and ensure that it is not the result of treatable mental illness or inadequate treatment of symptoms that can be palliated. In addition, the clinician can advise a patient of his options and what to expect if he does decide to stop eating and drinking. If a patient decides to pursue VSED, the clinician can support the patient and his family emotionally through this process, and assist in palliating symptoms such as physical pain, dry mouth, nausea and vomiting, and agitation. Several observational studies suggest that death from lack of hydration and nutrition in this setting usually is peaceful and comfortable if pharmacologic treatment is provided to treat uncomfortable symptoms (Ganzini et al. 2003).

Empirical evidence suggests that many patients with advanced illness express a desire to hasten death. The majority of these patients have advanced cancer or severe neurological disease such as amyotrophic lateral sclerosis, but some have complex constellations of chronic illness that severely compromise their independence and quality of life.

Breitbart and colleagues (2000) administered a self-report measure called Schedule of Attitudes toward Hastened Death to 92 terminally ill cancer patients and found that 17% had a high desire for hastened death. Likewise, in a survey of 69 patients with advanced cancer, 58% of the participants believed that, if legal, they might request a hastened death and 12% would have made a request at the time of the interview (Wilson et al. 2000). In another survey of 988 terminally ill patients, 10.6% reported seriously considering euthanasia or PAD for themselves (Emanuel, Fairclough, & Emanuel 2000).

These studies are supported by evidence that clinicians frequently receive requests from patients for PAD. Of 828 clinicians over a range of specialties responding to a questionnaire in the state of Washington before PAD became legal in that state, 26% had been asked at least once for PAD or euthanasia (Back et al. 1996). In a study by Meier and colleagues published in 1998, 11% of 1,902 clinicians surveyed said there were circumstances in which they would be willing to hasten a patient's death by prescribing medication and 18.3% had received a request from a patient for assistance with suicide since starting practice. In a more recent study in France, 342 out of 789 palliative care organizations reported a total of 783 requests for hastened death during the year 2010 (Ferrand et al. 2012).

Although there is strong evidence for the desire to hasten death and for requests for PAD among patients with advanced illness, there is sparse evidence to suggest how often patients raise or discuss the specific possibility of VSED as an option with their clinicians or how many are aware that VSED is an option. In a series of studies conducted in Oregon between 1997 and 2001, Ganzini and colleagues examined the experience of hospice nurses and social workers with patients who requested hastened death. Forty-five percent of 179 nurses and social workers reported caring for one or more patients who had explicitly requested a prescription for lethal medication (Ganzini et al. 2002). Forty-one percent of 307 nurses reported caring for a patient who voluntarily chose to stop eating and drinking (Ganzini et al. 2003).

A convincing body of evidence suggests that, although physical pain can be a contributing factor, patients with advanced illness who consider taking measures to hasten their own death are most often motivated by other reasons (Breitbart et al. 2000; Emanuel et al. 2000; Ganzini et al. 2003). The reasons most frequently cited for such requests include actual or feared loss of independence, poor quality of life, readiness to die, loss of dignity, feeling that continued existence is pointless, and desire to have some control over the circumstances of one's own death (Ganzini et al. 2002, 2003). As Quill and colleagues (1992) noted, many people fear the "prospect of losing control and independence and of dying in an undignified, unesthetic, absurd, and existentially unacceptable condition."

VSED as a Legal and Ethical Last Resort Distinct from PAD

As a starting premise, any intervention that is specifically intended to or likely to hasten death should be considered only as a last resort. Early and optimal palliative care should be the standard of care in all communities and should include the management of physical pain, depression, anxiety, and spiritual and existential issues including loss of meaning and dignity. When a patient with advanced illness indicates a desire to hasten death, the physician and other caregivers should first seek to address all potential sources of suffering, ideally in consultation with palliative care specialists and mental health professionals if there is serious concern that treatable mental illness may be contributing to the desire to hasten death.

The palliative care movement embraces the notion that the entire life cycle, including the dying process, presents opportunities for meaning and personal growth (Block 2001). Many have argued, specifically in the context of PAD, that intentionally hastening death in a patient with advanced illness runs contrary to this deeply embedded spirit and detracts from the goal of optimal palliative care for all patients (Foley 1997; Byock 2012; Emanuel 2012). It is a reality, however, that certain competent patients will persist in desiring a hastened death notwithstanding best efforts to palliate their suffering. When this happens, VSED is the least ethically and legally controversial option.

Legally and ethically VSED is distinct from PAD. Because both actions involve the intentional hastening of death, one could argue that drawing an ethical line between them is therefore arbitrary. However, VSED can be distinguished practically and ethically from PAD on the grounds that VSED involves a *refusal* of an intervention while PAD involves a *request* for lethal medication (Bernat 1993; Miller & Meier 1998). An informed patient with capacity to understand the consequences of his or her decisions has the right to refuse unwanted medical intervention (Cruzan 1990; Meisel 1992; Bernat et al. 1993; Miller & Meier 1998). That right is based on respect for individual autonomy and bodily integrity, which forbids a competent patient from being forcibly treated against his will, and the right to refuse intervention holds even if that refusal will have the effect of hastening death (Vacco v. Quill 1997). There is no corresponding right to receive an intervention such as the prescription of a lethal dose of medication. As Miller and Meier (1998) put it, "refusal of a carefully considered request for clinician-assisted suicide interferes with a patient's self-determination but does not amount to a personal assault."

In supporting a patient who elects VSED, a clinician is respecting the patient's right to refuse an intervention. There is a well-recognized ethical distinction between respecting a patient's right to refuse treatment and providing the actual means by which a patient may hasten his own death, between "letting a patient die and making that patient die" (Vacco v. Quill 1997). This distinction most often has been discussed in the setting of distinguishing PAD from the withdrawal of life-sustaining treatment such as mechanical ventilation, dialysis, or artificial nutrition and hydration (Alpers & Lo 1997; Vacco v. Quill 1997; Miller, Fins, & Snyder 2000). There is broad consensus that declining these types of life-sustaining medical interventions is not a suicidal act and a clinician's participation in the discontinuation of such treatments is therefore not considered PAD (Fosmire v. Nicoleau 1990; Vacco v. Quill 1997).

Some argue that, based on the bedrock bioethical principle that a clinician must honor a patient's valid refusal of an intervention, the practice of patients voluntarily stopping eating and drinking near the end of life "avoids moral controversy altogether" (Bernat et al. 1993, p. 2723). Under this logic, food and fluids are an intervention that patients are as free to reject as life-sustaining interventions such as mechanical ventilation, hemodialysis, chest compressions or antibiotics (Truog & Cochrane 2005). Clinicians are "morally and legally prohibited from overruling the rational refusal of therapy by a competent patient even when they know that death will result" (Bernat et al.1993). On the contrary, they are permitted, and arguably professionally obligated, to provide appropriate palliative care for any pain and suffering that may accompany the refusal of such therapy.

Others less comfortable with the notion of VSED might argue, however, that the consumption of food and fluids by a patient who is physically able to take them by mouth is not properly designated "medical care" or a "medical intervention" because even completely healthy patients ultimately would die if they did not eat and drink. They might further argue that refusal of food and fluids by one who is able to take them by mouth is therefore suicide, that suicide is immoral and that clinicians should not facilitate suicide in any way.

It is true that the refusal to take food and fluids by mouth is not precisely equivalent to the refusal of interventions that we typically consider to be "life-sustaining." Whereas we routinely respect a patient's right to refuse life-sustaining medical interventions, we do not routinely allow people to commit suicide or compromise their health by starvation and dehydration without intervening. Patients with life-threatening anorexia nervosa or severe depression, and prisoners who undertake hunger strikes, for example, sometimes are fed against their will. They are not generally considered to have a categorical right to refuse food and fluids (although it is not ethically uncontroversial to force feed adult anorexics and some argue that at least some patients with eating disorders should have their refusals of food and fluids respected based on principles of autonomy and self-determination [Draper 2000; Campbell & Aulisio 2012]).

Regardless, however, VSED by patients with advanced illness can be distinguished from self-starvation and dehydration by patients with anorexia based on the concept of rationality. A patient's decision can be considered "rational" if it does not cause harm to the patient without sufficient reason, such as avoiding a greater harm. Although rationality is by nature subjective and depends on how each individual ranks harms and benefits, rankings of harms and benefits that result in a person suffering great harm without an adequate reason, and which would be viewed as irrational by almost everyone in that person's culture, can generally be counted as irrational (Bernat et al. 1993). An otherwise healthy anorexic who weighs the benefits of not eating more highly than the risk of death from starvation arguably is acting irrationally in ranking priorities in that order. Given the irrationality of such a patient's thought process, which suggests a failure to appreciate the consequences of his actions, the otherwise healthy anorexic patient might also be said to lack decision-making capacity. It is much more difficult to argue that a patient with terminal cancer or another advanced illness who ranks weeks to months of physical and existential suffering as worse than immediate death is acting irrationally or lacks decision-making capacity.

Likewise, we think that the argument that VSED is suicide and therefore immoral can be rejected based on similar grounds. It is arguably true that a patient who elects VSED "introduces the fatal cause," begging the question of whether it is a form of suicide (Cantor & Thomas 2000). However, although suicide is defined by most sources as voluntary and intentional self-killing (Merriam-Webster 2012) without any reference to rationality or justification, one of the primary reasons that many consider suicide morally objectionable is that they view the individual who commits suicide as acting under an irrational assumption that his situation will never improve to the point where taking his own life would no longer seem preferable to continuing to live (Schwartz 2007). One who commits suicide typically is considered to be acting irrationally in prioritizing immediate death over continued life. As Judith Schwartz (2007) has suggested, suicide implicates tragedy, waste, and the possibility of regret.

This moral objection cannot reasonably be applied to a patient who is in the final stages of life and has no realistic prospect of continued life without significant suffering. One might acknowledge that hastening one's own death in the setting of advanced illness accompanied by significant suffering is suicide, but argue that it is nevertheless a rational act under those circumstances and therefore not immoral. One could also argue that suicide is by definition an irrational act and so the rational prioritization of immediate death over continued suffering is not accurately characterized as suicide. This distinction is largely semantic, however. Whether or not VSED is classified as a form of suicide, it is not categorically irrational for a terminally ill or chronically ill patient to hasten death in order to relieve intractable suffering of a physical or psychosocial nature or to end an existence that the patient finds intolerable.

Potential Benefits of VSED over Other Methods of Hastening Death

VSED has several potential benefits over other forms of hastening death. First, the fact that VSED is a process that requires time can be viewed as an advantage. Although getting through the initial days to weeks of consciousness without eating and drinking can require determination and resolve by the patient, it has the attendant benefit of providing a natural period for grieving, reconciliation and saying goodbye to loved ones. It also provides an opportunity for a patient to reverse the process if he has a change of heart once the process is underway.

It is generally understood that patients who refuse nutrition and hydration and receive adequate palliative care for symptoms die peacefully and do not suffer (Printz 1992; Bernat et al. 1993; Eddy 1994; Quill et al. 1997). This may be in part because ketones and other metabolites that accumulate during the starvation process are thought to have sedative and anesthetic effects (Elliott, Haydon, & Hendry 1984). If symptoms do become difficult to manage, administration of deep sedation to manage them is an option (Rady & Verheijdge 2012). The hospice nurses in Oregon surveyed by Ganzini and colleagues who had cared for a patient choosing VSED "rated the last two weeks of life as peaceful with low levels of pain and suffering" (Ganzini 2003, p. 362) and rated most deaths as "good." VSED avoids some of the complications that can occur when patients attempt suicide by lethal ingestion, including vomiting and inability to swallow enough pills (Emanuel 2012).

An additional benefit of VSED is to allow the clinician in his final interactions with the patient to act as a caregiver rather than an agent of the patient's death. Many object to PAD on the grounds that a clinician should never be in the role of facilitating the death of a patient and that to involve clinicians in such an enterprise distorts the role of the clinician in society, compromises professional integrity, and ultimately undermines public trust in the profession (American Medical Association 1996; Curlin et al. 2008). Others have attempted to extend similar arguments to VSED, suggesting that if a clinician believes that VSED is a form of suicide, he should not support VSED as an acceptable alternative because, in doing so, he would be collaborating in wrongdoing (Jansen & Sulmasy 2002). One might further argue that supporting a patient's decision to stop eating and drinking is in conflict with a clinician's professional commitment to healing and supporting a patient through his natural lifespan.

On the contrary, respecting a patient's refusal of intervention; supporting and caring for a patient and his family through the dying process by treating unpleasant symptoms; and helping to provide the patient with a peaceful, dignified death can be viewed as an extension of the healing and caring role (Jacobs 2003). In addition, a clinician faced with a patient insistent on stopping eating and drinking has essentially no ethically acceptable option other than to support the patient in his or her choice. It would be morally repugnant for a clinician to attempt to involuntarily hospitalize or force feed a patient with a terminal illness against the patient's will, and it would be a violation of the covenant between clinician and patient for a clinician to abandon a patient in need toward the end of life. The only possible option other than supporting the patient through the process of VSED would be to find another clinician willing to do so, and this is likely to prove quite difficult in the setting of advanced illness and an established therapeutic relationship.

Just as supporting a patient through VSED is less morally ambiguous than participating in PAD, it likely is considered legal in all states. Laws against assisted suicide are commonplace. The California Penal Code Section 401, for example, provides that "every person who deliberately aids, or advises, or encourages another to commit suicide, is guilty of a felony." Although a law such as this theoretically could be used against a clinician who encouraged a patient in a decision to hasten his death by cessation of eating and drinking, the authors are not aware of any case in which this has happened, and the provision of support and palliative care to a patient going through the process of VSED clearly does not fall within the spirit or intention of the statutes governing assisted suicide. It seems extremely unlikely that a court ever would intervene to force nutrition and hydration on a competent patient with advanced illness who refused them.

Finally, even in states where PAD is legal, there are noteworthy bureaucratic hurdles involved in the process. Because VSED involves refusal of an intervention rather than affirmative action on the part of the clinician to hasten death, it can be a decision and a process that takes place between a patient, the patient's loved ones, and the patient's clinician, avoiding the involvement of third parties and outside regulators.

Potential Disadvantages

There also are potential disadvantages to VSED. First, it takes much resolve by the patient to persist through the first few days of the process without eating or drinking. Any attempt to offer the patient food or water might be seen as unwelcome pressure on the patient to reconsider, but failure to offer might also be perceived as endorsing the choice to hasten death (Bernat et al. 1993; Miller & Meier 1998). Some might argue that requiring a terminally ill patient to demonstrate the resolve required to maintain the decision to stop eating and drinking and to endure several days of lingering in a semiconscious state is cruel and demeaning if there are options available for hastening death that might entail less suffering, such as palliative sedation. On this note, many patients in the study conducted by Ganzini and colleagues (2003) favored PAD over VSED as a means of hastening death based on the belief that clinicians have the expertise required to peacefully end life.

Another potential concern about VSED as a means of hastening death is the effect that it might have on family members and nonfamily caregivers. A more prolonged process arguably provides a natural window for grieving, making peace, and saying goodbye. On the other hand, it may be difficult for certain family members or other loved ones to witness the slow decline of a loved one over a period of several days to weeks. There may also be caregivers who are morally opposed to VSED and need to be educated about the rights of the patient.

Standards and Safeguards

Although it ultimately is a competent patient's prerogative to decide whether to stop eating and drinking, physicians and other clinicians who are privy to a patient's desire to hasten his death have a responsibility to implement safeguards to avoid coercion and uninformed or impulsive decision making. If a patient expresses a desire to stop eating and drinking, notwithstanding a clinicians' efforts to address any identifiable sources of suffering, the clinician should seek to ensure that the patient (1) has a desire to hasten death that is stable over time; (2) does not have a treatable mental illness that might be influencing the decision to hasten death; (3) is fully informed about his disease processes and prognosis; (4) is not being pressured to hasten his death; and (5) has the capacity to understand the consequences of the decision to undertake VSED. The last three of these criteria, taken together, are the elements of informed consent.

One serious concern is that a patient who expresses a desire to hasten his death might be going through a low period and that the desire may not be stable over time. There is evidence to suggest that the desire of terminally ill patients to hasten death does not remain stable over time (Chochinov et al. 1995). In one study of terminally ill patients conducted by Emanuel and colleagues (2000), for example, half of those who seriously considered PAD or euthanasia later changed their minds. The clinician caring for such a patient should ideally have many visits with the patient over a period of time to ensure that the expression of a readiness to die is enduring.

Others have expressed legitimate concern that the desire to hasten death might be a sign of depression in terminally ill patients and that it would be wrong to allow patients with untreated depression to hasten their own death. It is notoriously difficult to identify depression in medically ill patients and to distinguish depression from hopelessness or demoralization. The hallmarks of clinical depression include hopelessness about the future and loss of appetite, two features that are often present in terminally or chronically ill patients. It can be very difficult to separate out a potentially irrational wish for death precipitated by clinical depression from a rational wish to die rather than endure a life one understandably finds unbearable (Chochinov et al. 1997; Block 2000; Breitbart et al. 2000; Cohen et al. 2000; Werth 2004).

There is robust evidence that depression is strongly correlated with desire to hasten death. In a study of 92 terminally ill cancer patients, Breitbart and colleagues (2000) found that desire for hastened death was significantly associated with both a clinical diagnosis of depression and hopelessness (without a clinical diagnosis of depression). In a prospective cohort study of 138 terminally ill cancer patients, Dutch researchers found that depressed patients were four times more likely to request euthanasia or physician-assisted suicide (van der Lee et al. 2005). Similarly, in a study of 988 terminally ill patients, those with depressive symptoms were 25% more likely than those without to consider euthanasia or PAD and were over five times as likely as those who were not depressed to change their mind about desiring a hastened death (Emanuel et al. 2000). In one cross-sectional survey of 58 Oregonians ill with cancer or amyotrophic lateral sclerosis who had requested or expressed interest in aid in dying, 15 met criteria for depression and 13 met criteria for anxiety. Of that cohort, 3 depressed participants died by lethal ingestion (Ganzini, Goy, & Dobscha 2008).

All patients who express a wish to hasten death by any means should be evaluated for depression and anxiety and those who appear to be suffering from a treatable mental illness should be encouraged to try a course of treatment prior to making a definitive decision about hastening death. In cases in which it is difficult to determine whether a patient is depressed, the treating clinician should pursue consultation by a mental health professional. In jurisdictions in which PAD is legal, these requirements generally are codified as part of the rules governing the legal implementation of PAD (e.g., Oregon Death with Dignity Act, 127.825 §3.03). With VSED, because the patient rather than the clinician controls the means of hastening death, the clinician cannot strictly require that such steps to rule out and treat depression be taken as a precondition to taking action to hasten death. Nevertheless, clinicians may be in a position to encourage a patient to take seriously the possibility that mental illness is influencing her or his thinking and to trial a course of treatment. Ultimately, if a patient rejects this suggestion, but still has capacity to understand the implications of his decision to stop eating and drinking, a clinician would be obligated to respect that refusal.

Another relevant apprehension about any method of hastening death in the setting of advanced illness is the possibility that a vulnerable patient will feel pressured into hastening death by financial considerations or anxiety that he is a burden on loved ones or society. This pressure is of particular concern if a clinician is the one to mention the possibility of hastening death, as opposed to the patient initiating the conversation voluntarily.

The prospect of undue influence raises the question of how the prospect of VSED should be handled in routine palliative care. For example, should VSED be a routine part of discussions about palliative care in terminally ill patients? Or should those involved in the care of such patients discuss it only if a patient voluntarily and consistently expresses a desire to hasten death? Or should clinicians raise the option of VSED only if a patient specifically asks about it? Some might argue that routine discussion by clinicians of VSED as an option is contrary to the role of the clinician as healer and that, given the authority many patients assign to clinician suggestions, the mere raising of the possibility of VSED would make some patients feel pressured into following through (Jansen & Sulmasy 2002). Under this logic, discussion of VSED would be appropriate only if the conversation were initiated by the patient.

Other commentators have suggested that discussing the possibility of VSED with a patient as a mode of hastening death poses a smaller possibility of undue influence than discussing the possibility of PAD (Bernat et al. 1993; Miller & Meier 1998), in part because the affirmative act of prescribing lethal medication might be viewed as legitimization by the medical profession in a way that supporting a patient through VSED may not. It may also be that, because VSED is carried out over a period of days to weeks instead of in a discrete action, offering the possibility of a change of heart, it is less likely to result in pressure on the patient. Realistically, however, it is possible that any given patient to whom a clinician mentions the possibility of a hastened death might interpret this as a suggestion and feel pressure to avail herself of the option of hastening death in order to unburden others.

On the other hand, we know that many terminally ill patients consider and take action to intentionally hasten death by stopping eating and drinking. Some of those patients might undertake the process without optimal support and palliative care, and suffer unnecessarily as a result. If the option were normalized and demystified as a part of overall conversations about options at the end of life, patients likely would feel more free to discuss it openly, be more likely to be evaluated for depression or other potentially treatable mental illnesses, and be less likely to feel that they were alone or being singled out or coerced into considering into ending their lives. Just knowing that there is an option to exert some control over the circumstances of one's death might comfort patients, even if few ever chose to take advantage of that option.

Likewise, if VSED were a more universally acknowledged option for patients with advanced illness who express a readiness to die, it might relieve pressure from physicians who may be asked to provide lethal medication in violation of state law and feel pressure to do so in order to help a suffering patient. Finally, if VSED were a part of the conversation about legitimate palliative care options for patients who have an enduring readiness to die notwithstanding provision of thorough palliative care, more clinicians might be educated about how to provide optimal support and treatment of symptoms through that process. All clinicians involved in these conversations should take particular care to reassure patients that the decision to stop eating and drinking is intensely personal and that the clinician's willingness to discuss it is in no way intended to suggest that the patient should pursue it.

Another challenge is whether and how to delineate boundaries between patients who might express a desire for VSED. Generally, we think of palliative options of last resort applying to patients who are terminally ill (i.e., have a prognosis of 6 months or fewer to live). However, patients who are chronically but not terminally ill, either with one primary disorder such as ALS or another devastating neurological disorder, or with a constellation of medical problems that markedly compromises independence or quality of life (similar to Mrs. M. in case #2 laid out in the introduction to this chapter), may also seek to hasten death (Eddy 1994; Mackenzie 2012). Furthermore, some patients who are given a particular diagnosis they find unbearable and who do not wish to live through the process of treatment and likely inevitable physical decline might also wish to hasten death. Consider, for example, a young patient in her late forties recently diagnosed with metastatic ovarian cancer but otherwise doing fairly well physically with an overall prognosis that is unfavorable but not clear in terms of time. She has always been extremely independent and active and finds the mere prospect of the medicalization of her life and slow physical decline so untenable that she wishes to stop eating and drinking now.

Some scholars argue that any patient who is informed and understands the consequences of voluntarily stopping eating and drinking should have the right to make that decision free of intervention (Truog & Cochrane 2005). There may be, however, some situations in which a clinician is faced with a seriously medically ill patient who has decisional capacity but whose desire to stop eating and drinking in an effort to hasten death seems so premature or irrational that the clinician feels compelled to aggressively discourage the patient from taking steps to hasten death. Although it is difficult to imagine a scenario under which it would be ethically appropriate to actually force a competent patient with terminal illness or complex chronic medical conditions to accept nutrition and hydration via a feeding tube or otherwise, individual clinicians need to use prudence and judgment regarding whether and how vigorously to attempt to dissuade such patients from proceeding with VSED and when to insist on psychiatric intervention.

Some invoke the danger of the "slippery slope" and the difficulty of drawing clear lines to argue that clinicians simply should not support any method of hastening death. The mere prospect that some patients might feel an element of pressure, or that there could be outliers at the extreme who seek to undertake VSED when many people would judge that decision to be irrational, does not mean that we should dismiss or discourage the practice of VSED. As Marcia Angell wrote in support of PAD in 1997, "the question is not whether a perfect system can be devised, but whether abuses are likely to be sufficiently rare to be offset by the benefits to patients who otherwise would be condemned to face the end of their lives in protracted agony" (p. 52).

Conscientious Objection

Although VSED is legal, certain individual clinicians might have specific moral or religious objections to the practice of VSED and on that basis refuse to support any patient who is considering it. In the case of PAS, states that have legalized the practice have provided explicitly that physicians who have moral objections to the practice are not obligated to participate in it (ORS 127.885 §4.01). There is a generally recognized right among clinicians to decline to provide certain other medical services based on conscientious objection, which historically has focused largely on activities such as abortions and prescription of emergency contraception (Dickens 2001; Curlin et al. 2007; Wicclair 2011).

Many states have conscience clauses that protect clinicians who invoke moral or religious objection in declining to provide a particular service (e.g., Michigan Conscientious Objector Policy Act, 2004). There is, however, an ongoing vigorous debate about the propriety of clinicians prioritizing their own personal values over the provision of legal medical care, with some arguing that a clinician's individual values should not be permitted to interfere with the quality and availability of legal medical care and that conscientious objections to providing such care should be honored only when there are readily available alternative care providers (Charo 2005; Savulescu 2006).

It may be extremely difficult for a clinician to smoothly transition care of a terminally ill patient who is intent on VSED and, particularly where the clinician and patient have had a longstanding relationship, such a transition has the potential to cause harm to patients at an extremely vulnerable time if not done in a timely and compassionate manner. If a clinician with a patient who wishes to pursue VSED has a moral or religious objection to the practice, he should attempt to transition care of the patient to another clinician who feels able to fully support the patient and provide appropriate palliative care. If this proves difficult or impossible, the clinician's duty not to abandon the patient should prevail.

Conclusion

Many patients with advanced illness express a desire to hasten death, driven largely by factors such as loss of independence and dignity, unacceptable quality of life, meaningless of life, and the desire to control the circumstances of death. Clinicians caring for a patient with advanced illness who is considering hastening his own death should take steps to address identifiable sources of suffering, to ensure that the patient does not feel pressured or unduly influenced into ending his life, and to evaluate and treat depression or other mental illness that might be influencing the patient's desire to die. When a competent patient is steadfast in his readiness to die notwithstanding provision of optimal palliative care, the clinician should address the option of VSED. If the patient elects to proceed with VSED, the clinician should remain involved, providing support for the patient and his family and palliative care as necessary to ensure a peaceful death.

References

Alpers, A., and B. Lo. 1997. Does it make clinical sense to equate terminally ill patients who require life-sustaining interventions with those who do not? *JAMA*, June 4;277(21):1705–8.

American Medical Association. 1996. Opinion 2.211. Physician-assisted suicide. Accessed at http://www.ama-assn.org/ama/pub/physician-resources/medical-ethics/code-medical-ethics/opinion2211.page. November 28, 2012.

Angell, M. 1997. The Supreme Court and physician-assisted suicide—the ultimate right. *N Eng J Med*, Jan 2;336(1):50–3.

Back, A.L., J.I. Wallace, H.E. Starks, R.A., and A.L. Pearlman. 1996. Physician-assisted suicide and euthanasia in Washington state: patient requests and clinician responses. *JAMA*, Mar 27;275(12):919–25.

Bernat, J.L., B. Gert, and R.P. Mogielnicki. 1993. Patient refusal of hydration and nutrition: an alternative to physician-assisted suicide or voluntary active euthanasia. *Arch Intern Med*, Dec 27;153(24):2723–8.

Block, S.D. 2000. Assessing and managing depression in the terminally ill patient. *Ann Intern Med*, Feb 1;132(3):209–18.

Block, S.D. 2001. Perspectives on care at the close of life. Psychological considerations, growth and transcendence at the end of life: the art of the possible. *JAMA*, Jun 13;285(22):2898–905.

Breitbart, W., B. Rosenfeld, H. Pessin, M. Kaim, J. Funesti-Esch, M. Galietta, C.J. Nelson, and R. Brescia. 2000. Depression, hopelessness and desire for hastened death in terminally ill patients with cancer. *JAMA*, Dec 13;284(22):2907–11.

Byock, I. 2012. Physician-assisted suicide is not progressive. *The Atlantic*, October 25.

Campbell, A.T., and M.P. Aulisio. 2012. The stigma of "mental" illness: end stage anorexia and treatment refusal. *Int J Eat Disord*, Jul;45(5):627–34.

Cantor, N.L., and G.C. Thomas. 2000. The legal bounds of clinician conduct hastening death. *Buffalo Law Rev*, Winter;48(1):83–173.

Charo, R.A. 2005. The celestial fire of conscience—refusing to deliver medical care. *N Engl J Med*, June 16;352(24):2471–73.

Chochinov, H.M., K.G. Wilson, M. Enns, N. Mowchun, S. Lander, M. Levitt, and J.J. Clinch. 1995. Desire for death in the terminally ill. *Am J Psychiatry*, Aug;152(8):1185–91.

Chochinov, H.M., K.G. Wilson, M. Enns, and S. Lander. 1997. "Are you depressed?" Screening for depression in the terminally ill. *Am J Psychiatry*, May;154(5): 674–6.

Cohen, L.M., M.D. Steinberg, K.C. Hails, S.K. Dobscha, and S.V. Fischel. 2000. Psychiatric evaluation of death-hastening requests: lessons from dialysis discontinuation. *Psychosomatics*, May-Jun;41(3):195–203.

Cruzan v. Director, Mo. Dept. of Health, 497 U.S. 261, 278 (1990).

Curlin, F.A., R.E. Lawrence, M.H. Chin, and J.D. Lantos. 2007. Religion, conscience, and controversial clinical practices. *N Engl J Med*, February 8 356(6):593–600.

Curlin, F.A., C. Nwodim, J.L. Vance, M.H. Chin, and J.D. Lantos. 2008. To die, to sleep: US physicians' religious and other objections to physician-assisted suicide, terminal sedation, and withdrawal of life support. *Am J Hosp Palliat Care* 25:112–20.

Dickens, B.M. 2001. Reproductive health services and the law and ethics of conscientious objection. *Med Law*, 20(2):283–93.

Draper, H. 2000. Anorexia nervosa and respecting a refusal of life-prolonging therapy: a limited justification. *Bioethics*, Apr;14(2):120–33.

Eddy, D.M. 1994. A piece of my mind: a conversation with my mother. *JAMA*, Jul 20;272(3):179–81.

Elliott, J.R., D.A. Haydon, and B.M. Hendry. 1984. Anaesthetic action of esters and ketones: evidence for an interaction with the sodium channel protein in squid axons. *J Physiol*, 354:407–18.

Emanuel, E.J., D.L. Fairclough, and L.L. Emanuel. 2000. Attitudes and desires related to euthanasia and physician-assisted suicide among terminally ill patients and their caregivers. *JAMA*, Nov 15;284(19): 2460–8.

Emanuel, E.J. 2012.Four myths about doctor-assisted suicide. *New York Times*, Oct 27.

Ferrand, E., J.F. Dreyfus, M. Chastrusse, F. Ellien, F. Leimaire, and M. Fischler. 2012. Evolution of requests to hasten death among patients managed by palliative care teams in France: a multicentre cross-sectional survey. *Eur J Cancer*. Feb;48(3):368–76.

Foley, K.M. 1997. Competent care for the dying instead of physician-assisted suicide. *N Eng J Med*, Jan 2;336(1):54–7.

Fosmire v. Nicoleau, 75 N.Y.2d 218, 227 (1990).

Ganzini, L., T.A. Harvath, A. Jackson, E.R. Goy, L.L. Miller, and M.A. Delorit. 2002. Experiences of Oregon nurses and social workers with hospice patients who requested assistance with suicide. *N Engl J Med*, Aug 22;347(8):582–8.

Ganzini, L. E.R. Goy, L.L. Miller, T.A. Harvath, A. Jackson, and M.A. Delorit. 2003. Nurses' Experience with hospice patients who refuse food and fluids to hasten death. *N Engl J Med*, Jul 24;349(4):359–65.

Ganzini L., E.R. Goy, and S.K. Dobscha. 2008. Prevalence of depression and anxiety in patients requesting clinicians' aid in dying: cross sectional survey. *BMJ*, Oct 7;337:a1682. doi: 10.1136/bmj.a1682.

Jacobs, S. 2003. Death by voluntary dehydration—what the caregivers say. *N Engl J Med*, Jul 24;349(4): 325–6.

Jansen, L.A., and D.P. Sulmasy. 2002. Sedation, alimentation, hydration, and equivocation: careful conversation about care at the end of life. *Ann Intern Med*, Jun 4;136(11):845–9.

Mackenzie, S. 2012. It was a good death, the kind most people would choose. *The Guardian*, Friday 7 September 2012.

Meisel, A. 1992. The legal consensus about foregoing life-sustaining treatment: its status and its prospects. *Kennedy Inst Ethics J.* Dec;2(4):309–45.

Merriam-Webster. Accessed at http://www.merriam-webster.com/dictionary/suicide. November 28, 2012.

Michigan Conscientious Objector Policy Act. HB-5006 (2004). Accessed at http://www.legislature.mi.gov/documents/2003-2004/billengrossed/house/htm/2003-HEBH-5006.htm. November 28, 2012.

Miller, F.G., and D.E. Meier. 1998. Voluntary death: a comparison of terminal dehydration and physician-assisted suicide. *Ann Intern Med*, Apr 1;128(7)559–62.

Miller, F.G., J.J. Fins, and L. Snyder. 2000. Assisted suicide compared with refusal of treatment: A valid distinction? *Ann Intern Med*, Mar 21;1323(6):470–5.

Oregon Death with Dignity Act. ORS Chapter 127 §§ 800–995. Oregon State Legislature (2011 Edition). Accessed athttp://www.leg.state.or.us/ors/127.html. November 28, 2012.

Printz, LA. 1992. Terminal dehydration, a compassionate treatment. *Arch Intern Med*, Apr;152(4):697–700.

Quill, T.E., C.K. Cassell, and D. E. Meier. 1992. Care of the hopelessly ill—proposed clinical criteria for physician-assisted suicide. *N Engl J Med*, Nov 5;327(19):1380–4.

Quill, T.E., B. Lo, and D.W. Brock. 1997. Palliative options of last resort. a comparison of voluntarily stopping eating and drinking, terminal sedation, physician-assisted suicide, and voluntary active euthanasia. *JAMA*, Dec 17;278(23):2099–104.

Rady, M.Y., and J.L. Verheijde. 2012. Distress from voluntary refusal of food and fluids to hasten death: what is the role of continuous deep sedation? *J Med Ethics* Aug;38(8):510–2. Epub 2011 Oct 29.

Savulescu, J. 2006. Conscientious objection in medicine. *BMJ*, February 4;332:294–7.

Schwartz, J. 2007. Exploring the option of voluntarily stopping eating and drinking within the context of a suffering patient's request for a hastened death. *J Palliat Med*, Dec;10(6):1288–97.

Truog, R.D., and T.I. Cochrane. 2005. Refusal of hydration and nutrition: irrelevance of the "artificial" vs "natural" distinction. *Arch Intern Med*, Dec 12–26;165(22):2574–6.

Vacco v. Quill 117 S.Ct. 2293 (1997).

Van der Lee, M.L., J.G. van der Bom, N.B. Swarte; A.P. Heintz; A. de Graeff; J. van den Bout. 2005. Euthanasia and depression: a prospective cohort study among terminally ill cancer patients. *J Clin Oncol* Sep 20;23(27):6607–12. Epub 2005 Aug 22.

Werth, J.L. 2004. The relationships among clinical depression, suicide, and other actions that may hasten death. *Behav Sci Law*, 22(5):627–49.

Wicclair, M.R. 2011. Conscientious Objection in Health Care: An Ethical Analysis. Cambridge: Cambridge University Press.

Wilson, K.G., J.F. Scott, I.D. Graham, J.F. Kozak, S. Chater, R.A. Viola, B.J. de Faye, L.A. Weaver, and D. Curran. 2000. Attitudes of terminally ill patients toward euthanasia and clinician-assisted suicide. *Arch Intern Med*, Sep 11;160(16):2454–60.

16

Physician-Assisted Death
Timothy E. Quill and Franklin G. Miller

Physician-assisted suicide and voluntary active euthanasia have been topics of intense controversy in the medical profession, within bioethics, and among the public over the past 25 years. With physician-assisted suicide (PAS), a physician prescribes a lethal dose of medication that is self-administered by a patient who has requested the means to end his or her life; in voluntary active euthanasia (VAE), a physician administers a lethal dose of medication in response to a request for help in ending life by a competent patient.

This chapter is divided into six sections, each addressing an important moral question that relates to the practices of PAS and VAE. Both of us believe that these practices can be morally justified in some circumstances and should be legally available with suitable regulatory safeguards, at least in some jurisdictions, as a last resort for mentally competent, terminally ill patients who have access to palliative care and hospice, and for whom standard palliative measures are insufficient to adequately relieve their suffering [1]. Those who are morally opposed to these practices under any circumstances believe that they are inherently unethical for physicians, and that the risks of legalization far outweigh the benefits under all circumstances [2].

Each section of this chapter will begin by posing a clinical or policy question, and illustrate it with an example in which this question was encountered in clinical practice. The subsequent discussion will include relevant clinical and ethical issues, and it will close with how the actual situation was resolved by those involved. There will be no attempt in this chapter to exhaustively explore every moral question potentially raised by these practices or these cases, but rather to consider some of the more central moral questions in this domain that have emerged from our work as a palliative care clinician (TQ) and an ethicist (FM). The case illustrations are based on real clinical experiences, but the personal details have been altered to make the cases unidentifiable.

Before immersing ourselves in these clinical questions, we wanted to briefly explore how language has been used and manipulated by those on both sides of the controversy about the morality of these practices. Public debate has been plagued by vague, confusing, or misleading language to describe a physician's role in helping suffering patients to die. This is particularly true with the label of physician-assisted *suicide*, because the word "suicide" has so many meanings that seem to miss the mark in terms of describing this practice [3]. There has been less controversy over the language to describe physician-administered lethal medication (euthanasia). The Webster's definition of suicide is "the act or an instance of taking one's own life voluntarily and intentionally especially by a person of years of discretion and of sound mind," which sounds accurate and morally neutral, but it then suggests that the practice "may have psychological origins such as difficulty coping with depression or other mental disorders" (www.merrian-webster.com/dictionary/suicide). The multiple layers of potential meanings include heroic suicides (jumping on a bomb to save one's troop mates) or suicide bombers (detonating explosives carried on one's own body to martyr oneself and to kill and terrorize one's enemies). But when one looks at the synonyms for "suicide," the terms that emerge include "self-destruction," "self-slaughter," and "self-murder," all of which seem to miss the mark in terms of accurately describing this practice.

Advocates of legalization of this practice as a last resort prefer the more morally neutral terms "physician-assisted death" or "physician aid-in-dying," which have much less negative perceptions [4-6], and in public polling these terms are much more likely to be positively endorsed as a last resort option [1]. However, this language also suffers from being rather vague, such that one cannot be sure exactly which end-of-life practices are being included and excluded. The laws allowing this practice under highly restricted circumstances in Oregon, Washington, Montana, and Vermont use this language in part to stay out of the conundrum associated with the "suicide" label, but also because the public acceptability of the practice drops by about 10 percentage points if the language of suicide is used.

Philosophers generally prefer to use the term "physician-assisted suicide" because of its literal accuracy, and because they view the term as morally neutral. It is also the preferred term used by opponents of legalization because of the negative connotations of the term "suicide," and its association with clinical depression and panic disorder. Clinicians occasionally encounter patients who are "suicidal" as a symptom of mental illness, and they properly go to great lengths, including involuntary hospitalization, to prevent the associated self-destruction. Most clinicians on both sides of the end-of-life choices debate would acknowledge that most terminally ill, suffering patients who are considering a hastened death are a different population from a meaning standpoint, and that the word "suicide" misses the mark in a vast majority of these cases. In fact, most terminally ill, suffering patients who are considering this option view ending their lives as a way to preserve what remains of their integrity as persons, and to avoid the disintegration that sometimes accompanies the last phase of dying [7]. (To take some of the political noise out of the debate, consider the messages given surrounding how clinicians are encouraged to approach those terminally ill patients wanting to stop a life support—the generally agreed upon strategy is to carefully evaluate the patient to be sure you understand the meaning of the request and to look for alternate ways to better address the associated suffering, but ultimately to listen to the patient who should be in charge of his life and his body.)

For the purposes of this chapter, we will call the practice of physician prescription of lethal medication physician-assisted suicide because it accurately describes the practice, and because at the clinical level the relative discomfort that it engenders is probably useful to work through upfront for anyone who is considering this practice in earnest, whether a patient or a partner in the process (family member or clinician). We also want readers to understand and work through some of the moral implications of the language they choose to use in describing the practice.

How Much and What Kind of Suffering Is Required?

CASE #1 PRESENTATION

AA was an 80-year-old woman with long-standing chronic obstructive lung disease who now has stage IV non–small cell lung cancer. She was hospitalized for the second time in the past 4 weeks with severe dyspnea (shortness of breath). She was recovering to the extent that her dyspnea was now tolerable, but she dreaded the suffering anticipated with her next exacerbation. She had decided against cardiopulmonary resuscitation and intubation at the time of her cancer diagnosis, but now was very fearful about how bad her shortness of breath might get before she finally died. She was not afraid of death, but she was terrified about the suffering she would experience just before death given her recent experience in the hospital. AA was a woman who always liked to be in charge of her life, and she wanted to know what options she might have for a "preemptive strike" rather than waiting for the next exacerbation.

CASE #2 PRESENTATION

BB was a 60-year-old man who received surgery and radiation therapy for a brain tumor 20 years earlier. He did very well with this treatment, and led a full and active life for the next 15 years. Unfortunately, over the last 5 years he began to develop a slowly progressive neuromuscular disease that was thought to be a delayed effect of his previous cancer treatment. He was fully intact cognitively and very capable of making decisions for himself, but his motor function was progressively becoming limited such that he was dependent on others for assistance with all of his activities of daily living. His physical symptoms were minimal in terms of pain or dyspnea, but he hated his increasing weakness, debility, and dependence with no end in sight other than more loss of function. Although not currently seeking death, he asked his doctor if he was willing to assist him with physician-assisted suicide (PAS) at some time in the future before he became too weak to take the medication himself.

DISCUSSION

Both of these patients had challenging medical situations, and their requests for some kind of assistance with determining the timing and circumstances of their deaths were certainly understandable. AA would be a more paradigmatic case in the sense that she was clearly terminally ill (stage IV lung non–small cell lung cancer, minimal pulmonary reserve, and several recent hospitalizations), her suffering was more physical than psychological (severe dyspnea is one of our more challenging symptoms to relieve), and her terminal event would likely involve another episode of severe shortness of breath from which she would not bounce back. Her questions for her clinical team were whether she had to wait for the next exacerbation to be allowed to escape through her death, and, if she had to wait, how much dyspnea would she have to experience before they would be willing to provide her with heavy sedation. She was not afraid of death per se, but was terrified about what degree of suffering she would experience before dying. The medical team also understood that her time was very limited no matter what they did, but they were uncertain about how much leeway they could give AA in choosing the timing and circumstances of her death, and with what kinds of options they could provide her.

BB's case posed a different set of clinical and ethical questions. He clearly had a terminal illness, but because its pace was very slow it was not at all certain that he would die within the next 6 months. Furthermore, his suffering was as much psychosocial and existential as physical. He had no severe physical symptoms other than progressive weakness and a growing inability to manage even basic bodily functions, both of which he found unacceptable. He was certainly sad about his condition, but he was not clinically depressed and his concerns and experiences were grounded in the reality of his situation. His increasing suffering was clearly understandable, but we also know that many patients adapt to physical limitations that they never could have imagined accepting before becoming ill. Furthermore, he was not asking for assistance in dying right now, but he was exploring the options he might have in the future.

KEY ETHICAL ISSUES

If severe and unrelievable suffering is the central moral requirement to allow access to last-resort options that might end in death, then the distinction between physical and psychosocial suffering would seem to be relatively unimportant [7]. The fact that AA's suffering was dyspnea and fear would make it no more compelling that BB's suffering, which was based on progressive debility and dependence. In both cases the suffering was severe, and posed a direct threat to each person's sense of self. Although physicians in general have more expertise assessing and addressing physical suffering than psychosocial or existential suffering, this does not mean that such suffering does not "count" as much; rather, they may need to get additional help addressing the dimensions of suffering around which they lack expertise.

When patients are fearful about future suffering and want to know their options for potentially escaping through death, this suggests that autonomy and choice are particularly important to them [8]. These issues head the list of motivating factors for patients who are seeking the potential of PAS in Oregon and Washington [8], and also are key values for those seeking PAS or voluntary active euthanasia (VAE) in the Netherlands [9]. Many believe that it is better to let death happen than to make it happen; however, there is no consensus over what constitutes a "good death." Many patients who gain access to potentially lethal medication with knowledge of how to use it if needed never actually take the overdose, suggesting that for them the possibility of being in control of one's death may in some circumstances be more important than the reality.

The degree of terminality (prognosis of less than 6 months in Oregon, Washington, Montana, and Vermont) is more of a practical safeguard than a matter of ethical principle—it limits the number of patients potentially eligible for assisted death. AA would clearly meet these terminality standards, and BB would probably not. Yet BB's losses and degree of suffering were no less profound, and his future prospects were daunting and (to him) potentially far worse than death. Although policy considerations might justify limiting legislation permitting PAS or VAE to those who are terminally ill, irreversibly suffering patients who are not terminally ill will still need other last resort options [10, 11].

The possibility of implementing PAS or VAE may be much more important than the reality for many patients. AA was directly confronting the reality of imminent severe suffering, and she was pursuing the possibility of PAS in earnest to be used in her immediate future. BB, on the other hand, was more interested in the potential reassurance of a future escape. If he could be reassured that an escape would be possible, he might be able to live more securely and focus his energies on other more immediate matters [12]. In Oregon, where PAS is legal, one in six terminally ill patients talks to his or her family about the possibility, one in 50 talks to his or her doctor, and only one in 500 to 1,000 actually carries out the practice [13]. Nonetheless, if a clinician does reassure a patient that she or he will be responsive to a request for PAS or VAE in the future, the clinician should have thought through and potentially explored with the patient in very explicit terms what that response might look like.

When discussing the potential of PAS or VAE in the future or exploring a real-time request, the clinician caring for the patient must ensure that all palliative care alternatives have been optimized within the limitations set by the disease and the patient's preferences and values. Physician-assisted suicide or voluntary active euthanasia, whether in the legal or illegal environment, should never be activated because of inadequate palliative care, and the same should be said for other more legally accepted last resort options such as stopping life supports, palliative sedation, or voluntarily stopping eating and drinking. A central, required part of the evaluation whenever any last resort option is being considered is to insure that standard palliative treatments have been optimized.

CONCLUSION OF THE CASES

After extensive discussion with the physician and her family, AA was provided with the means to carry out PAS in a state in which the practice was illegal. The patient felt reassured to have the prescription, but knew that if she waited too long she could end up in the hospital since her breathing exacerbations came on quickly and severely. About 2 weeks later, the patient took the medication all at once in the presence of her family, and died peacefully within several hours. The family was grateful to the physician for helping, but they did not openly discuss what had happened with anyone outside their immediate family. The physician felt he had been morally and clinically responsible in the case, but was very anxious about the legal repercussions should the process have been discovered. He signed "metastatic lung cancer" as the sole cause of death on the death certificate.

BB's request for medication that could be used for PAS was turned down by his clinician because of the lack of a clearly terminal condition, and because of the relative absence of physical suffering. The clinician empathized with BB's predicament, and proposed the "option" of voluntarily stopping eating and drinking in the future when and if BB was sure he was ready. The clinician also offered to explore the possibility of admitting him to an inpatient palliative care or hospice unit if and when he made that decision, because the professional caregivers who provided 24 hour per day home care for him were not accepting of that future option. If his suffering became severe in this process, he was promised the option of heavy sedation to relieve such symptoms.

Armed with this potential escape, BB chose to live another 18 months before activating this last resort option. He did not feel trapped during this time because he knew an escape was within his control. When he decided he was ready, he went through another full evaluation, including an independent psychologist and a medical ethics consult, before he was admitted to an inpatient palliative care unit where he began the process of voluntarily stopping eating and drinking. The reasons for his decision and the process of evaluation were shared with the staff on the unit, and all were eventually supportive. His dying took about 2 weeks, much of which was very meaningful to him, his family, and his caregivers. He required proportional palliative sedation for his last few days because of agitated terminal delirium. A "neuro-degenerative syndrome" was written as the cause of death on his death certificate, and family and staff involved all felt able to discuss openly their reaction to the process that he (and they) went through.

Is There a Moral Bright Line Between Withdrawing Life-Sustaining Treatment and Physician-Assisted Suicide or Voluntary Active Euthanasia?

CASE #3 PRESENTATION

Debbie, aged 50, was thrown from her horse in a horse-show event. After being resuscitated and flown by helicopter to an academic medical center, she was diagnosed as sustaining a high-level spinal cord injury, which left her quadriplegic and ventilator-dependent. She underwent extensive rehabilitation and eventually returned to her horse farm in Kentucky, where she lived with the help of her partner and paid caregivers. However, 2 years after her accident, Debbie decided that, in view of her total physical dependence and absence of privacy, her life was no longer worth living. She was able to arrange admission to an academic medical center for the purpose of stopping her ventilator. Heavily sedated before the ventilator was withdrawn, Debbie died within a short period of time.

CASE #4 PRESENTATION

Hans, a 55-year-old man living in Amsterdam, sustained a spinal cord injury in a bicycle accident, making him quadriplegic. Initially needing mechanical ventilation, he was able to breathe spontaneously after being weaned off the ventilator. After rehabilitation, Hans returned to living at home with the support of his wife. Four years later, however, he found his life intolerable and asked his general physician to administer a lethal dose of medication, which is legal in the Netherlands. After careful evaluation, including consultation with another physician, Hans's physician agreed to perform VAE.

KEY ETHICAL ISSUES

Since the mid 1970s, patients in the United States have had a legal and ethical right to refuse life-sustaining treatment, such as mechanical ventilation, dialysis, or artificial nutrition and hydration. In traditional medical ethics, there is a sharp distinction between stopping life-sustaining treatment on the one hand and either PAS or VAE on the other. Although there is a solid moral justification for the former, the latter is never justified. It is doubtful, however, that this ethical stance and/or line of reasoning can hold up under critical scrutiny.

Are there any grounds for drawing a moral bright line between the cases of Debbie and Hans? The issues relevant to answering this question are complex and contested. Here we will simply suggest why we think the answer to this question is "No." Death was the result of stopping life-sustaining treatment in Debbie's case and of administering lethal medication in the case of Hans. Is there a morally relevant difference of *intention* between these two cases? Both Debbie and Hans found their lives intolerable and sought death with the help of clinicians. Whether there might a difference in intentions on the part of the clinicians in these two cases is less clear. Certainly, a physician who administers lethal medication intends to help the patient die. Yet it also seems reasonable to suppose that the clinicians who agreed to stop Debbie's ventilator intended to help her die. In a brief delivered to the US Supreme Court relating to the issue of whether terminally ill patients have a right to PAS, five distinguished philosophers wrote the following about the issue of intention: "Whether a doctor turns off a respirator in accordance with the patient's request or prescribes pills that a patient may take when he is ready to kill himself, the doctor acts with the same intention: to help the patient die" [14]. Some may dispute this and insist that the intent of clinicians in cases of withdrawing life-sustaining treatment is merely to respect the patient's right to refuse treatment, not to help in causing the patient's death. Nevertheless, we see no reason to suppose that an explicit intent by a caring clinician to help a suffering patient achieve a wished-for death is inherently unethical. Moreover, the values that justify refusal of life-sustaining treatment—patient well-being and respect for patient autonomy—are just as operative in the case of Debbie as in that of Hans [15].

Are the Differences Between Physician-Assisted Suicide and Voluntary Active Euthanasia Important?

CASE #5 PRESENTATION

CC was a 65-year-old man with stage IV esophageal cancer who had been extensively treated in the past with surgery, radiation, and chemotherapy. He had a temporary feeding tube during the initial phase of treatment, but now did not want it reinserted. He weighed 80 pounds, and was having progressive difficulty swallowing. He was told that no further surgery, radiation, or stenting would be possible. He was enrolled in hospice, and his physical symptoms were well managed. He was a long-standing member of the Hemlock Society, and believed that he and others should be able to control the timing and manner of his own death. He lived in Oregon, so PAS was potentially available, but he was now unable to swallow the amount of medication needed to successfully end his life. He wondered what his options were, and in particular whether his doctor would be willing to provide voluntary active euthanasia.

DISCUSSION

The clinical evaluation of patients potentially receiving PAS or VAE (or other last resort medical interventions that will likely result in an earlier death) should be roughly the same: (1) Does the patient have full decision-making capacity, and is he or she aware of all alternative approaches? (2) Is the patient's suffering being fully addressed with all reasonably available palliative treatments? (3) Is the patient's illness fully defined, including its degree of reversibility? And (4) is the degree to which the patient is terminally ill fully understood [10]? Some last resort options are restricted to those with full decision-making capacity (PAS, VAE, voluntarily stopping eating and drinking), whereas others might be available to patients who are suffering severely but have lost the ability to make their own decisions (palliative sedation, stopping or not starting life-sustaining therapies, aggressive symptom management). We do not consider here the controversial question of whether active euthanasia by injecting lethal medication may be justified under some circumstances for patients who lack decision-making capacity.

Voluntary active euthanasia and physician-assisted suicide are similar in several ways. In both interventions the physician is intentionally contributing to a consenting patient's earlier death. The agreed-upon end point for both is a peaceful death that is desired by the patient. The patient should be the central decision maker for both practices, and the physician, professionally committed to preserving life, may be a hesitant partner but should also have the right not to participate if he could not morally abide by the practice. If the physician chooses to participate, he is a morally responsible agent contributing to an intended earlier death.

There are also potentially important moral and clinical differences between PAS and VAE. The patient is the final actor in PAS. On the positive side, this is an added safeguard in terms of voluntariness, although not a guarantee, because patients with compromised decision-making capacity may be capable of self-administering lethal medication. On the other hand, the physician typically is not present in cases of PAS (especially in an illegal environment), and is thereby unavailable to ensure final consent and to be able to assist if complications arise (such as the patient being unable to swallow all of the medication or perhaps the medication not producing the desired effect).

The physician is the final actor in VAE, albeit at the patient's behest. In VAE, the physician administers both the sedating medication as well as the lethal injection. Inevitably, the timing of the patient's death will be the result of some negotiation between patient preference and physician availability (not dissimilar to the timing of life support cessation procedures). Voluntary active euthanasia is much more psychologically and morally taxing for physicians than PAS, because the proximity between the physician's action and the patient's death could not be more direct [16]. (Yet there is often also a close proximity between withdrawing mechanical ventilation and the patient's death, which may also be psychologically taxing although legally permitted.)

KEY ETHICAL ISSUES

Clinicians have a clear moral responsibility in both PAS and VAE for their role in intentionally causing or at least contributing to the patient's death. This responsibility holds for other last resort practices that knowingly contribute to an earlier death, but is more clear and direct in PAS and especially in VAE.

The psychological differences between PAS and VAE also have moral implications for both patients and physicians. In some ways, PAS is harder psychologically on patients and families who have to finally act in isolation. The physician is usually not present when the lethal medication is ingested, so he is removed from the associated uncertainty and finality. He is still morally responsible for his participation and facilitation, but it is potentially harder psychologically on patients and families than VAE (which some might view as an important safeguard). Voluntary active euthanasia might be slightly easier psychologically and practically on patients and families, because the physician has the medical "tools" to be sure that the intervention is "successful." The patient and family also have the comfort of knowing that a person in a position of authority and power supports the process in real time. Voluntary active euthanasia is clearly harder on physicians, as the proximity between their action and the patient's death could not be clearer.

The timing of VAE, like the practice of stopping a life support, inevitably will depend to some degree on the clinician's schedule and availability. With PAS, once a patient goes through the evaluation process and obtains the potentially lethal medication, she or he may use that medication (or not) at a time of her or his own choosing. Voluntary active euthanasia, on the other hand, is a scheduled event in which the physician comes to the patient's residence prepared with the proper medication at a preset time, and then administers the medication. Although patients are offered the opportunity to change their minds, a lot of set up and expectation would need to be countered to allow this to happen.

Finally, the laws governing PAS and VAE are very different in the United States. (See chapter 17 for an analysis of the legal situation in the United States as well as the Netherlands and Western Europe.) Physician-assisted suicide is now legal in four US states provided one adheres to defined safeguards, but even in states where it is illegal, the practice is not likely to be actively prosecuted even if discovered provided it is not publicized. Voluntary active euthanasia, on the other hand, is clearly illegal throughout the United States, and it is likely to be prosecuted if discovered. This is illustrated by the actions of Jack Kevorkian, who openly flaunted the laws prohibiting PAS by assisting well over 100 cases and being unsuccessfully prosecuted several times. On the other hand, his one case of VAE resulted in his being successfully prosecuted and then jailed for several years. This is not to say that PAS can be openly practiced in states where it is illegal or where its legal status is uncertain. Several physicians have found their license in jeopardy over cases in which some variant of PAS has been suspected. Even though they were not legally convicted, their professional lives were turned upside down and threatened. So the practice of PAS is likely to remain deeply underground in states where it is currently illegal or its legal status is uncertain, which is potentially bad for both patients and clinicians.

CONCLUSION OF THE CASE

Even though PAS was legal in his home state of Oregon, CC could not take advantage of the law because he would be unable to reliably swallow enough medication. His doctor was hesitant to provide VAE given the status of the law, even though he was not morally opposed to the practice (at least in principle). The patient was not symptomatic enough to receive aggressive palliative sedation (to unconsciousness), and he wanted to stay as alert as possible until the very end. He was offered the option of stopping eating and drinking, but he thought that would be too hard to do because he already felt thirsty and hungry much of the time. He decided to hold off on any major decision with his doctor's reassurance that with any serious exacerbation he would receive very aggressive symptom management, including heavy sedation if needed. About a month later he developed aspiration pneumonia. He was admitted to an inpatient hospice unit, antibiotics were withheld, and he was treated symptomatically with opioids for his dyspnea and additional sedation for his delirium until he died. His family and his hospice team felt that his wishes had been honored within the limits of current laws.[1]

Are the Differences between Palliative Sedation to Unconsciousness and Physician-Assisted Suicide/Voluntary Active Euthanasia Important?

CASE #6 PRESENTATION

DD was a 75-year-old man with a progressive brain tumor that had been treated with surgery, radiation, and chemotherapy. He had recurrent and intractable partial complex seizures that were manifest by his feeling terrified and confused. When he was seizing, he felt as if he was living in a nightmare from which there was no escape. When he was seizure free, he lived in extreme fear of the episodes recurring. He begged for his clinicians to put him "out of his misery." He was on multiple anti-seizure medications, steroids, and antipsychotics, and multiple consulting teams were trying (unsuccessfully) to help him. The clinicians felt this was a palliative care emergency, but were uncertain how to respond.[1]

DISCUSSION

At the time this case was transpiring, the full range of last resort options hand not been fully articulated [10]. Proportionate palliative sedation was beginning to be described as a last resort option as long as death was in no way intended [17]. The fact that this man would have preferred euthanasia, and let it be known, made the practice of palliative sedation potentially much more controversial, but the physician's intention arguably would count more than the patient's intention in this situation. If the clinicians were to honor his request for sedation with knowledge that he desired death to come as soon as possible, it would have been absurd to potentially prolong his dying process by providing artificial hydration and nutrition.

DD's suffering was extreme, and all who cared for him were searching for better ways to address it. He was having terrifying hallucinations caused by his partial complex seizures, and when not seizing he lived in extreme fear of the "living nightmares" recurring. Using the minimal amount of sedation possible ran the risk of having him experience the terror while being too sedated to verbally report. The clinical team debated whether it would be permissible to offer him the "option" of heavy sedation to unconsciousness given the fact it was so close to euthanasia (although clearly different in important ways).

Although there are similarities between proportionate palliative sedation (PPS) and palliative sedation to unconsciousness (PSU) on the one side, and VAE and PAS on the other, there are also clear differences [10]. The main difference is that the clinician and patient intention in both VAE and PAS is to hasten a wished for death at the patient's explicit behest, whereas with PSU and in particular PPS, the clinician's intention *may* be more uncertain and ambiguous. If the physician's intent is purely to relieve suffering and not in any way to hasten death, then the practice might still be justified using the principle of double effect [18]. On the other hand, such clarity of intention becomes harder for clinicians to sustain when a patient expresses a clear desire for an earlier death, and sees this intervention as the best available means of achieving that end. Purity of intent is also harder to justify if other potentially life prolonging therapies are simultaneously discontinued, and the patient's eventual death becomes more of a certainty [19].

Physician-assisted suicide and voluntary active euthanasia require a high degree of mental clarity from the patient to allow for valid consent. In DD's case, that clarity was intermittently present, but not sustained. The clinicians had no doubt about his wishes when he was mentally clear, but when he was having partial complex seizures he was terrified but in no way able to make decisions of this complexity. Proportionate palliative sedation and palliative sedation to unconsciousness on the other hand can be used in circumstances in which capacity is lost or uncertain. This allows clinicians to address a much broader range of clinical circumstances and types of suffering, including those patients who have clearly lost decision-making capacity and also have lost the ability to self-administer medication. Proportionate palliative sedation tends to use the least amount of sedation necessary to achieve the needed relief, whereas with PSU unconsciousness is the intended endpoint. Palliative sedation to unconsciousness should be reserved for the more extreme cases, and should be much more rarely used.

KEY ETHICAL ISSUES

Palliative sedation has been given wide legal support after the 1997 US Supreme Court decision addressing PAS [20, 21]. While the court refused to make any binding decision with regard to the legal permissibility of PAS, leaving it to the "laboratory of the states," the decision was clear in legally permitting use palliative sedation "even to the level of unconsciousness" if needed to relieve otherwise intractable suffering.

There is wide ethical consensus about the moral permissibility of PPS and even PSU provided that neither the patient nor the physician are explicitly intending the patient to die sooner as a result of the practice [22]. However, the criteria for pure intentions (relief of suffering and not intending an earlier death) are sometimes unrealistic and ethically unnecessary in our opinion [19].

There might be some circumstances in which simultaneous provision of food and fluids might be justified, especially in cases on the mild end of the PPS spectrum; however, in circumstances in which more heavy PPS or PSU is warranted because suffering is severe and irreversible, then in our opinion the simultaneous provision of artificial hydration and nutrition makes no sense medically and should be avoided unless it is clearly requested by the patient or family for religious or ethical reasons.

There are many similarities between PSU and VAE, but the differences are also important [10]. Specifically, in both circumstances the patient is sedated to unconsciousness, but in VAE this is followed by an explicitly intended lethal injection. In PSU, the patient is heavily sedated but then dies from some combination of dehydration, hypoventilation from the heavy sedation, and additional adverse effects of the underlying disease. In VAE, the immediate cause of death is a lethal injection that follows the heavy sedation. Both practices might potentially be ethically justified as a last resort response to extremes of suffering, and the physician is morally responsible as a partner in both processes.

CONCLUSION OF THE CASE

DD remained desperate to find a way to escape his suffering, and all involved agreed that his circumstances required some kind of aggressive palliative response. The clinicians felt they could justify offering him PSU to allow him to escape his suffering. His anti-seizure medications and analgesics would be continued, and he would be sedated until he was unconscious and then not provided any life-prolonging treatments, including artificial hydration and nutrition, during the process. That evening during a lucid interval this option was posed to the patient, who immediately consented. He was offered to take some time to say goodbye to his family before the clinicians started the process, but he implored them to start as soon as possible as his life seemed to him to be a "living hell." His family supported his decision, and he was heavily sedated that evening. He remained quiet in his appearance for the next 72 hours when he died with family in attendance. The staff felt anxious that what they were doing was on the edges of the law and of accepted practice, but they felt good about their efforts to try to address this man's extreme situation.

Are Other Legally Available Last Resort Options Besides Physician-Assisted Suicide and Voluntary Active Euthanasia Adequate?

CASE #7 PRESENTATION

EE was a patient with amyotrophic lateral sclerosis who desperately wanted to have the option of physician-assisted suicide in the future should his suffering become unacceptable. His doctor was not morally opposed to the practice, but they lived in a state in which PAS was illegal and he was very concerned about the prospect of breaking the law. He proposed other "last resort" options to the patient, including the possibility of voluntarily stopping eating and drinking and of providing sedation if symptoms became severe and otherwise untreatable. The patient appreciated learning about the other legally permitted options, but he still wanted to stay in control of the process by having access to the possibility of PAS, and was willing to work through underground channels to obtain a potentially lethal prescription if the physician did not want to participate.

CLINICAL ISSUES

As previously stated, patients who desire and receive PAS tend to be relatively control-oriented in comparison with those who do not, and their suffering tends to be based more on debility, dependence, and tiredness of dying than uncontrolled pain or other more severe, immediately compelling physical symptoms [8]. The marked disproportion between the public support for potential legal access to PAS and the number who actually activate it suggests that the possibility of this kind of escape is much more important than the reality. There is also little or no evidence that patients in Oregon or Washington are requesting this option because they do not have access to adequate healthcare in general or adequate palliative care in specific (http://public.health.oregon.gov/). The vast majority is already enrolled in hospice, and uncontrolled pain is rarely the main motivating factor. In fact, many patients who desire this option are sufficiently reassured by a potential escape that is under their own control that they never actually take the potentially lethal medication even after they gain access to it.

In practice, the option of PAS is not nearly as flexible as other last resort options such as palliative sedation or voluntarily stopping eating and drinking [10, 11]. Physician-assisted suicide requires that the patient be not only mentally competent, but also physically capable of self-administering a relatively large amount of medication. Patients who have severe neurological conditions or those whose disease affects the ability to swallow or digest may not be able carry out this option. For such patients, the possibility of palliative sedation or of voluntarily stopping eating and drinking might be more realistic alternatives, but such practices require prolonged periods of increased debility and dependence, and also require that the patient spend his last hours and days sedated and potentially out of control of his or her mental faculties—just the kind of status that such control-oriented patients are trying to avoid. In that sense, PAS is sometimes viewed as a preemptive strike to avoid the very last phase of debility and dependence imposed by one's illness.

KEY ETHICAL ISSUES

There is much debate about how much control and choice physicians and society in general should allow dying patients [1, 2]. We certainly give individuals considerable leeway in terms of how much and what kinds of potentially life-extending treatments they receive. We also give those who are being kept alive on life-prolonging therapies almost complete authority to stop such treatments if they no longer meet their goals, even if their desire is to die sooner. In fact, the odds of ending up in a situation in which suffering is significantly increased to the point where it is unacceptable may well be higher in part as a result of patients choosing treatments that help them live even a little longer. One could argue that a "natural death" is hard to find in the developed world, and that it is unfair to suddenly prohibit options for an easier death after we have medically altered the final course of life so substantially.

There is also a fairness issue in that we are able to give those on life supports considerable authority in terms of determining the timing of their own deaths, but those not on life supports who might be suffering as much or more have much more restricted options. In our opinion, the psychological and clinical evaluation of those who are requesting that life supports be stopped should be similar to the evaluation of those requesting PAS, because death will be the likely result of both interventions [10]. But if there are no reasonable medical or palliative alternatives to help a patient escape unacceptable, severe suffering, then in our opinion clinicians should help such patients escape their suffering in the most humane way that is currently available.

Medical responses to requests for PAS in the United States vary considerably depending on whether one lives in one of the four states in which it is legally sanctioned or whether one lives on one of the remaining 46 states. In the legal environment, a request for PAS leads to a careful evaluation according to agreed-upon criteria that include assessments of competency, terminality, and adequacy of palliative treatments (http://public.health.oregon.gov/). If criteria are met and confirmed by a second physician, this evaluation is followed by a 14-day waiting period, after which one can receive the potentially lethal medication. (About one-half of the patients in Oregon who receive this medication actually take it, and for the others it presumably serves as a safety net against unacceptable suffering.) In the rest of the country, such patients' requests are either rejected because of the legal prohibition or the process moves underground. If the request is rejected, other last resort alternatives should be proposed and discussed in detail (sedation, stopping eating and drinking), although knowledge of these alternatives among clinicians not to mention patients is not consistent. When the response moves underground, clinicians secretly give whatever information they have about gaining access to potentially lethal medication, sometimes including a referral to an advocacy organization such as Compassion and Choices, which can help patients and families navigate this very uncertain terrain (http://www.compassionoforegon.org/). The secret practice is generally reserved for the affluent and well connected, and is very uncertain and unpredictable in terms of access, evaluation, and effectiveness.

RETURN TO THE CASE

EE was very well connected, and he was able to gain access to a potentially lethal prescription of barbiturates through an alternate pathway that included a family member making a trip to another country. He did not tell his doctor about his prescription, nor did he tell his hospice workers. He felt very reassured by the prescription, and knew that eventually he would probably become too weak to use it if he did not act in a timely way. He eventually became too weak and had too much difficulty swallowing to reliably take the medication all at once. He would clearly have preferred VAE had it been available, but he did not even raise this question with his clinical team for fear of frightening them away from finding some way to help. Although he thought it was absurd to have to "starve himself to death," he eventually decided to stop eating and drinking, which was the "least worst" option legally available to him. He told his physician, hospice team, and family about his plan, and all accepted and supported his decision. He secretly kept his stash of barbiturates nearby as a "security blanket," and died about 2 weeks after starting his fast, receiving mild sedation at home.

Is Self-Administration a Guarantee of Voluntariness?

CASE #8 PRESENTATION

FF, a longtime member of the Hemlock Society, developed metastatic lung cancer. She lived in a state in which PAS was illegal, but she was able to obtain a prescription for barbiturates to take at a time of her own choosing. Her family was aware of her plan and of her stock of potentially lethal medications, but she and they did not want to compromise her doctor (or her options) by telling her about the plan. As she got sicker and death approached, FF became acutely delirious and agitated. This was just the kind of "out of control" death she had feared. Her family wanted to help her out, but did not know how to proceed.

CLINICAL ISSUES

About 50% of terminally ill patients lose decision-making capacity before death [23]. This statistic clearly underscores the importance of advance care planning, because families will be thrust into the role as surrogate decision makers, being asked as much as possible to represent the patient's values and preferences rather than their own. This situation is particularly challenging for those patients and families who might be in various stages of planning for the possibility of PAS as a last resort option, whether it be in the legal or illegal environment. Such patients may have already stockpiled or had legally prescribed potentially lethal medication, and decisions would need to be faced by surrogates about whether or not to use that medication. For many patients such as FF, losing control of one's mental capacities before death is their worst nightmare. Staying in control of their life and death is at the core of the desire for PAS in many cases.

Furthermore, the presence of full decision-making capacity is one of the main safeguards of any attempt at regulating PAS. The laws governing the practice in Oregon, Washington, Montana, and Vermont all require that the patient be decisionally capable. A second opinion is always required from another physician, and if capacity is still in question, a further evaluation by a psychiatrist or psychologist is required. Of course in the illegal environment, no such second opinions are obtained, as they would be tantamount to an admission of a plan to break the law. To make matters more complex, decision-making capacity may well be present at the time of initial prescribing, but then many patients store the medications to take at a later time of their own choosing. Hopefully the prescribing physicians remain actively engaged with the patient and family so they can jointly face the kinds of challenges potentially faced by patients like FF who lose decision-making capacity as death approaches. Because losing mental capacity before death is often the biggest fear of such patients, a plan for how to address such situations other than PAS should be in place.

KEY ETHICAL ISSUES

Self-administration by a mentally competent patient is one of the main safeguards of the practice of PAS. There was no doubt in this family's mind that FF would want an escape through death in her current clinical situation, but there was no way she could reliably confirm those wishes in her delirious condition. On the other hand, some patients do change their minds, and some find reassurance in the availability of a potentially lethal medication that they never take. In the absence of a physician who is fully aware of the plan and the situation, families are often making such decisions on their own. These decisions often leave families feeling "damned if they do and damned if they don't," and unable to share their concerns because of the legal uncertainty of their situation.

Ideally, such daunting decisions should be make conjointly with the physician and the medical team. Physician and family should jointly establish whether the patient has decision-making capacity. A relatively high level of capacity would be needed for such major life and death decisions such as PAS or voluntarily stopping eating and drinking, and second opinions by those with expertise in capacity determination (usually psychiatrists or psychologists) may be needed in uncertain situations.

If decision-making capacity is lost, family and physician may potentially activate other last resort options to address intractable symptoms. The potential options for patients who have lost decision-making capacity include aggressive symptom management, withholding or withdrawing potentially life-prolonging therapies, proportionate palliative sedation, or palliative sedation to unconsciousness. Families should use substituted judgment in making these decisions, thereby trying to make decisions as the now-incapacitated patient would under the current circumstances.

Voluntarily stopping eating and drinking, PAS, and VAE are all inappropriate when a patient loses capacity, because each of these interventions requires a high level of patient consent in a legal or illegal environment. In circumstances in which a dying patient loses capacity for decision making and is severely symptomatic, the clinician and surrogate decision makers will need to choose among aggressive symptom management, stopping or not starting life supports, and various levels of palliative sedation individually or in combination as last resort options.

RETURN TO THE CASE

The family contacted the hospice program and the patient's doctor to report that FF was acutely agitated, and implored them to "do something" because this kind of suffering was her worst nightmare. The team offered to admit the patient to their acute palliative care unit and manage her symptoms aggressively. The family prompted them that FF had said repeatedly that she would rather be sleepy than to be "out of her mind," and that she had implored them not to let her be agitated or out of control. The family did not tell the hospice team or the doctor about FF's plan to activate PAS for fear that would make them reluctant about providing aggressive sedation. The team treated the patient with a rapidly escalating palliative sedation, and over the course of 24 hours the patient was progressively sedated to unconsciousness. She eventually appeared to be comfortable and her agitated behavior disappeared completely. Artificial hydration and nutrition were offered, but the family declined knowing the patient would not want such treatment. The patient died peacefully 7 days later.

Final Thoughts

Physician assisted suicide, voluntary active euthanasia, and voluntarily stopping eating and drinking are potential palliative options of last resort that could be activated by mentally competent patients who are suffering unacceptably in ways that more standard palliative interventions cannot adequately relieve. There are potentially important practical, moral, and legal similarities and differences among these practices that clinicians, patients, and families should be aware of before activating any of them. These possibilities are ethically "off the table" for patients who lack decision-making capacity, because they each require valid consent of a decisionally capable patient to be activated no matter what the legal environment. For severely suffering patients who lack decision-making capacity, other last-resort options are permissible, including more aggressive pain and symptom management, cessation of life-prolonging therapies, and varying levels of sedation. Clinicians who care for seriously ill patients should be fully aware and capable of delivering standard palliative measures, which are highly effective in most cases, but they must also become knowledgeable about potential last-resort options that they can personally support so they can have a plan for how to approach those infrequent but challenging cases in which suffering persists unacceptably despite their best efforts.

Note

1. This case was from the 1980s, when the full range of last-resort options was not as clearly worked out.

References

1. Quill, T.E. and Battin, M.P., ed. Physician-Assisted Dying: The Case for Palliative Care and Patient Choice. 2002, Johns Hopkins University Press: Baltimore, MD.

2. Foley, K, and Hendin, H., ed. The Case Against Assisted Suicide: For the Right to End of Life Care. 2002, Johns Hopkins University Press: Baltimore, MD.

3. Daube, D., The linguistics of suicide. Suicide Life Threat Behav, 1977. **7**(3): p. 132–82.

4. Battin, M.P., et al., Legal physician-assisted dying in Oregon and the Netherlands: evidence concerning the impact on patients in "vulnerable" groups. J Med Ethics, 2007. **33**(10): p. 591–7.

5. Quill, T.E., Physician-assisted death: progress or peril? Suicide Life Threat Behav, 1994. **24**(4): p. 315–25.

6. Miller, F.G., et al., Regulating physician-assisted death. N Engl J Med, 1994. **331**(2): p. 119–23.

7. Cassel, E.J., The nature of suffering and the goals of medicine. N Engl J Med, 1982. **306**(11): p. 639–45.

8. Back, A.L., et al., Physician-assisted suicide and euthanasia in Washington State. Patient requests and physician responses. JAMA, 1996. **275**(12): p. 919–25.

9. van der Maas, P.J., [Medical decisions around life's end, the study by instruction of the Commission Remmelink]. Ned Tijdschr Geneeskd, 1990. **134**(37): p. 1802–5.

10. Quill, T.E., B. Lo, and D.W. Brock, Palliative options of last resort: a comparison of voluntarily stopping eating and drinking, terminal sedation, physician-assisted suicide, and voluntary active euthanasia. JAMA, 1997. **278**(23): p. 2099–104.

11. Quill, T.E., B.C. Lee, and S. Nunn, Palliative treatments of last resort: choosing the least harmful alternative. University of Pennsylvania Center for Bioethics Assisted Suicide Consensus Panel. Ann Intern Med, 2000. **132**(6): p. 488–93.

12. Quill, T.E., Doctor, I want to die. Will you help me? JAMA, 1993. **270**(7): p. 870–3.

13. Tolle, S.W., et al., Characteristics and proportion of dying Oregonians who personally consider physician-assisted suicide. J Clin Ethics, 2004. **15**(2): p. 111–8.

14. Dworkin R, N.T., Nozick R, Rawls J, Thomson JJ, et al, Assisted Suicide: The Philosophers' Brief. New York Rev Books, 1996 (March 22).

15. Miller, F.G. and Truog, R.D., Death, Dying and Organ Transplantation: Reconstructing Medical Ethics at the End of Life. 2012, New York: Oxford University Press.

16. Meier, D.E., A.L. Back, and R.S. Morrison, The inner life of physicians and care of the seriously ill. JAMA, 2001. **286**(23): p. 3007–14.

17. Cherny, N.I. and R.K. Portenoy, Sedation in the management of refractory symptoms: guidelines for evaluation and treatment. J Palliat Care, 1994. **10**(2): p. 31–8.

18. Quill, T.E., Principle of double effect and end-of-life pain management: additional myths and a limited role. J Palliat Med, 1998. **1**(4): p. 333–6.

19. Quill, T.E., The ambiguity of clinical intentions. N Engl J Med, 1993. **329**(14): p. 1039–40.

20. Court, U.S.S., Vacco v. Quill. Wests Supreme Court Report, 1997. **117**: p. 2293–312.

21. Court, U.S.S., Washington v. Glucksberg. Wests Supreme Court Report, 1997. **117**: p. 2258–93.

22. Jansen, L.A. and D.P. Sulmasy, Sedation, alimentation, hydration, and equivocation: careful conversation about care at the end of life. Ann Intern Med, 2002. **136**(11): p. 845–9.

23. Starks, H., et al., Why now? Timing and circumstances of hastened deaths. Journal of Pain & Symptom Management, 2005. **30**(3): p. 215–26.

17A

Lessons from Legalized Physician-Assisted Death in Oregon and Washington

Linda Ganzini

Four states have defined a legal pathway for their residents to choose physician-assisted death (PAD). The Oregon Death with Dignity Act was passed by citizen's initiative in 1994 and, after a series of legal challenges, enacted in 1997. In 2008, through a voter-initiated referendum, Washingtonians passed an almost identical law (Pisto & Sanford, 2010). In 2009, the Montana Supreme Court held that a terminally ill, mentally competent patient's consent to physician aid-in-dying protected the physician against a charge of homicide (Supreme Court of the State of Montana, 2009). In 2013, Vermont became the fourth state to legalize PAD, the first to use the traditional legislative process. (http://healthvermont.gov/family/end_of_life_care/patient_choice.aspx). No other form of PAD—that is physician prescription and patient consumption of medications for the sole purposes of causing death—is legal in the United States at this time, though studies support that in other states physicians prescribe medications to hasten death. In this chapter I review the epidemiology of PAD in states where it is illegal, death with dignity laws in Washington and Oregon, and the evolution of palliative care and hospice in these states.

Epidemiology of Assisted Death in the United States

Physician-assisted suicide (PAS) is the term most often used in early literature to refer to self-administration, usually orally, of lethal medications both illegally and under death with dignity laws. This chapter uses the term PAD or physician aid-in-dying unless citing studies wherein the authors originally used the term PAS. Active voluntary euthanasia refers to physician-administered lethal medications, usually parentally, at a competent patient's request; nonvoluntary euthanasia is physician-administered lethal medication to a patient who lacks ability to consent, such as an unconscious patient.

   Large, well-done surveys and studies of the prevalence and correlates of PAD were completed over a decade ago. Meier and colleagues (1998) received 1,902 surveys from US physicians in ten specialties likely to care for patients at the end of life. Since entering practice 3.3% had written a prescription to be used to hasten death and 4.7% had administered at least one lethal injection. Physicians who wrote prescriptions for lethal medications were more likely to be male and to be less religious as measured by frequency of prayer. Physicians who had given lethal injections were more likely to live in the west, be Jewish or not religiously affiliated, and less likely to be Catholic. Physicians were more likely to honor requests if the patient was in severe pain or discomfort, had a life expectancy of less than 1 month, and was not depressed (Meier et al., 2003). Emanuel and coauthors (1998) completed phone interviews with a national sample of 355 oncologists of whom 10.7% had participated in PAS or euthanasia. Those who had performed PAS or euthanasia were less religious and more likely to receive requests. In 37 of 38 cases described, the patients were experiencing unremitting pain and such poor physical functioning they could not perform self-care. Emanuel and co-investigators (2000) also prospectively interviewed 988 terminally ill patients and their caregivers from five metropolitan and one rural area twice over 15 months. During the first interview, 10.6% of patients seriously considered euthanasia or PAS for themselves. At follow-up, half had changed their minds but almost an equal number newly considered wanting these interventions. Caregivers of 256 decedents reported one patient died by PAD, one unsuccessfully attempted suicide, and one persisted in her requests for PAD although her family and physicians refused. No new national data on prevalence of or circumstances around PAD has been published in the last decade.

Before enactment of Oregon's law, a survey in 1995 found that 7% of Oregon physicians had ever complied with a request for PAS (Lee et al., 1996). Back and coauthors published a survey in 1996 of 828 Washington physicians. Ninety-nine (12%) physicians had received a request for PAS in the previous year and 32 had complied. These data suggest that a significant minority of physicians in Oregon and Washington were willing to participate in aid-in-dying even before legalization.

Legalized Physician-Assisted Death in Oregon and Washington

The Oregon and Washington Death with Dignity laws are virtually identical (Oregon Public Health Division, 2012; Pisto & Sanford, 2012, Washington State Department of Health, 2012). They allow a competent adult with a life expectancy of less than 6 months to obtain, from a physician, a lethal dose of medication that may be voluntarily self-administered to cause death. The laws include a series of safeguards. Individuals must make two oral requests and one written request over a period of 15 days to lessen the risk of impulsive and ill-considered decisions. Both an attending physician (the physician who will ultimately prescribe the lethal medication and simultaneously become responsible for care of the patient's terminal disease) and a second consulting physician must confirm that the patient has a disease that within reasonable judgment is likely to cause death within 6 months. The physicians must also agree that the patient is capable (i.e., competent) to make such a decision and that the decision is voluntary. Individuals must be informed of interventions that might acceptably address their suffering and desire for hastened death such as hospice and comfort care. The attending or consulting physician must refer the patient to a mental health professional if there is concern that the desire for hastened death stems from impaired judgment resulting from mental illness such as depression. The physician must request, but not require, that the patient notify her or his family of the request for aid in dying.

Neither the Oregon nor the Washington law allows lethal injection and individuals cannot acquire a lethal prescription through advance directive for future states of mental incapacity. In both states physicians who prescribe must notify their respective state public health departments, who collect and publish data yearly. In Oregon, failure by the physician to comply with all aspects of the laws' requirements may be reported to the state licensing board, which can take action against the physician. Several Oregon physicians have been investigated, though for relatively minor problems in documentation. Differences between the Oregon and Washington laws are minor—in fact, the authors of the Washington law in many places adopted almost identical wording as the Oregon law (Pisto & Sanford, 2010). For example, although using the same definitions, the Oregon law uses the term "capable" and Washington law uses the term "competent." The Washington law explicitly defines the term "self-administer" and added a provision regarding safe disposal of unused medications.

Sources of Information about Physician-Assisted Death in Washington and Oregon

The authors of the laws included the requirement that healthcare providers report prescriptions and information verifying that they have complied with the law's provisions. Both states must make information available to the public regarding compliance with the law in an annual statistical report (Oregon Public Health Division, Washington State Department of Health 2012). These reports include the number of prescriptions written, demographic information on patients who have died of PAD, hospice enrollment, insurance status, and complications. In Oregon, through 2005, published data compared patients who died by lethal prescription with all other Oregon deaths. The states do not gather information on patients who request but do not receive prescriptions. Although these reports lack depth, they are comprehensive in including every individual who received a prescription under the law, and therefore do not have the response biases found in other research about the practice of PAD from Oregon and Washington. In contrast, there is almost no information about PAD from Montana; the pathway through which it became legal did not result in any reporting requirements. In addition, there is no information about assisted death that might occur outside the law since legalization, nor is there any information about the incidence of and circumstances around euthanasia.

Other information about PAD comes from groups of researchers in each state. Before enactment of Oregon's law, investigators in Washington began qualitative studies of Washington and some Oregon patients who accessed illegal lethal prescriptions (Back et al., 2002; Pearlman et al., 2005, Stark et al., 2007). Soon after the law was passed, I and others at Oregon Health and Science University began to plan for studies to examine the law as it unfolded. Our questions were pragmatic in nature, informed by our work as healthcare professionals who anticipated caring for requesting patients. We were additionally involved in developing policies and guidelines around PAD at our institutions, medical centers, and professional societies. As such, our lines of inquiry were less couched in the language of ethics and law than the practical issues of how better care might be delivered (The Task Force, 2008). Other investigators in both states have added studies of important depth particularly to understanding how hospice organizations have balanced ethical concerns when caring for patients who died by PAD, patients' understanding of their options, and differing professional groups' responses to legalization (Mesler & Miller, 2000; Ogden & Young, 2003, Silveira et al., 2000; Campbell & Cox, 2010, 2012).

Oregon, with over 15 years of data, offers the most comprehensive information on legalized PAD (Oregon Public Health Division, 2013). Through 2012, 673 Oregonians have died by PAD under Oregon's law, approximately two in 1,000 deaths in that state. They are almost equally divided between men and women; racially 98% were white and 1% were Asian; and their median age was 71 years. Overall, 90% had been enrolled in hospice (97% in 2012) and 2% lacked medical insurance. The most common terminal diseases were cancer (80%) and amyotrophic lateral sclerosis (7%). Ninety-four percent of individuals informed their family of the decision and 95% died at home. After taking the medications, most commonly secobarbital or pentobarbital, patients became unconscious on average within 5 minutes and died within a median of 25 minutes. Complications included regurgitation in 22 patients and regaining of consciousness after ingestion of medication in 6 patients; for some it was minimal level of awareness with death occurring within a few days, whereas another individual awoke after 3 days and lived for 3 more months. In some cases, regaining of consciousness was attributed to incomplete consumption of the medication, regurgitation, or medication tolerance. None reattempted PAD. Washington's data is comparable, though with a somewhat lower rate of hospice enrollment—83% in 2011. Compared with all other deaths in Oregon (data available through 2005), those who die by PAD are less likely to be over the age of 85 years; more likely to be divorced or never married; more highly educated—particularly more likely to have a bachelor's degree or higher; and more likely to have cancer. In Oregon the risk of choosing PAD is comparatively very high in patients with ALS (rate ratio 31, 95% confidence interval 14.4-73.5) and HIV (rate ratio 25.1, 95% confidence interval 6.9-80.4), though these diseases constitute a small proportion of PAD deaths (Oregon Department of Human Services, 2006).

Safeguards in the Death with Dignity Laws

Critics have suggested the need for additional safeguards in the laws in Oregon and Washington. For example, intolerable suffering is a requirement for legal euthanasia in the Netherlands, but not in Oregon. Because patients in Oregon often request prescriptions before they develop symptoms such as pain, critics have charged that voters were misled to support PAD by the specter of patients with physical suffering for which there were no other alternatives save death (Foley & Hendin, 2002). Some Oregon physicians have expressed discomfort with the apparent lack of suffering that many Oregon patients have exhibited at the time of their first request (Dobscha et al., 2004). In Oregon and Washington there is no requirement that either the primary or the consulting physician have expertise in the terminal disease, to assure there are palliative alternatives or if the estimates of prognosis are well informed. Patients may be competent at the time they receive the prescription but there are no safeguards to assure they are competent at the time they take the prescription—this is of concern because most patients with diseases such as advanced cancer begin to develop episodes of confusion in the weeks before death. Finally, critics have contended that physicians often do not know the patients to whom they prescribe well enough to be sure they are eligible for the law. Because many physicians decline to participate in the law—only a third are willing to participate—or work for healthcare systems that contractually preclude them from participating, patients of these physicians must find a new physician late in the course of their terminal illness if they wish to access a lethal prescription (Ganzini et al., 2001). Among patients who requested but did not receive a prescription, the physician was unwilling prescribe 55% of the time (Ganzini et al., 2000).

There have also been concerns about whether safeguards in the law are adequately complied with or enforced. Some patients who have received prescriptions have not used them and gone on to live longer than 6 months, bringing into question the accuracy of physician assessment of prognosis.

A major source of concern is around the adequacy of the mental capacity safeguard. Patients assessed to have a mental illness or depression influencing their judgment about hastened death are disqualified under the law, or as stated in the measure, "If in the opinion of the attending physician or the consulting physician a patient may be suffering from a psychiatric or psychological disorder or depression causing impaired judgment, either physician shall refer the patient for counseling. No medication to end a patient's life in a humane and dignified manner shall be prescribed until the person performing the counseling determines that the patient is not suffering from a psychiatric or psychological disorder or depression causing impaired judgment" (Oregon Public Health Division, 2012). Persons qualified to perform the counseling are licensed psychologists and psychiatrists.

Although "depression" is not defined in the law, this is accepted to refer to "clinical depression" or, in psychiatric nomenclature, major depressive disorder. During an episode of major depressive disorder a patient has pervasive low mood;

inability to experience pleasure; has sad, blue or depressed feelings most of the time over weeks, so persistently that everyday functioning is impacted. Other symptoms include hopelessness, a belief of burdening others, guilt, poor self-esteem, and desire to die. This type of depression differs from a less severe but diagnosable mood disorder such as dysthymia (chronic mild depression), and understandable and normal grief, sadness, and dysphoria experienced by many with a terminal illness. Major depressive disorder can be reliably diagnosed in between 10% and 25% of patients with advanced cancer (Hotopf et al., 2002).

There are several important arguments for excluding patients with clinical depression from being eligible for PAD. Depressed persons view their future through a lens of pessimism, hopelessness, and apathy. Major depressive disorder can render a person unable to enjoy life or experience pleasure, personal worth, or hope for recovery. Depressed persons therefore can make decisions that are potentially inauthentic and not true to their values, life philosophy, or personality, even if the decisions otherwise appear competent and voluntary. In fact, depression may not prevent expression of an articulate and coherent analysis of the benefits and rationale for PAD (Ganzini & Dobscha, 2003). Depressed patients particularly have more variability and instability in their desire for death (Emanuel et al., 2000; Ganzini et al., 2006).

What is known about the relationship of depression and desire for hastened death comes from decades of research on suicide. Very few other measurable risk factors are as strong as depression in predicting suicide through the life cycle in both physical health and disease. Among patients with cancer who suicide, 80% have a mental disorder with major depressive disorder along with substance abuse as the most common (Henriksson et al., 1995). Among patients with advanced cancer and HIV, surveys that measure desire for hastened death find a strong and consistent association with major depressive disorder, depressive symptoms and hopelessness (Breitbart, et al., 2000; Rosenfeld et al., 2006). For example, in a study of 98 patients admitted to a US hospice inpatient unit those with major depressive disorder were four times more likely to have an elevated desire for hastened death. (Breitbart et al., 2000). Among 200 inpatients with advanced cancer, a depression syndrome was diagnosed in 59% of patients with a serious and pervasive desire to die, but only 8% without such a desire (Chochinov et al., 1995). Suicide prevention interventions are effective, and treatment of depression reduces hopelessness and suicidal thoughts and ideation among older primary care patients (Bruce et al., 2004). Depression treatment will improve mood, outlook, and function even in a situation where low mood might be an understandable response to a disheartening situation such as terminal illness. Among elderly patients, up to two-thirds will remain well for several years following depression treatment; one-quarter to one-third will remain depressed, relapse, or die (Murphy, 1994).

There are also arguments for not having an absolute ban on patients with depression accessing lethal prescriptions. Depression compounds suffering at the end of life and is not always treatable in the shortened time period before death.

Many patients who request PAD have only weeks of remaining life, yet most antidepressant treatment regimens are not effective until 1 or 2 months of treatment. Successful treatment of major depressive disorder increases interest in life-sustaining treatments in only a minority of patients and only those with the most severe mood symptoms (Ganzini et al., 1994). Oregon law does not exclude all depressed patients—only cases in which depression is impairing judgment around desire for death. Although mental health professionals have expertise in diagnosis of mental disorders, determining whether the disorder influences desire for hastened death is difficult and there are no published standards or guidelines for this assessment. Understanding whether depression influences the decision for PAD requires knowing an individual over time while both depressed and euthymic. Ninety-five percent of Oregon psychiatrists were somewhat or very confident in the context of a long-term relationship in which they could determine whether a mental disorder, such as depression, was influencing the decision for PAD; but only 6% were very confident that in a single evaluation they could make this assessment (Ganzini et al., 1996). Moreover, ethical views on PAD may influence these assessments where standards are lacking. In a national study of forensic psychiatrists, those ethically opposed to PAD advocated for higher thresholds for competence—including that the finding of depression should result in automatic finding of incompetence, and more extensive reviews of the decision—for example, more than one forensic examiner or judicial review (Ganzini et al., 2000). As such, the determination of whether depression is influencing the decision about PAD may reflect more about the mental health professionals' ethical and moral views of PAD than any reliable or valid mental health assessment technique or psychiatric expertise. In the national survey of forensic psychiatrists, 42% did not agree that major depressive disorder should automatically render a patient incompetent to choose assisted suicide, supporting that some experts believe that clinical depression should not necessarily exclude every terminally ill person from pursuing PAD (Ganzini et al., 2000).

The prevalence of depression in individuals in Oregon who actually request PAD does not appear to be markedly higher than the prevalence of depression in terminally ill patients who have not made such requests. In a survey of physicians' experiences with Oregonians who requested PAD, 20% of requesting patients were assessed as depressed (Ganzini et al., 2000). In a study of Oregonians who requested PAD and underwent rigorous assessment for depression, 26% met criteria for major depressive disorder (Ganzini et al., 2008). As previously noted, studies of the prevalence of depression in patients with terminal illness who are not seeking PAD report proportions of 10% to 25% (Hotopf et al., 2002). Hospice social workers and nurses rated depression as a relatively unimportant reason that Oregonian hospice patients requested PAD. In fact, among 21 reasons, hospice social workers who have substantial experience in evaluating the psychosocial state of patients at the end of life rated depression as the least important (Ganzini et al., 2002).

Though the burden of depression may be lower than anticipated among patients pursuing PAD, some depressed patients may access lethal prescriptions.

In our study of 58 Oregonians who requested PAD, 18 received lethal prescriptions, including three patients who had met very rigorous criteria for depression. All three died by lethal ingestion within 2 months of the research interview, though in one case the depression was successfully treated before death and in the other two cases the patients denied that depression was influencing their decision (Ganzini et al., 2008). This finding supports the need for more active and systematic screening and surveillance for depression to determine which patients should be referred for mental health evaluation. Despite this finding, the proportion of Oregon and Washington PAD decedents referred for mental health evaluation has remained very low and critics have called for mandatory mental health evaluation in all cases (Oregon Public Health Division, 2012). It is unknown how many patients were referred to mental health professionals who found the patient ineligible for a prescription—the health department data of these states only include information on persons who received prescriptions. With aforementioned problems with mental health evaluation, it remains unclear if mandatory psychiatric assessment would balance the protection of vulnerable persons with advancing patient autonomy, or if it would cast mental health professionals in the role of ethics consultants (Sullivan et al., 1998).

Physician-Assisted Death, Hospice and Palliative Care

From the outset, legalization of PAD posed challenges to the burgeoning end-of-life care movement on several levels. By the time the Act was implemented in 1997, Oregon had a well-developed hospice system, though hospital-based palliative care was otherwise in its infancy—as it was throughout the United States. Based on studies of interest in assisted suicide, it was anticipated that up to 10% of all terminally might request a lethal prescription (Emanuel et al., 2000). Comparing the costs of expanding and improving the quality of hospice and palliative care with the minimal costs of a lethal prescription provoked fears of subtle pressure for PAD, undermining and diverting attention and resources from the development of palliative care. Passage of the Oregon Death with Dignity Act occurred in the backdrop of the beginnings of reorganization of healthcare into managed care with the goal of curtailing escalating healthcare costs. The ease of prescribing a single lethal prescription led to fears that physicians' efforts to learn about the more difficult aspects of end-of-life care and pain management might be eroded (Goy et al., 2003).

This did not happen, in part because PAD was ultimately very rare—increasing slowly from one to two in 1,000 deaths over the 15 years of legalization. The uncommonness of PAD may stem from several factors. First, studies that led to projections of higher rates were based on surveys of preferences and interest, but subsequent studies showed that only a fraction of those who indicated interest on a survey actually made requests. Only 1% of Oregonians who die each year make explicit requests for PAD; only one in 10 who make explicit requests die by lethal prescription (Ganzini et al., 2000). Second, obtaining the prescription requires a fair degree of foresight, planning, and determination to push against a variety of obstacles. Barriers included that many patients are unable to find a willing physician—only a third of physicians indicated willingness to prescribe, and physicians in rural areas are particularly unwilling. Patients at times die or lose capacity before completing the requirements (Ganzini et al., 2000). Patients who do consider PAD on the basis of physical symptoms often are late in the course of their illness and less likely to live through the waiting period. Tolle and coauthors (2004) found an association between symptom distress in the last week of life and consideration of PAD. Physicians are very reluctant to prescribe to patients if there are family members with objections (Ganzini et al., 2003). Third, palliative interventions, particularly referrals to hospice, did result in some patients rescinding their request for lethal prescriptions, particularly for patients who had not yet experienced the benefits of hospice (Ganzini & Dobscha, 2004).

Advocates for palliative care were able to use the specter of bad publicity around patients choosing PAD because of denial of care effectively with the administrators of hospital systems, who over time added palliative care services; insurers, all of whom included hospice in their benefits packages; and the state, which maintains end-of-life care as a high priority in its landmark Medicaid system, the Oregon Health Plan. During the 3 years of preparation allowed between passage of the law and implementation, Oregon healthcare leaders came together to develop educational programs for which one of the most important messages was "refer to hospice, find palliative care alternatives." The message was effective. Through 2012, 90% of Oregonians who died by lethal prescription were hospice-enrolled. In a survey of over 2,600 Oregon physicians in 1999, 30% agreed they made higher rates of hospice referrals the previous year compared to 5 years earlier; only 2% of surveyed physicians indicated they had made fewer referrals. Among the over 2,000 who had cared for at least one terminally-ill patient in the previous year, 76% reported they had made efforts to improve their knowledge of the use of pain medications "somewhat" or "a great deal" and 79% reported that their confidence in prescribing pain medications had improved (Ganzini et al., 2001). Hospice professionals concurred. In a 2001 survey of 237 hospice nurses and social workers, 67% ranked Oregon physicians as more competent in caring for hospice patients than five years earlier, 4% viewed them as less competent; 77% viewed them as more willing to refer to hospice over the previous 5 years, and only 3% viewed them as less willing (Goy et al., 2003). These improvements occurred against the backdrop of national advances in palliative care and cannot necessarily be attributed to legalization of PAD. Yet the concern that PAD would undermine end-of-life care is entirely unsupported.

Another challenge to palliative care is that PAD requests often are motivated by concerns not easily ameliorated by hospice care. In the arguments around legalization, the role of pain was central—proponents of legalization argued that not all pain could be effectively treated, and the opponents of legalization argued that good palliative care and pain treatment would make PAD unnecessary. A surprising finding from studies of Oregonians pursuing PAD was the relative lack of importance of pain in a request for PAD. For example, patients pursuing a lethal prescription rated experienced pain as completely unimportant as a reason for the request, though fears of pain in the future were more important (Ganzini et al., 2009). Because most patients receive the prescription before they actually experience substantial pain, there is not much of a role for expert pain management in reducing prescriptions—though it is possible that pain management may delay taking of the lethal medication or result in a patient with a prescription never needing to use it.

The reasons individuals give for wanting access to PAD—wanting to maintain independence, control, self-care, and high quality of life—represent states that hospice has fewer means of addressing than traditional symptom management (Ganzini et al., 2009). These individuals highly value control and dislike dependence on others; this often represent a strong enduring value, a philosophy and defining lifelong personality attribute. These characteristics of control, self-sufficiency, self-reliance, and independence represent a challenge in hospice. Patients accurately foresee that the dying process will not allow them to maintain these cherished attributes and abilities, that they ultimately will become dependent on others. Entry into hospice underscores these fears—in fact, in the early years after the law passed many PAD patients "fired" their hospice nurse before getting through the intake process. Further, hospice represents more care to patients who wish to avoid being dependent on others. Compassion and Choices of Oregon, anticipating this resistance to hospice, emphasizes that patients have ultimate control over how much hospice is involved and that good symptom management is the best method of maintaining independence (Ganzini, 2010).

For hospices, PAD patients can present a variety of challenges both for individual practitioners and at a policy level. For individual practitioners, those opposed to PAD may believe they have fallen short when their patients choose to take the lethal medication. Or as one hospice nurse said, "I felt like a failure at controlling her symptoms because that's my job to keep people comfortable and when the choose PAS, they're deciding that they're not comfortable" (Harvath et al., 2006). Hospice nurses with discomfort around PAD struggle to maintain boundaries and not be drawn in; for example, being asked to manage a symptom such as nausea to help prepare a patient to take the medication. Many believe that a natural death offers opportunity for growth and spiritual transformation for both the patient and family that is missed when the patient chooses PAD (Harvath et al., 2006). But overall in Oregon, 48% of hospice nurses, 72% of hospice social workers, and even 40% of hospice chaplains support legalization (Ganzini et al., 2002; Carlson et al., 2005). Twelve percent of hospice nurses and 2% of hospice social workers would transfer a patient to another hospice provider if they knew the patient had requested a lethal prescription, supporting that most nurses and social workers who opposed PAD would still continue to care for the patient (Ganzini et al., 2002). One percent of hospice social workers and 6% of hospice nurses believed that a patient requesting PAD should be discharged from hospice (Miller et al., 2004).

Hospices vary along a continuum of policies regarding several aspects of involvement in PAD. First, for every patient there is the choice to not ever tell their hospice providers of their plans to obtain or use a lethal prescription. Because their relationship with their physician is separate from the hospice, it is possible to obtain the medication and use it without hospice providers knowing. Ninety-five percent of PAD deaths occur at home, hospice nurses visit only a few hours each week, and a PAD death is most often indistinguishable from other deaths. Campbell and Cox (2010, 2012), outlined a variety of organization positions and policies of the over 60 Oregon hospices around PAD. Oregon hospices will not discharge a patient who entertains the goal of PAD, yet no hospice will provide a patient with the lethal medication or assist in the self-administration. Within these boundaries hospices vary in the degree to which they allow staff to discuss PAD, notify the attending physician of the patient's interest in PAD, refer the patient to an advocacy organization for more information, or allow hospice staff presence before or during ingestion of the medication. For example, hospices range from the minority of mostly religiously-based hospices that view PAD as incompatible with hospice care, who will not provide information about patients' choices and ask patients to respect their hospice's position; to those that have specific personnel who adopt a posture of neutrality in talking to the patient and family; and those that emphasize respect for patient self-determination, allow hospice personal to discuss this option, refer the patient to PAD advocacy organizations for more information, and attend the PAD death.

Final Thoughts

There are many challenges to research in this area. The study of illegal PAD outside of Oregon and Washington is fraught with ethical and legal challenges and the study of PAD in Oregon and Washington is less attractive to national funders because of lack of generalizability. Access to requesting patients in my studies was possible through a successful collaboration with Compassion and Choices of Oregon, an advocacy organization which gives information or attends the deaths of three quarters of Oregonians who die by PAD. However, a more recent study I proposed on whether receiving a prescription resulted in reduction of anxiety and increased sense of peace was not allowed by their parent organization, Compassion and Choices. As to whether other states should legalize PAD, studies that examine how they differ from the Pacific Northwest may be difficult and further unbiased research on patients in the United States requesting PAD and their families may face potentially insuperable hurdles.

During the last 15 years only four states have legalized PAD, whereas attempts to approve legalized physician aid-in-dying in numerous US states have failed, most recently in 2012 in Massachusetts, one of the most liberal states in the country. Whether advocates for legalized PAD will prevail either in referenda or legislatures or the courts in other states is unknown. Most untoward consequences predicted by legalization in Oregon were unfounded, yet voters in others states are either worried about whether PAD can be introduced with a minimum of problems in their states, or simply do not see the need for this type of legislation. The desire for PAD had highlighted the heterogeneity of patient's values and goals at the end of life. For those who place a high value on staying in control, dying at home, and avoiding dependence on others, hospice and palliative care are challenged to move away from a limited focus on symptom control, family, and spiritual needs. Further research on meeting the needs of these types of patients at the end of life would have universal value.

Acknowledgement and Disclaimer

This material is the result of work supported with resources and the use of facilities at the Portland Veterans Affairs Medical Center.

The views expressed in this chapter are those of the author and do not necessarily reflect the position or policy of the Department of Veterans Affairs or the United States government.

References

1. Back AL, Starks H, Hsu C, Gordon JR, Bharucha A, Pearlman RA. Clinician-patient interactions about requests for physician-assisted suicide: a patient and family view. Archives of Internal Medicine 2002;162:1257–65.
2. Back AL, Wallace JI, Starks HE, Pearlman RA. Physician-assisted suicide and euthanasia in Washington State: patient requests and physician responses. Journal of the American Medical Association 1996;275:919–25.
3. Breitbart W, Rosenfeld B, Pessin H, Kaim M, Funesti-Esch J, Galietta M, Nelson CJ, Brescia R. Depression, hopelessness, and desire for hastened death in terminally ill patients with cancer. Journal of the American Medical Association 2000;284:2907–11.
4. Bruce ML, Ten Have TR, Reynolds CF 3rd, Katz II, Schulberg HC, Mulsant BH, Brown GK, McAvay GJ, Pearson JL, Alexopoulos GS. Reducing suicidal ideation and depressive symptoms in depressed older primary care patients: a randomized controlled trial. Journal of the American Medical Association 2004;291:1081–91.
5. Campbell CS, Cox JC. Hospice and physician-assisted death: collaboration, compliance, and complicity. Hastings Center Report 2010;40:26–35.
6. Campbell CS, Cox JC. Hospice-assisted death? A study of Oregon hospices on death with dignity. American Journal of Hospice Palliative Care 2012;29:227–35.
7. Carlson B, Simopolous N, Goy ER, Jackson A, Ganzini L. Oregon hospice chaplains' experiences with patients requesting physician-assisted suicide. Journal of Palliative Medicine 2005;8:1160–6.
8. Chochinov HM, Wilson KG, Enns M, Mowchun N, Lander S, Levitt M, Clinch JJ. Desire for death in the terminally ill. American Journal of Psychiatry 1995;152:1185–91.

9. Dobscha SK, Heintz RT, Press N, Ganzini L. Oregon physicians' responses to requests for assisted suicide: a qualitative study. Journal of Palliative Medicine 2004;7:451–61.

10. Emanuel EJ, Daniels ER, Fairclough DL, Clarridge BR. The practice of euthanasia and physician-assisted suicide in the United States: adherence to proposed safeguards and effects on physicians. Journal of the American Medical Association 1998;280:507–13.

11. Emanuel EJ, Fairclough DL, Emanuel LL. Attitudes and desires related to euthanasia and physician-assisted suicide among terminally ill patients and their caregivers. Journal of the American Medical Association 2000;284:2460–8.

12. Foley K, Hendin H. The Oregon experiment. In: Foley K, Hendin H, eds. The Case against Assisted Suicide. Baltimore: The Johns Hopkins University Press; 2002:144–74.

13. Ganzini L. Strange death bed fellows. Hastings Center Report 2010;40:3.

14. Ganzini L, Beer TM, Brouns M, Mori M, Hsieh Y-C. Interest in physician-assisted suicide among Oregon cancer patients. Journal of Clinical Ethics 2006;17:27–38.

15. Ganzini L, Dobscha SK. Clarifying distinctions between contemplating and completing physician-assisted suicide. Journal of Clinical Ethics 2004;15:119–22.

16. Ganzini L, Dobscha SK. If it isn't depression. Journal of Palliative Medicine 2003;6:927–30.

17. Ganzini L, Dobscha SK, Heintz RT, Press N. Oregon physicians' perceptions of patients who request assisted suicide and their families. Journal of Palliative Medicine 2003;6:381–90.

18. Ganzini L, Fenn DS, Lee MA, Heintz RT, Bloom JD. Attitudes of Oregon psychiatrists toward physician-assisted suicide. American Journal of Psychiatry 1996;153:1469–75.

19. Ganzini L, Goy ER, Dobscha SK, Prigerson H. Mental health outcomes of family members of Oregonians who request physician aid in dying. Journal of Pain and Symptom Management 2009;38:807–15.

20. Ganzini L, Goy ER, Dobscha SK. Oregonians' reasons for requesting physician aid in dying. Archives of Internal Medicine 2009;169:489–92.

21. Ganzini L, Goy ER, Dobscha SK. Prevalence of depression and anxiety in patients requesting physicians' aid in dying: cross sectional survey. British Medical Journal 2008;337:a1682.

22. Ganzini L, Goy ER, Miller LL, Harvath TA, Jackson A, Delorit MA. Nurses' experiences with hospice patients who refuse food and fluids to hasten death. New England Journal of Medicine 2003;349:359–65.

23. Ganzini L, Goy ER; Dobscha SK. Why Oregon patients request assisted death: family members' views. Journal of General Internal Medicine 2008;23:154–7.

24. Ganzini L, Harvath TA, Jackson A, Goy ER, Miller LL, Delorit MA. Experiences of Oregon nurses and social workers with hospice patients who requested assistance with suicide. New England Journal of Medicine 2002;347:582–8.

25. Ganzini L, Lee MA, Heintz RT, Bloom JD, Fenn DS. The effect of depression treatment on elderly patients' preferences for life-sustaining medical therapy. American Journal of Psychiatry 1994;151:1631–6.

26. Ganzini L, Leong GB, Fenn DS, Silva JA, Weinstock R. Evaluation of competence to consent to assisted suicide: views of forensic psychiatrists. American Journal of Psychiatry 2000;157:595–600.

27. Ganzini L, Nelson HD, Lee MA, Kraemer DF, Schmidt TA, Delorit MA. Oregon physicians' attitudes about and experiences with end-of-life care since passage of

the Oregon Death with Dignity Act. Journal of the American Medical Association 2001;285:2363–9.

28. Ganzini L, Nelson HD, Schmidt TA, Kraemer DF, Delorit MA, Lee MA. Physicians' experiences with the Oregon Death with Dignity Act. New England Journal of Medicine 2000;342:557–63.

29. Ganzini L, Silveira MJ, Johnston WS. Predictors and correlates of interest in assisted suicide in the final month of life among ALS patients in Oregon and Washington. Journal of Pain and Symptom Management 2002;24:312–7.

30. Goy ER, Jackson A, Harvath TA, Miller LL, Delorit MA, Ganzini L. Oregon hospice nurses and social workers' assessment of physician progress in palliative care over the past five years. Palliative and Supportive Care 2003;1:215–9.

31. Harvath TA, Miller LL, Smith KA, Clark LD, Jackson A, Ganzini L. Dilemmas encountered by hospice workers when patients wish to hasten death. Journal of Hospice and Palliative Nursing 2006;8:200–9.

32. Henriksson MM, Isometsa ET, Hietanen PS, Aro HM, Lonnqvist JK. Mental disorders in cancer suicides. Journal of Affective Disorders 1995;36:11–20.

33. Hotopf M, Chidgey J, Addington-Hall J, Ly KL. Depression in advanced disease: a systematic review Part 1. Prevalence and case finding. Palliative Medicine 2002;16:81–97.

34. Lee MA, Nelson HD, Tilden VP, Ganzini L, Schmidt TA, Tolle SW. Legalizing assisted suicide: views of physicians in Oregon. New England Journal of Medicine 1996;334:310–5.

35. Meier DE, Emmons CA, Litke A, Wallenstein S, Morrison RS. Characteristics of patients requesting and receiving physician-assisted suicide. Archives of Internal Medicine 2003;163:1537–42.

36. Meier DE, Emmons CA, Wallenstein S, Quill T, Morrison RS, Cassel CK. A national survey of physician-assisted suicide and euthanasia in the United States. New England Journal of Medicine 1998;338:1193–201.

37. Mesler MA, Miller PJ. Hospice and assisted suicide: the structure and process of an inherent dilemma. Death Studies 2000;24:135–55.

38. Miller LL, Harvath TA, Ganzini L, Goy ER, Delorit MA, Jackson A. Attitudes and experiences of Oregon hospice nurses and social workers regarding assisted suicide. Palliative Medicine 2004;18:685–91.

39. Murphy E. The course and outcome of depression in late life. In: Schneider LS, Reynolds III CF, Lebowitz BD, Friedhoff AJ, eds. Diagnosis and treatment of depression in late life: results of the NIH Consensus Development Conference. Washington, DC: American Psychiatric Press; 1994:81–98.

40. Ogden RD, Young MG. Washington State social workers' attitudes toward voluntary euthanasia and assisted suicide. Social Work in Health Care 2003;37:43–70.

41. Oregon Department of Human Services. Eighth Annual Report on Oregon's Death with Dignity Act. http://public.health.oregon.gov/ProviderPartnerResources/EvaluationResearch/DeathwithDignityAct/Documents/year8.pdf. Eighth Annual Report on Oregon's Death with Dignity Act. March 9, 2006. Last accessed January 31, 2013.

42. Oregon Public Health Division. Oregon's Death with Dignity Act—2011. http://public.health.oregon.gov/ProviderPartnerResources/EvaluationResearch/DeathwithDignityAct/Documents/year14.pdf. March 2012. Last accessed January 31, 2013.

43.. Pearlman RA, Hsu C, Starks H, Back AL, Gordon JR, Bharucha AJ, Koenig BA, Battin MP. Motivations for physician-assisted suicide. Journal of General Internal Medicine 2005;20:234–9.

44. Pisto LA, Sanford ST. 2012. Implementing Washington's Death with Dignity Act: Legal and Policy Issues. Two Down, More to Come? Or Is This The End of the Line? In: http://www.healthlawyers.org/Events/Programs/Materials/Documents/AM10/pisto_sanford.pdf (Accessed today October 21).

45. Rosenfeld B, Breitbart W, Gibson C, Kramer M, Tomarken A, Nelson C, Pessin H, Esch J, Galietta M, Garcia N, Brechtl J, Schuster M. Desire for hastened death among patients with advanced AIDS. Psychosomatics 2006;47:504–12.

46. Silveira MJ, DiPiero A, Gerrity MS, Feudtner C. Patients' knowledge of options at the end of life: ignorance in the face of death. JAMA 2000;284:2483–8.

47. Starks H, Back AL, Pearlman RA, Koenig BA, Hsu C, Gordon JR, Bharucha AJ. Family member involvement in hastened death. Death Studies 2007;31:105–30.

48. Sullivan M, Ganzini L, Youngner SJ. Should psychiatrists serve as gatekeepers for physician assisted suicide? Hastings Center Report 1998;28:14–22.

49. Supreme Court of the State of Montana. Robert Baxter, Stephen Speckart, M.D., C. Paul Loehnen, M.D., Lar Autio, M.D., George Risi, Jr., M.D. Compassion & Choices v. State of Montana and Steve Bullock. In: DA 09-0051 2009 MT 449, 2009.

50. The Task Force to Improve the Care of Terminally-Ill Oregonians, Dunn P, Reagan B, Tolle SW, Foreman S. The Oregon Death with Dignity Act: A Guidebook for Health Care Professionals. (2008) http://www.ohsu.edu/xd/education/continuing-education/center-for-ethics/ethics-outreach/upload/Oregon-Death-with-Dignity-Act-Guidebook.pdf. Last accessed February 26, 2013.

51. Tolle SW, Tilden VP, Drach LL, Fromme EK, Perrin NA, Hedberg K. Characteristics and proportion of dying Oregonians who personally consider physician-assisted suicide. Journal of Clinical Ethics 2004;15:111–8.

52. Washington State Department of Health. Washington State Department of Health 2011 Death with Dignity Act Report; 2012.

17B

Physician-Assisted Death in Western Europe: The Legal and Empirical Situation

Heleen Weyers

The aim of this chapter is to provide a brief review of the legal and empirical situation of physician assisted death in Western Europe and its consequences. In 2008 we (John Griffiths, Maurice Adams and Heleen Weyers) published a book[1] in which we provide detailed information on the situation in the Netherlands and Belgium and more general information about England and Wales, France, Italy, the Scandinavian countries (Denmark, Norway, and Sweden), Spain, and Switzerland. This chapter consists mainly of extracts of this book[2] with some addition on the situation in Germany.

In this chapter I deal with the legal situation of euthanasia and assistance with suicide of the 11 countries, with the frequencies of medical behavior that potentially shortens life in some of them, and with the results of the control system of euthanasia of the Netherlands and Belgium. I end this chapter with some reflections on intended and unintended consequences of legalization of euthanasia and assisted suicide.

A FEW WORDS ON TERMINOLOGY

"Euthanasia" in the strict sense, and in the Dutch and Belgian context the only, refers to a situation in which a doctor ends the life of a person who is suffering "unbearably" and "hopelessly"—that is, without prospect of improvement—at the latter's explicit request. Euthanasia usually is carried out by administering a lethal injection. When a distinction is made between the two, "euthanasia" is reserved for killing on request as opposed to "assistance with suicide." In the Netherlands and Belgium the two are generally treated together. In *Euthanasia and Law* we followed this practice and used the single term "euthanasia" to cover both where the distinction is not relevant.

Euthanasia is a form of a death that is an outcome of medical behavior performed by a doctor expecting that the behavior will lead to the earlier death of the patient. Besides euthanasia, four other types of this behavior are distinguished: honoring a patient's refusal of treatment, withholding or withdrawing "futile" life-prolonging treatment ("abstention"), pain relief with life-shortening effect, and termination of life without an explicit request.[3] All of this behavior together we call medical behavior that potentially shortens life (MBPSL).

Legal Situation

In all the countries we have studied except in the Netherlands and Belgium, euthanasia is illegal (either murder or a lesser offense of homicide on request).[4] However, except in Italy, France, and England (and the Netherlands before the change of law) euthanasia seems rarely to be prosecuted.

Physician-assisted suicide is legal in the Netherlands and Belgium (where it is assimilated with euthanasia), and in Switzerland (where doctors are involved but the actual help is given by right-to-die societies). It is specifically illegal in Italy, Spain, Norway, and Denmark. It is also illegal in the United Kingdom. This prohibition in the United Kingdom, however, has become more theoretical with respect to non-doctors because of a new policy of the prosecutorial authorities.[5] Assisted suicide is in theory legal in France and Sweden; however, disciplinary action under the deontology code against doctors would be possible. In Germany assistance with suicide is also not prohibited, but a doctor is not allowed to prescribe a lethal drug and ought to rescue a patient who took such drugs.

Termination of life without request from the patient is illegal everywhere. Only in the Netherlands (and in highly unusual circumstances in England and Wales[6]) have the courts recognized the possibility of the defense of necessity[7] in the situation of neonatology.

In Belgium and the Netherlands euthanasia is legal under specific circumstances. The doctor who has carried out euthanasia should comply with the "criteria of due care"[8] and should report the case to the authorities. Reporting results in a review by specially installed committees, the Regional Review Committees. These committees judge whether a reported case of euthanasia fulfills the "due care" criteria. Only those cases in which a committee finds the doctor "not careful" are sent to the prosecutorial authorities.

There is a general agreement among the European countries we have studied that pain and symptom relief can be given even though it potentially will shorten the patient's life. However, the legal grounds on which this can be done are not clear. Two doctrines are available: the "doctrine of double effect" and the "medical exception." The first holds that potentially life-shortening pain relief is permissible so long as the doctor's intention is to relieve pain and not to shorten life.[9] Although it is widely supposed to have legal status, the only country in which the doctrine has been accepted for legal purposes is England. The second approach—"medical exception"—holds that doctors are authorized to do things that are otherwise forbidden, *so long as there is a medical indication for what they do.*[10] A gradual shift to medical indication as the criterion for distinguishing between pain relief and termination of life is visible in the Netherlands and Switzerland. If medically indicated, giving high doses of pain relief, even if they terminate the life of the patient, are seen as "normal medical treatment." Euthanasia never is.[11]

Furthermore, there is general agreement in Western European countries that life-prolonging treatment can be withheld or withdrawn if it either would be or has become "futile."[12] However, in most countries neither the criteria according to which treatment can be considered "futile" nor the decision-making procedure required before such a judgment is carried out, are well developed. In the Netherlands, Switzerland, Norway, and England treatment of patients in a permanent vegetative state can be withdrawn because it is deemed futile.

All Western European countries give at least lip service to the principle of informed consent. Although it is anchored in the European Convention on Human Rights, the idea that the patient has a right to refuse life-prolonging treatment is only gradually spreading. Belgium, England, Germany, the Netherlands, Sweden, and Switzerland accept the principle in all situations. In Denmark, treatment cannot be refused if life is at stake; in Norway not in an "emergency" situation. Recent law cases in Italy and Spain suggest that the law there seems to be developing in the direction of the European norm. Advance treatment directives are known in all countries, but in only some (Belgium, England, Germany, the Netherlands, and Switzerland) do they have a strong legal status. Nevertheless, the legally binding character of a patient's advance written refusal of treatment seems gradually to be becoming accepted in the other countries too. The role of representatives of a noncompetent patient (appointed by a court or by the patient, or statutory "default" representatives) is legally well-defined in England, Belgium, Germany, the Netherlands, and Switzerland. Most other countries accept some form of "proxy decision making" based on the patient's "best interest" or "presumed will" if the treatment wishes of a noncompetent patient are not known, but the proxy generally only gives information that a doctor can take into account.

Continuous sedation until death (often called "terminal sedation") seems to be generally accepted as a legitimate form of pain and symptom relief. Apparently only in Norway and Sweden and in the Netherlands (and to a more limited extent in Switzerland) has it been subjected to specific regulatory attention. The legitimacy of withholding artificial nutrition and hydration from a sedated patient at the end of life is unsettled everywhere except in the Netherlands and England (TABLE 17B.1).

Empirical Data

COMPARATIVE DATA ON THE FREQUENCY OF MEDICAL BEHAVIOR THAT POTENTIALLY SHORTENS LIFE

In 2003 a comparative study (EURELD) on MBPSL practices was published in which Belgium, Denmark, Italy, the Netherlands, Switzerland, and Sweden took

TABLE 17B.1

Varieties of Medical Behavior That Potentially Shorten Life

General Category	Specific Category	Legitimating Principle	Legal Formulation
"Normal medical practice"	Honoring patient's refusal of treatment (current or in advanced treatment directives)	Autonomy	Patient's consent required for treatment
	Abstention: withholding or withdrawing "futile" life-prolonging treatment	Nonmaleficence	Medical exception
	Pain relief with life-shortening effect	Beneficence	Doctrine of double effect Medical exception
Termination of life	Euthanasia	Beneficence/autonomy	Euthanasia Law[13]
	Physician-assisted suicide	Beneficence/autonomy	Justification of necessity[14] Prosecutorial guideline[15] Restricted prohibition[16]
	Termination of life without an explicit request	Beneficence	Justification of necessity

part. A study by Seale using the same methodology was carried out in England some years later. We therefore can compare countries in which euthanasia has been legalized (at that time the Netherlands) and countries in which it is not (TABLE 17B.2).[17]

Medical behavior that potentially shortens life practice in the European countries covered in the studies seems on the whole rather similar. Only Italy, where rates for all MBPSL except pain relief with life-shortening effect and continuous sedation are much lower than in other countries, stands out as a consistent deviant. Setting aside Italy, the total rate of MBPSL is everywhere greater than 35% of all deaths. The highest rate of death caused by MBPSL occurs in the United Kingdom.

The Dutch rate of euthanasia/physician-assisted suicide is by far the highest in Europe. The Swiss have the highest rate of assisted suicide, and a surprisingly high rate of euthanasia (given the fact that it is illegal in Switzerland). The Belgian rate—at a time when euthanasia was still illegal—was also high by European standards.[20]

TABLE 17B.2

Frequencies of Euthanasia and Other Medical Behavior That Potentially Shortens Life in Some European Countries in 2001–2002 (Percentages of Death)

	NL[18]	BE	CH	DK	SW	IT	UK
Euthanasia	2.59	0.3	0.27	0.06	—	0.04	0.16
Physician-assisted suicide	0.21	0.01	0.36	0.06	—	0.00	0.00
Abstention (refusal or futility)	20	15	28	14	14	4	30.3
Pain relief with life-shortening effect	20	22	22	26	21	19	32.8
Termination of life without request	0.60	1.5	0.42	0.67	0.23	0.06	0.33
Total MBPSL	44	38	51	41	36	23	64
Terminal sedation (without artificial nutrition and hydration)[19]	3.7	3.2	2.9	1.6	1.8	3.0	?

Although the Netherlands is the only county in which termination of life without request from the patient was legal in certain circumstances at this time, it is not the country with the highest rate of this most controversial of MBPSLs: The Belgian rate is at least double the Dutch rate, and the Danish is slightly higher. In Switzerland, the United Kingdom, and Sweden termination of life without a request is also practiced rather often.

There is, of course, a whole host of questions surrounding these comparative results. Are the results reliable (samples, response rates)? Are the same things being counted in different countries? Are doctors equally honest in all countries? This is no reason to reject the results to date out of hand: They are, for the time being, the best we have.

In the meantime, the results do seem to justify the conclusion that medical practice at the end of life in countries in which euthanasia and assistance suicide are legal is not so very deviant from that in other European countries, except that small part of medical practice that shortens life.

EUTHANASIA AND PALLIATIVE CARE

Critics of the practice of euthanasia in the Netherlands and Belgium argue that the legal possibility of euthanasia closes off the development of palliative care. However, comparative research shows that palliative care is well developed in countries with legalized euthanasia or assisted suicide, or at least not less well developed than in other European countries (i.e., France, Germany, and Spain[21]). Belgium, the Netherlands, and Switzerland rank high in Europe for most structural and national palliative care indicators.[22] A literature review confirmed a degree of palliative care provision in Belgium and the Netherlands that is comparable with surrounding countries. The authors conclude that "there is evidence of advancement of palliative care in countries with legalized euthanasia, also after the legalization of euthanasia. The idea that legalization of euthanasia might obstruct or halt palliative care development thus seems unwarranted and is only expressed in commentaries rather than demonstrated by empirical evidence." [23]

Chronological Data on Medical Behavior That Potentially Shortens Life

The Netherlands disposes of national data on the frequencies of MBPSL spanning a period of more than two decades.[24] In TABLE 17B.3 we see that the frequency of euthanasia has always been fairly low. Termination of life without a request is declining since 1990. The total amount of MBPSL is increasing. The main reason is a steady increase of pain relief with life-shortening effect. The table further shows that not only euthanasia is carried out with the explicit intention to shorten life, but also half of the cases of abstention are decided with this (subjective) intention on the part of physicians.

TABLE 17B.3

Estimated Frequencies of Medical Behavior That Potentially Shortens Life in the Netherlands in National Studies: 1990, 1995, 2001, 2005, 2010 (Percentages of all Deaths)

	1990	1995	2001	2005	2010
Termination of life on request[25]	1.9	2.6	2.8	1.8	2.9
Termination of life without request	0.8	0.7	0.7	0.4	0.2
Pain relief with life-shortening effect	19	19	21	25	36
Accepting the risk[26]	15	16	19	24	35
Subsidiary intention	4	4	2	1	1
Withholding and withdrawing life-prolonging treatment	18	20	20	16	18
Accepting the risk	9	7	7	8	8
Explicit intention[27]	9	13	13	8	10
Continuous sedation				8[28]	13[29]
Total MBPSL	39	43	44	43	57

In Belgium less data are known. Three surveys of MBPSL practice are published. However, they only cover a part of Belgium—Flanders[30]—and they are of considerable lesser quality than the Dutch studies.

The Working of the Dutch and Belgian System of Control of Euthanasia

In Belgium and the Netherlands, medical behavior that potentially shortens life (MBPSL) can be legally divided into acts that fall under the "medical exception" and acts that do not. If "normal medical practice" causes the patient to die, the death is considered a "natural" one. Medical behavior under the scope of the medical exception is, therefore, not a subject of criminal law (if a doctor does not act according normal medical practice he or she will be subject of medical disciplinary law).

Termination of life (with or without explicit request) does not fall under the medical exception. A death resulting from this medical behavior is considered to be a death that requires further investigation. In cases of euthanasia a special form has to be filled in and sent to a Regional Review Committee.

The Dutch spent many years developing a system to control euthanasia. In 1990 the special reporting form was developed. In 1998 the first Review Committees were installed, at that time with only an advisory task. The Law of 2002, in addition to codifying the legislation of euthanasia, put the Dutch Review Committees on a firm statutory footing. More or less together with the coming into being of the Regional Review Committees, the Dutch Medical Association founded a special service: Support and Consultation in cases of Euthanasia in the Netherlands (SCEN).[31] The aim of the development of this control system is to stimulate transparency and complying with the "due care" criteria. The Belgians incorporated the idea of special forms and a review committee.[32]

There are three kinds of data that give an indication for the effectiveness of the control system: the number of reported cases, the national studies, and the annual reports of the Regional Review Committees.

Reporting

In the Netherlands, the number of reported cases increased almost every year between 1983 and 1999 (from 16 to 2,216). Between 1999 and 2003 there was a decline (to 1,815). Ever since, the numbers have risen. In 2011, 3,695 cases were reported. However, bare numbers on reported cases can indicate but not prove the success or failure of the control system.

According to the national surveys, the reporting rate increased from 18% in 1990, to 41% in 1995 and 54% in 2001 to 80% in 2005 and (more or less the same) 78% in 2010. The estimated reporting rates have given rise to much discussion. From the discussion it has become clear that, at least since the change of law in 2002, doctors report almost all the cases to the Review Committees that *they* consider to be euthanasia;[33] that is, cases in which the doctor administered an immediately lethal substance (not morphine) to a patient on request at a moment agreed on beforehand.[34]

Since the enactment of the Law of 2002 the number of reported cases in Belgium increased steadily from 258 cases in 2002–2003 to 1,133 cases in 2011.[35] Most of these cases were reported by Flemish doctors.[36] Establishing a sequence of reporting rates for Belgium is impossible, because there have been no nationwide studies on the subject. In 2007 Belgian researchers estimated the reporting rate in Flanders to be 53%.[37]

Complying with the "Due Care" Criteria

The Dutch law on euthanasia contains two "substantial due care" criteria and three "procedural" ones. According to the substantial criteria, the patient must have made a voluntary and well-considered request and the patient's suffering must be unbearable and hopeless. The procedural criteria prescribe that the doctor and the patient were convinced that there was no reasonable alternative in light of the patient's situation; that the doctor consulted at least one other, independent physician; and that the doctor terminated the patient's life or provided assistance with suicide with due medical care and attention.

Most cases that reach the Dutch Regional Review Committees appear to be unproblematic in terms of compliance with the established legal criteria. For example, in 2005 the committees sought further information from the reporting doctor in about 6% of all cases (1.65% by telephone, 3.8% in writing, and 0.5% by summoning the doctor to a meeting of the committee in question). The additional information requested most often (one-third of such requests) concerned the consultation with another physician[38] or the patient's suffering[39]; one-fifth of the requests concerned the way the euthanasia was carried out,[40] and one-tenth the voluntariness of the request.[41]

In most cases to which the committees give special attention, they ultimately conclude that the doctor had acted "carefully." Since the Law of 2002, 56 cases have been adjudged "not careful" and referred to the prosecutorial authorities for further consideration; that is, less than 0.3%.[42]

Defects in consultation (timing, independence) are by far the most common reason that the committees come to the conclusion that the doctor was "not careful." Then next most common defects were determinations of "unbearable suffering" and the way the euthanasia was carried out. To date there have been no prosecutions in the cases found to be "not careful."

With respect of the compliance with the "due care" criteria, it is important to notice that SCEN seems to be developing in the direction of before-the-fact control of euthanasia: reviewing the doctor's proposed course of conduct before he or she carries it out.[43] The annual reports of the Regional Review Committees give the impression that the committees are increasingly inclined to regard a report of euthanasia that is accompanied by the report of a SCEN consultant[44] as requiring less attention than other cases. If this is true and becomes known among doctors, one can expect them to be increasingly prepared to make use of SCEN consultants because this will more or less guarantee that they will not experience an unpleasant in depth review later on.

To date no case has been adjudged "not careful" by the Belgian Review Committee. According to the 2010 report, 85% of submissions were approved by the committee without further analysis. In the remaining 15%, the Committee pointed out small mistakes of interpretation concerning the procedure or incomplete answers (4%), or asked the physician for further information (11%).[45]

Evaluation of the Dutch System of Control

Regarded as the results of an experiment in legal control, the data on the reporting rates are impressive. A new policy concerning behavior that the state cannot observe directly, that requires expenditure of time and energy and involves some unpleasantness, and that requires people concerned to run a risk of external criticism or even legal sanctions, started with an effectiveness of about zero, as one would expect. In the Netherlands and in Flanders almost all euthanasia cases that doctors consider to be euthanasia are now reported.

The data on compliance of the "due care" criteria are also very promising. A skeptical person might counter that doctors only send in trouble-free cases or that the Committees are too lenient. The national surveys show the first to be not true. There is no proof for a "lying doctor" hypothesis. It is hard to prove that the Regional Review Committees are too lenient. A comparison between the activities of the Dutch prosecutorial authorities and these committees might help. Between 1991 and 2003 the prosecutorial authorities discussed 226 cases (of 20,600 reported). In almost all these cases the prosecutorial authorities decided without further investigation not to prosecute: further investigation has been carried out in 37 cases. The least that can be concluded is that the prosecutorial authorities did not put more "sanction pressure" than do the Regional Review Committees.

Furthermore, before jumping to the conclusion that these systems have little teeth, one should consider that the legal obligation to report is itself a form of prospective control: knowing that one will have to report colors the behavior that will be reported. The reporting system might thus induce doctors either not to perform euthanasia where the rules do not allow it, or to perform it in the right way. As noted, SCEN is also very important in this respect.

Within the control system itself, doctors are sometimes required to provide more information and explain their behavior in person to the committees. In practice, many doctors apparently experience this as a significant sanction. That the cases judged "not careful" in the Netherlands have not been prosecuted does not mean that nothing at all is done. There have been discussions between doctors and prosecutors and medical inspectors.

One of the most important advantages of the Regional Review Committees is the transparency of what they do. Before 1998, when decision making on reported cases was entirely in the hands of prosecutorial authorities, practically nothing was known publicly about what they did, or how, or why. The annual reports of the Review Committees are a rich source of both quantitative and qualitative information.

After Legalization

RECENT DEVELOPMENTS

Legalization did not silence the debate on euthanasia in the Netherlands. On the contrary, further legal development has undeniably taken place as a direct consequence of legalization. Almost all of it has been in the direction of clarifying and tightening the requirements of "due care." The issues that provoked a lot of public debate most recently are "euthanasia and tired of life," "euthanasia and demented patients," and the "euthanasia clinic" of the Dutch Association for Voluntary Euthanasia.

The rulings of the Dutch courts did not make a distinction between somatically based and nonsomatically based suffering and neither does the Law of 2002. A ruling of the Supreme Court (1994[46]) made explicit that nonsomatically based suffering (suffering from psychiatric disorders) can support a valid request for assistance with suicide—that for the purpose of the "justification of necessity," the source of a patient's suffering is irrelevant.[47] The decision of the Supreme Court could be seen as having opened the way to a legal development that would accept assistance with suicide to persons whose suffering has no "medically" recognized character at all, somatic or otherwise. However, in a more recent case (2002[48]), the Supreme Court held that in a case the patient's suffering is predominantly based on things other than "medically classifiable" disorder, the doctor exceeded the scope of his professional competence in assisting a suicide. The Supreme Court's emphasis on the "medical" character of legally justifiable euthanasia was explicitly embraced by the government and many members of Parliament in the proceedings leading to the Law of 2002. More recently, the Regional Review Committees received a couple of cases that at first sight resemble the 2002 case. They were concluded to be "careful." In the opinion of the Committees "the cause of the hopeless and unbearable suffering could be traced back predominantly to a medically classified disease."[49]

With respect to dementia, two different issues are at stake: euthanasia in an early stage of dementia and euthanasia at a late stage of dementia. In the first case the question is whether the requirement of unbearable suffering is fulfilled, in the second whether an advance written request is sufficient.[50] The Regional Review Committees have taken the position that in principle both situations can lead to the decision that the doctor acted "carefully." With respect to the early stages of dementia, the Review Committees observed in the reported cases that those patients suffer from a special and painful combination of early stages of dementia and insight in their future (often from previous experiences with family members). This combination enables them competently to assess themselves and their future, and make clear that their suffering is unbearable.[51] In 2011 the Regional Review Committees for the first time approved a case to be "careful" in which a doctor reported euthanasia on a patient with advanced dementia. The patient had an advanced written request and the doctor and the patient discussed this request many times in the years before the euthanasia was carried out. In 2012 the Regional Review Committees decided another case of euthanasia in which the advanced written request stands for the oral request to be "not-careful." The difference between the cases is that the second one lacked proof of the repeated discussion.

In 2009 The Dutch Association for Voluntary Euthanasia started a new initiative: a euthanasia clinic. When this clinic started to function in 2012, the association tried to address the problem that some patients cannot find a doctor willing to carry out their euthanasia.[52] Before the Law of 2002 it was generally supposed that euthanasia must (at least "in principle") be carried out by the doctor responsible for the patient's treatment. No such limitation is explicitly included among the requirements of "due care" in the Law of 2002. The Regional Review Committees take the position that what is decisive is whether "the doctor has such a relationship with the patient as to permit him to form a judgment concerning the requirements of due care." A couple of euthanasia cases carried out by doctors of the clinic have been discussed by the Regional Review Committees and they decided that these cases were "careful."

ARE THE DUTCH SLIDING DOWN A SLIPPERY SLOPE?

Do these and former developments lead to the conclusion that the Netherlands has entered an unavoidable slippery slope? On an empirical level—the scope of this chapter—two slippery slope arguments can be distinguished: a "legal control variant" and a "legal change variant."

The legal control variant of the slippery slope argument against euthanasia is that in practice legal control of euthanasia will not be able to prevent the nonvoluntary medical killing of the vulnerable. To test the assertion empirically, one would need to be able to compare the frequency of nonvoluntary termination of life before and after legalization, and the situation in places where it is legal with that in places where it is not. However, there is very little reliable evidence on either point. We simply do not know how much nonvoluntary termination of life there was in the Netherlands before the legalization of euthanasia, and the only evidence for the years after legalization suggest a modest decline. Nor, is it the case, as we have seen before in the EURELD-study, that there is more nonvoluntary termination of life in the Netherlands than in countries where euthanasia remains illegal. Furthermore, there is no evidence that members of any of the supposedly vulnerable groups die more frequently from euthanasia than anyone else.

There is another way to approach the legal control variant: by looking not at the actual results of legal control, about which not very much is known, but at the amount of control activity itself. As we have seen before, the legalization of euthanasia led to an outburst of regulation and other control activity in Belgium and especially in the Netherlands, unequaled in any other country. This concerns not only euthanasia itself, but also includes other sorts of medical behavior that potentially shortens life that are traditionally been regarded as "normal medical practice" not requiring any regulation—such as continuous sedation and abstention.[53] The result of all this is that end-of-life practice of Dutch doctors is much more transparent and exposed to far greater regulatory pressure and concrete social control than it ever was before.[54]

In the case of the "legal change variant" of the slippery slope argument against the legalization of euthanasia, the prediction is that if once we allow practice A we will sooner or later find ourselves allowing a more problematic practice B.[55] The proponents of the slippery slope argue that after the legalization of euthanasia in the Netherlands there have been relevant legal developments that have not taken place in other countries and that can be seen as proofs of a slippery slope: acceptance of physician-assisted suicide in the case of persons who are not in the "terminal phase" and whose suffering is not somatically based; acceptance of physician-assisted suicide in the case of persons not suffering from any "medical" condition, and acceptance of termination of life in the case of noncompetent patients (in particular severely defective newborn babies).

However, those who think there has been a "slide" in the direction of accepting physician-assisted suicide in the case of nonsomatic suffering and patients outside the "terminal phase" are simply unaware of the facts of Dutch legal development.

Neither in the case law that over a period of more than 20 years led to the recent Dutch legislation, nor in the Law of 2002 itself, have restrictions limiting access to those in the terminal phase of illness or those with exclusively somatically based suffering. Therefore, there has never been a possibility of such a slide. From the beginning of the discussion, these situations were seen as falling under practice A.

With regard to persons who are "tired with life": The Dutch Supreme Court has held that such a case does not fall within the scope of the legalization of euthanasia and the Dutch Parliament has held this position too.[56] This "slide" therefore turned out not to be inevitable at all: It has not taken place and it is not clear that it ever will.

The third example of the slippery slope is more interesting. Dutch courts have held that there can be circumstances that justify termination of life in the case of newborn babies. And it is undeniably the case that the form that legal regulation is assuming—for example, the "due care" criteria that apply in such cases—has been heavily influenced by the earlier development of euthanasia law. But what does this prove? Medical practice in the case of very ill newborn babies is largely similar in the Netherlands and in Flanders. The fact that termination of life takes place at about the same rate in both countries, whereas at least some of it is legal in one and all of it is on the face of things illegal in the other suggest that the legal variable may not be very important as a determinant of the way doctors treat severely defective newborn babies. Quantitative comparisons with other European countries suffer from a variety of methodological and conceptual difficulties but do tend to the direction of a generally similar conclusion. The question to be answered is: Where is the sliding part in the Netherlands? Some part of all the termination of life that is in fact taking place is now explicitly recognized as calling for formal regulation. Substantive criteria, procedural requirements, and a control system are all in place.

In conclusion, legal control over euthanasia and other MBPSL is certainly not perfect in the Netherlands (or Belgium or Switzerland). However, it is better than in other countries for which information is available, and it has been getting more encompassing, more refined, and in practice more effective in the decades since euthanasia became legal.

Notes

1. John Griffiths, Heleen Weyers and Maurice Adams, *Euthanasia and Law in Europe*, Oxford and Portland: Hart Publishing, 2008.
2. All references to *Euthanasia and Law in Europe* are left out.
3. We consider continuous sedation until death (often labeled as "terminal sedation") to be a combination of pain relief and abstention.
4. Luxemburg followed the Dutch and Belgian example in 2009. However, almost nothing is known about euthanasia in this country. The Luxembourgian law very much resembles the Belgian law.

5. Penny Lewis, "Informal legal change on assisted suicide: the policy for prosecutors," *Legal Studies* 2011, Vol. *31*, no 1: 119–134.

6. In the well-known case of the conjoined twins.

7. According to the courts, a doctor confronted by a patient who is suffering very severely and cannot be helped in another way can be regarded as caught in a situation of conflict of duties. On the one hand, there is the duty to respect life. On the other hand, there is a duty to reduce suffering. If, in this situation of necessity, the doctor chooses a course of action that is justifiable, the doctor is not guilty of an offense. In the conjoined twin case the British court concluded separating the twins was justifiable. In the Dutch cases regarding severely defective newborn babies the courts also took this conclusion. (In the Netherlands before the change of law in 2002, the defense of necessity was the legal ground that made euthanasia legal.)

8. The "due care" criteria in Belgium and the Netherlands are more or less the same (the Belgian law is more detailed). In the Dutch law the next five criteria are mentioned: The patient's request was voluntary and carefully considered; the patient's suffering was unbearable and there was no prospect of improvement; the doctor and the patient were convinced that there was no reasonable alternative in light of the patient's situation; the doctor consulted at least one other, independent physician who must have seen the patient and given a written opinion on the "due care" criteria; the doctor terminated the patient's life or provided assistance with suicide with due medical care and attention. The "due care" criteria are developed in the 1980s in concerted action between courts, prosecutorial authorities, the Dutch doctor's association and legal, ethical, and medical scholars.

9. There is a latent doctrinal tension between the subjective conception of "intent" as used in the doctrine of double effect (purpose or motive) and the objectified intent that is generally used in the criminal law (knowledge and acceptance of consequences).

10. In principle, intentionally causing injury or death is an offense under one or more of a number of provisions of every criminal code. Nevertheless, in everyday medical practice behavior regularly occurs that is more or less certainly known and expected to have such a result: the dentist who causes pain by drilling in one's teeth, the surgeon who amputates a leg, the oncologist who administers chemotherapy. Although such behavior violates the literal terms of the criminal law, it also falls within the scope of the legal authority to practice medicine. As such it is taken to be covered by an implicit "medical exception" to the criminal offenses that protect life and bodily integrity. The death of a patient because of such "normal medical practice"; for example, during an open-heart surgery or as a result of intensive use of pain killing drugs—is considered a natural death.

11. In the first edition of *Euthanasia and Law* we argued that from the perspective of legal control it would be better to let euthanasia also fall under the medical exception.

12. A lot of attention has been paid to define "medical futility." According to Moratti, it is general accepted that "futility" can "best be operationalized through a procedure regulating the allocation of decision-making power among the various actors involved in the decision-making process, giving, under specific circumstances, the last word to doctors" (Sofia Moratti, *"Medical futility" in Dutch neonatology*, Dissertation, University of Groningen 2009).

13. Belgium (2002), the Netherlands (2002), and Luxemburg (2009).

14. The Netherlands before the change of law in 2002. In principle, this is possible in many countries.
15. The United Kingdom.
16. Switzerland.
17. In Belgium legalization was forthcoming.
18. NL: the Netherlands; BE: Belgium; CH: Switzerland; DK: Denmark; SW: Sweden; IT: Italy; UK: United Kingdom.
19. These data are presented here separately from the other MBPSL data because it is not clear whether or to what extent they are included within the data given for pain relief with life-shortening effect or abstention.
20. This percentage is doubtful and probably should be higher: Termination of life on request was estimated 1.2% in 1998 and 1.9% in 2007 (Tinne Smets *et al*, "Reporting of euthanasia in medical practice in Flanders, Belgium: cross sectional analysis of reported and unreported cases," *BMJ* 2010—http://www.bmj.com/content/341/bmj.c5174). The researchers do not give an explanation why 2001 differs that much from 1998.
21. The United Kingdom is considered as a country of reference rather than of comparison, understanding that it has the greatest degree of palliative care development.
22. Indicators are among others: palliative care beds, attendance at EAPC conferences, and publications on palliative care.
23. K. Chambaere *et al*, Palliative Care Development in Countries with a Euthanasia Law. Report for the Commission on Assisted Dying Briefing Papers. Submitted October 4th, 2011 (http://www.commissiononassisteddying.co.uk/wp-content/uploads/2011/10/EAPC-Briefing-Paper-Palliative-Care-in-Countries-with-a-Euthanasia-Law.pdf).
24. The results are based on large, carefully composed samples and generally high rates of response. The EURELD study and Clive Seal's study are based on this Dutch methodology.
25. From the studies we know that more than 80% of the patients who die from euthanasia have cancer. The estimated shortening of life is in 46% less than 1 week and in 46% 1 week to 1 month.
26. The research distinguished three modalities of intentions: explicit intention of shortening life, "partly with the intention of shortening life" (that is, a subsidiary intention associated with a primary intention of relieving suffering) and "taking into account that the life of the patient might be shortened by the pain relief" ("accepting the risk").
27. The study shows that hastening death is intentional in 45% of all cases of abstention.
28. Agnes van der Heide *et al, Euthanasie en andere medische beslissingen rond het levenseinde. Sterfgevallenonderzoek 2012,* [Euthanasia and other medical decisions at the end of life, death certificate study] Den Haag: ZonMw.
29. Idem ditto.
30. Tinne Smets *et al*, "Reporting of euthanasia in medical practice in Flanders, Belgium: cross sectional analysis of reported and unreported cases," *BMJ* 2010 (http://www.bmj.com/content/341/bmj.c5174).
31. SCEN provides independent and trained consultants to improve the quality of the euthanasia practice.
32. The most important difference between the Netherlands and Belgium is that in Belgium there is one national committee of nine members, in the Netherlands there

are five Regional Review Committees of three members. The Belgian service of consultants is a voluntary service and not a paid one as is the Dutch.

33. A finding of Donald Van Tol, *Grensgeschillen: een rechtssociologisch onderzoek naar het classificeren van euthanasia en ander medisch handelen rond het levenseinde* [Boundary disputes: a legal-sociological study of the classification of euthanasia and other medical behaviour at the end of life] Dissertation, University of Groningen, 2005.

34. The researchers in the 2005 national study confirm Van Tol's explanation for the reporting rate. A question was added to the death-certificate study in which the doctor was asked to classify what he or she did. In about one-fourth of all cases in which the researchers classified the doctor's behavior as termination of life (euthanasia, assisted suicide, or termination of life without a request), the doctor classified it differently—usually as palliative or terminal sedation or as pain relief. As supposed by Van Tol and another scholar (Den Hartogh), not their "intention" but the drug used is largely determinative of the doctors' classification: In 99% of all cases in which muscle-relaxants are used, the doctor's classification was "termination of life"; if morphine or benzodiazepines were used, such a classification was given in only 1% of all cases (in the case of morphine, the classification "pain relief" was usually chosen; in the case of benzodiazepines "palliative/terminal sedation").

35. 259 cases (2002-2003) to 349 (2004), 393 (2005) 429 (2006) 495 (2007) 655 (2008) 953 (2010) and 1133 (2011) Source: Annual reports of the Review Committee. Belgian researchers concluded that physicians who perceived their case as euthanasia reported it in 93% of cases (Tinne Smets *et al*, "Reporting of euthanasia in medical practice in Flanders, Belgium: cross sectional analysis of reported and unreported cases," *BMJ* 2010—http://www.bmj.com/content/341/bmj.c5174).

36. Recent research suggests that termination of life in request occurs less in Wallonia than in Flanders, at least with respect to general practitioners (Lieve van den Block *et al*, "Euthanasia and other end-of-life decisions: a mortality follow back study in Belgium," *BMC Public Health* 2009—http://www.bmj.com/content/339/bmj.b2772).

37. Tinne Smets *et al*, "Reporting of euthanasia in medical practice in Flanders, Belgium: cross sectional analysis of reported and unreported cases," *BMJ* 2010—http://www.bmj.com/content/341/bmj.c5174.

38. Consultation currently takes place in virtually all cases reported to the Regional Review Committees. The problems with consultation regard independence of the consultant and the timing of the consultation. The consultant must be independent both of the doctor and of the patient. Especially in the first years of the existence of the Review Committees there were doctors who reported that they had consulted close colleagues. Based on this finding the Dutch Medical association expanded SCEN (which originally existed of GPs) to nursing home doctors and medical specialists.

With respect to timing, the consultation should not be too early—in those cases the consultation can only be provisional, nor too late—in those cases the patient might not be capable of communication.

39. The cases discussed regard patients who became comatose before the euthanasia was carried out.

40. The issue most often discussed is the necessary amount of drugs to induce the unconsciousness of the patient.

41. Sometimes there is no written request (such a request is not obliged by the law); sometimes there had been a very short period between the first concrete request and the carrying out of euthanasia; and sometimes there are doubts whether the request was well considered (for example, in cases of dementia and psychiatric disorders).

42. Since 2002, 21,434 cases have been reported.

43. B. Onwuteaka-Philipsen *et al, Evaluatie Wet toetsing levensbeëindiging op verzoek en hulp bij zelfdoding* [Evaluation of the Termination of Life on Request and Assisted Suicide (Review Procedure) Act of 2002] Den Haag: ZonMw, 2007.

44. A SCEN consultant was involved in almost 90% of all cases of euthanasia (B. Onwuteaka-Philipsen *et al, Evaluatie Wet toetsing levensbeëindiging op verzoek en hulp bij zelfdoding* [Evaluation of the Termination of Life on Request and Assisted Suicide (Review Procedure) Act of 2002] Den Haag: ZonMw, 2007.

45. Smets *et al* concluded that unreported cases were generally dealt with less carefully than reported cases: A written request for euthanasia was more often absent, other physicians and caregivers specialized in palliative care were consulted less often, the life-ending act was more often performed with opioids or sedatives, and the drugs were more often administered by a nurse. (Tinne Smets *et al*, "Reporting of euthanasia in medical practice in Flanders, Belgium: cross sectional analysis of reported and unreported cases," *BMJ* 2010—http://www.bmj.com/content/341/bmj.c5174).

46. The Chabot case.

47. This position goes back to the State Commission of Euthanasia in 1985. The Court held that the wish to die of a person suffering from a psychiatric sickness or disorder can be legally considered the result of an autonomous (competent and voluntary) judgment.

48. The Brongersma case. The patient—ex-senator Brongersma—had been very active politically and socially engaged. But in recent years his physical condition had begun to deteriorate. The consequence was increasing social isolation. The patient found his situation unbearable and sought his general practitioner's (GP's) help to end his life (a suicide attempt had failed). The GP had a number of discussions with the patient and had two independent consultants examine and talk to the patient. The consultants confirmed his view. In his report the GP characterized the reasons for Brongersma's request as: "lonely, feeling of senselessness, physical deterioration and a long-standing wish to die not associated with depression." To a question concerning Brongersma's suffering the GP reported: "the person in question experienced life as unbearable." And to a question whether there were treatment alternatives, he answered: "No, the person in question 'weighted the pros and cons,' and there was no disease [to treat]."

49. Regionale Toetsingscommissies Euthanasie, Jaarverslag 2010 [Regional Review Committees, Annual Report 2010].

50. The Law of 2002 makes explicit for the first time that an advanced written request for euthanasia, made by a patient of 16 or older who is currently not competent but who was competent at the time he or she made the written request, can satisfy the requirement of a voluntary request.

51. Regionale Toetsingscommissies Euthanasie, Jaarverslag 2000, 2004–2010 [Regional Review Committees, Annual Report 2000, 2004–2010].

52. There is no right to euthanasia or assistance with suicide in the Netherlands, Belgium, Luxembourg, and Switzerland. National research shows that one-third of the explicit

requests for euthanasia are granted. That there is a need for such a clinic is showed by the fact that in the first 3 months of its existence there were 254 applications.

53. As we have seen, the Netherlands (and England) made clear on which ground futile medical treatment can be withheld and withdrawn in comatose patients; the Netherlands is one of the five European countries (together with Belgium, England, Germany, and Switzerland) in which advance treatment directives have a strong legal status and in which the role of the representatives of a noncompetent patient is legally well defined; and the Netherlands is one of the four countries (together with Norway, Sweden, and to a more limited extent Switzerland) in which continuous sedation has been subjected to specific regulation.

54. A spokesman of the Belgian Order of Physicians, which opposes legalization of euthanasia, stated in the Belgian Senate that legalization was not necessary because Belgian doctors practiced euthanasia whenever they thought it appropriate and never experienced any interference from the legal authorities. What the law really proposed to do, he argued, was to impose a legal regulatory system on the decision making of doctors and patients. Developments in Belgium and the Netherlands proved him absolutely right.

55. This argument resembles a conceptual variant of the slippery slope argument, but the strength of the empirical variant depends not on the proposition that people in the future will be unable to draw the relevant moral distinction, but on the prediction that they will in fact not do so.

56. In practice in turns out that most patients who are "tired of life" also have medical problems.

INDEX